Foundations of Neuroeconomic Analysis

Foundations of
Neuroeconomic Analysis

PAUL W. GLIMCHER
Center for Neuroeconomics
New York University

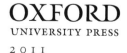

OXFORD
UNIVERSITY PRESS
2011

OXFORD
UNIVERSITY PRESS

Oxford University Press, Inc., publishes works that further
Oxford University's objective of excellence
in research, scholarship, and education.

Oxford New York
Auckland   Cape Town   Dar es Salaam   Hong Kong   Karachi
Kuala Lumpur   Madrid   Melbourne   Mexico City   Nairobi
New Delhi   Shanghai   Taipei   Toronto

With offices in
Argentina   Austria   Brazil   Chile   Czech Republic   France   Greece
Guatemala   Hungary   Italy   Japan Poland Portugal   Singapore
South Korea   Switzerland   Thailand   Turkey Ukraine   Vietnam

Copyright © 2011 by Paul W. Glimcher

Published by Oxford University Press, Inc.
198 Madison Avenue, New York, New York 10016
www.oup.com

Oxford is a registered trademark of Oxford University Press

Library of Congress Cataloging-in-Publication Data
Glimcher, Paul W.
Foundations of neuroeconomic analysis/Paul W. Glimcher.
p. cm.
ISBN 978-0-19-974425-1   1. Cognitive neuroscience. 2. Neuroeconomics.
3. Decision making. 4. Decision making–Physiological aspects. 5. Choice
(Psychology) I. Title.
QP360.5.G566 2011
612.8'233–dc22
2010013591

For Barbara

Preface

Nearly all of the ideas presented in this book had their inception at New York University's Center for Neuroeconomics. In the early part of the last decade NYU constructed what was, at the time, a unique interdisciplinary environment for studying how and why we choose. Psychologists, economists, and neuroscientists at all levels of training came together regularly to learn each other's trades, and to begin a new synthesis that has come to be known as *neuroeconomics*. In fairness, scholars at other universities also began to explore the connections between these three disciplines at this same time, but in 2005 and 2006 NYU's environment was unique for the depth and consistency of the interdisciplinary interaction it provided. This stems from the "first rule" of our Center, which is that you cannot dismiss any conclusion made by a scholar in another discipline until you first master the disciplinary source of that conclusion. The senior faculty here has always insisted that a mastery of neuroscience, for example, must *precede* any conclusions about the relevance of neuroscience to economics. Although this may sound obvious, we have found that it requires an enormous degree of tolerance and that it is a discipline of interaction practiced quite rarely in the academic world. For this reason, the first debts I must acknowledge are to the men and women of NYU's Center for Neuroeconomics, with whom I have interacted daily for half a decade. They have both enforced this discipline and provided the raw material for understanding from which this volume grew.

Although many people have participated in the life of the Center, two stand out for me as central figures who have shaped the ongoing thought at the Center in a general way, and have shaped my scholarship in particular. I want to acknowledge my debt to them. The first is Andrew Caplin.

In addition to being one of the world's leading microeconomic theorists, Andrew has taken the time to show me the beauty, poetry, and raw (often unappreciated) power of neoclassical economic thought. The second is Elizabeth Phelps. In addition to being one of the world's leading psychologists, Liz has taken the time to reintroduce me to the psychology I studied as a student. It is she who convinced me that neuroeconomics cannot survive without psychology, and I see the rich dose of classical psychology contained between the covers of this volume as her gift to me.

I also wish to thank my many students who contributed to this book. First I absolutely must thank Dan Burghart. He is a brilliant, and brilliantly trained, neoclassical economist who joined my laboratory a few years ago. More than anyone else he worked with me daily to try and understand how economics and neuroscience go together, and my debt to him is simply enormous. Dan, Dino Levy, and Kenway Louie served as a troika that read the book as I produced it. Dino served as the book's psychological critic and Kenway as its neurobiological critic. I am grateful for the many long hours that the four of us spent together trying to understand the relationship between psychology, neuroscience, and economics. To my many other students who read portions of the book I am also grateful. These include Eric DeWitt, Ifat Levy, Joe Kable, Mark Dean, Hannah Bayer, Robb Rutledge, Hiroshi Yamada, and Lauren Grattan.

Several of my closest colleagues also deserve my most profound thanks for taking the time to read my tangled Gordian knot of a first draft. First among these was my friend and colleague Antonio Rangel. Antonio is nothing less than a force of nature, and it was my good fortune that he took the time to help me along when I seemed most to have lost my way. Elke Weber, another friend and colleague, was of immeasurable help. I also thank Nathaniel Daw, Daeyeol Lee, and Mike Landy for their insightful comments.

I would also like to express my overall thanks to Samanta Shaw, who mothered the book through production, and Maggie Grantner, who mothered me and my lab through the sabbatical during which the book was written. Finally, I would like to thank Zoë Glimcher for her help with some of the more visually complicated and creative figures.

Contents

Introduction: Wherefore Neuroeconomics?

Posing the Problem

> I've studied now Philosophy,
> And Jurisprudence, Medicine,
> And even, alas, Theology:
> From end to end, with labor keen;
> And here, poor fool! with all my lore
> I stand, no wiser than before:
> I'm Magister—yea, Doctor—hight,
> And straight or cross-wise, wrong or right,
> These ten years long, with many woes,
> I've led my students by the nose,
> And see, that nothing can be known!
>
> —Goethe's Faust
> (Translation by Bayard Taylor, 1881)

A new academic discipline has emerged at the border of the social and natural sciences, a discipline calling itself neuroeconomics. Interdisciplinary research and controversy are nothing new in a university setting, but the birth of neuroeconomics—an attempted fusion of the neuroscience, psychology, and economics of decision making—has proved unusually acrimonious. Neuroeconomics is an effort to cross a sacrosanct border in the intellectual world. Unlike biochemistry's successful efforts to relate biology to chemistry in the 1950s, neuroeconomics is an effort to use natural scientific tools within the traditional boundaries of the social sciences, which has led to both confusion and controversy over the past decade.

Does a unique set of challenges preclude interdisciplinary fusion across the social-natural scientific frontier, or is building neuroeconomics simply a matter of integrating brain scanners and other neuroscientific tools into existing economic debates? If neuroeconomics were to become a stable interdisciplinary field at the border of the social and natural sciences, what could it tell us? Would relating the insights of neuroscience, psychology, and economics to one another yield new insights into how we make decisions?

Within this emerging field there has been an intense debate about how to answer these questions. Some scholars argue that the central contribution of neuroeconomics will be to add new methodological tools to the inquiries conducted by pre-existing disciplines. Others claim that only a detailed theoretical reconstruction of the parent disciplines could give rise to a truly valuable form of neuroeconomics, a novel discipline that could make new predictions that extend beyond the boundaries of existing theories.

Outside the emerging discipline, the debate has been even more contentious. While there is no doubt that neuroeconomics has rocketed into the public awareness at a rate completely out of proportion to its accomplishments, there is not even a consensus in the broader academic community about whether neuroeconomics has made *any* contribution. Some gifted scholars argue that the existing insights of neuroeconomics are, at best, trivial. Others contend that a carefully crafted interdisciplinary relationship has already revealed the basic mechanisms of human choice, and that an understanding of these mechanisms already constrains future economic thought. Yet others fear a reductionist effort by natural scientists to erode the relevance of the social sciences. Across neuroeconomics' parent disciplines of neuroscience, psychology, and economics, dispute about whether neuroeconomics has taught us anything seems to dominate interdisciplinary discourse on this subject.

What the debate has revealed are two separate questions, both of which neuroeconomics must answer. The first is largely philosophical: Should there be a distinct philosophical entity called neuroeconomics? The second is more practical: Is there anything like a standard theory of neuroeconomics and what, if anything, does the corpus of this theory tell us about human behavior that its parent disciplines have not already revealed?

I want to make it clear that I believe, on strictly philosophical grounds, that there can be an entity called neuroeconomics only if the discipline emerges synthetically from the unification of economics, psychology, and neuroscience. This is a point developed in detail in this book. I do not believe that the purely methodological use of brain scanners to provide social scientists with new measurements is interdisciplinary synthesis. Neuroeconomics as a philosophical entity has to emerge in the same way that physical chemistry, biochemistry, and neuroscience emerged during the past century. It has to be the product of a stable, philosophically driven effort to create interdisciplinary links within "the theory of knowledge." Admittedly this will be harder than it was for such fields as biochemistry, which united parent disciplines that were more closely related. But I believe not only that these deep conceptual links are possible, but that the foundations for most of them have already been laid. The first section of this book is an attempt to make these links explicitly within the framework of economics, psychology, and neuroscience.

The second goal of the volume is to reveal the depth and breadth of these existing links, to show what it is that neuroeconomics has already accomplished. We can already lay out quite a few facts about the fundamental mechanisms of human choice that have been gleaned by the parent disciplines of neuroeconomics. By stably linking these many pre-existing insights into a formally structured interdisciplinary theory, we can achieve an unexpectedly complete picture of how humans—and animals—choose. That set of arguments is presented in the second and third sections of this book and summarized in formal mathematical form in the penultimate chapter.

Philosophical Foundations

Over the past several years, a group of leading economists have proclaimed that neuroeconomics—the fusion of neuroscience, psychology, and economics—is *in principle* impossible. The Princeton economists Faruk Gul and Wolfgang Pesendorfer, for example, urged social scientists to pursue what they call a "Mindless Economics" (Gul and Pesendorfer, 2008). The Nobel Laureate Bob Lucas has even asked "Why *Neuro-Economics?*" (Lucas, 2008).

One starting point for many of these negative conclusions is a group of papers published by economists and psychologists that defines one philosophical view of what neuroeconomics is and how it should proceed empirically. The most widely read of these papers is probably Colin Camerer, George Loewenstein, and Drazen Prelec's 2005 paper, where the authors argue that the existing corpus of economic theory has failed to provide adequate predictive power; they suggest that by adding neuroscientific observations to economics—essentially by using brain scanners in economic experiments—pre-existing economic theories can be better assessed and improved. That paper argues that by directly incorporating natural scientific evidence into social scientific theories, social scientific theories will become more powerful.

For theorists such as Gul and Pesendorfer, however, economics is a science that by definition is concerned only with understanding choice. Understanding the brain mechanisms by which choice occurs, they point out, is irrelevant to economic theory. The corpus of economic theory, they stress, does not even include the objects of natural scientific study, objects like the "basal ganglia" or the "cerebral cortex." Instead economics rests on conceptual objects such as "choices," which they note are largely absent from natural scientific discourse.

They have argued that the absence of natural scientific objects from the tightly structured web of existing economic theory makes these objects irrelevant to economics. *There is no escaping the fact that they are right.*[1] Gul and Pesendorfer are correct in observing that if this were what neuroeconomics is about, neuroeconomics would at best offer trivial insights to economists. Economics is not about measurements; it is about predicting human behavior. Relating the theory of neuroscience to the theory of economics through purely empirical measurement will be as hopeless a task as the detractors of neuroeconomics fear. Gul and Pesendorfer go on, however, to argue that this means economics must remain unrelated to psychology and neuroscience. That is a much stronger, and much more speculative, statement.

Even a cursory review of the history of science and the philosophical foundations of the theory of knowledge suggests that in making this

---

1. At least with regard to positive economics, an area of economics that is the focus of this volume.

claim, Gul and Pesendorfer have gone too far. At this moment in history, it is certainly true that confusion seems to dominate the debate about reconciling the social and natural sciences. Many scholars seem not to understand how, at the level of the philosophy of science, these two disciplines could, even in principle, be related. But the history and philosophy of science provide clear signposts that show us how neuroeconomics should proceed to achieve successful linkages between its parent disciplines. These signposts suggest that the philosophical opposition of many social scientific scholars to linking the natural and social sciences is an ontological error.

A close relationship between the theory of economics, the theory of psychology, and the theory of neuroscience could be forged—but it would have to be forged by a partial reduction (and the word *partial* here is critical) of economics to psychology and thence to neuroscience. It would have to be accomplished by a set of interdisciplinary linkages like the ones that bonded physics to chemistry, chemistry to biology, and biology to psychology during the past century.

The key to understanding these historical linkages, and the key to charting the course of the emerging linkages that will relate the social and natural sciences, is a clear definition of the conceptual objects that make up a given science. Economics has been constructed from logical primitives such as utility, supply, demand, and choice. Neuroscience, at the other extreme, has been built from primitives such as brain activations, neurons, synapses, and neurotransmitters. How can we relate these seemingly unrelatable bodies of theory and their allied bodies of empirical measurements? They seem to have nothing in common. The answer to that question, the answer to Gul and Pesendorfer's question, is that we can intentionally forge links that conjoin these two different kinds of logical theories. We can directly incorporate conceptual objects from the social sciences downwards into the fabric of the natural sciences. For example, we can add objects such as "choices" (which come from the higher-level theory of economics) directly to (lower-level) neurobiological theories. Once such key concepts as "choice" are common elements in both sets of theories, once both theories engage at least a few common logical objects that of necessity have their origins in the higher-level theory, we can begin to link clusters of low-level concepts from neuroscience to high-level concepts in economics. Mean brain activation in the medial prefrontal cortex can be linked, through the common logical object of choice, to ideas such as expected utility. The linkages will of course not be perfect, but herein lies the greatest strength of the approach. As we adjust the conceptual objects in each discipline to maximize interrelations between disciplinary levels of analysis, we achieve both a formal reduction of the two theories and *a broadening of the predictive range of both theories*. By taking this approach, we eliminate the logical barrier to making economic predictions with neuroscientific theory, and we also eliminate the barrier to using observations of choice to infer neural function.

Once both economics and neuroscience take even a single common object—in this example, the concept of "choice"—as an object of study (and as we will see, it is critical that this be *exactly* the same concept and that this concept be anchored to the higher-level theory), then the linkage of fields as disparate as neuroscience and economics becomes the process of finding concepts from economics that can be linked to concepts (or concept groups) from neuroscience. This is a tried-and-true strategy in the history of science. It is exactly how chemistry and physics came to be closely related; it is also how biology and chemistry gave rise to biochemistry. But to understand how and why economics, psychology, and neuroscience are relatable, one has to truly understand the philosophical issues that must guide these linkages. Doubtless, many young scientists who support the fusion of the social and natural sciences will argue that actually understanding these metaphysical issues is irrelevant—far better, they will argue, to simply get to work on the daily empirical process. The consilience of knowledge is inevitable; digging through dusty debates about the theory of knowledge is a waste of time. These scholars need to recognize that the past decade has proven how mistaken they are in this belief. Literally hundreds of debates and dozens of papers have been produced, and thousands of scholars have drawn faulty conclusions, because of confusion about basic philosophical issues that lie at the root of this interdisciplinary endeavor.

Practical Neuroeconomics

Even among those who support interdisciplinary synthesis, however, it is often said that we simply do not yet know enough about the brain to constrain economic theories of human behavior. Even if we could philosophically link economics, psychology, and neuroscience at some conceptual level, these scholars argue, those linkages would be of little practical use in extending the predictive range of economic theories. In a similar way, many argue that economic theory is such a "dismal science" that its abstruse mathematical theories will never help to constrain neurobiological models of human behavior. As I hope to make clear in the pages that follow, no two statements could be farther from the truth.

What many economists do not realize is that the past decade has seen a revolution in the cognitive neurosciences. Detailed empirical datasets now tell us many fundamental things about how human minds work. These are not the kinds of insights one obtains from glancing through colorful pictures of brains in popular news magazines; these are insights produced by committed and mathematically sophisticated scholars. We know that there are things human brains can and cannot do. If economic theories about how people make choices should be constrained by what human brains actually can do, then quite a bit of contemporary neuroscience can be of use in the construction of economic theory. To a practicing economist that may seem an exorbitant claim on several levels, but it is the central claim developed formally in the pages that follow.

In a similar way, what many neuroscientists and psychologists may not realize is that the beautifully crafted mathematical tools of economic theory often can tell us when a statement about human brains is logically incoherent. When a neuroscientist or psychologist seeks to isolate measurements of risk aversion and utility in a behaviorally consistent chooser, he or she is attempting the impossible—in principle it is impossible to separate risk aversion and utility in such an actor. This is something economists have known for half a century.

What observations such as these imply is that knowing enough neuroscience, psychology, and economics—all at the same time—can provide scholars of human and animal choice with profound new insights. Combining the empirical and theoretical accomplishments of these disciples can yield significant added value. Neuroeconomics really can be (indeed it already is) more than simply the sum of its parts. This is the main point made in the second and third sections of this book.

The Structure of the Book

This book is composed of four parts. The first part lays the philosophical foundations for neuroeconomics. This section shows how and why the parent disciplines of economics, psychology, and neuroscience relate. It argues for fundamental changes in the core values of economics and ends by challenging the economist Milton Friedman's (1953) famous *as if* dictum on both philosophical and empirical grounds. It also makes clear why a few critical concepts need to be placed at the center of any future neuroeconomics.

The second and third sections of the book build on this foundation to develop a heavily constrained neuroeconomic theory of human (and animal) decision making. The second section presents an overview of what we already know about how the brain constructs, stores, and represents the values of choice objects. Further, it shows how existing economic theory can help us to constrain those notions in powerful and predictive ways. The second section is, in essence, a neuroeconomic *Theory of Choice*. The third section provides an overview of the neurobiological machinery for valuation (which turns out to be at least partially independent of the machinery for choice), a neuroeconomic *Theory of Value*. These two sections present all of the core evidence, from all three parent disciplines, for a fairly complete theory of decision making.

The final section of the book is composed of two chapters. The first summarizes, in fairly compact mathematical notation, everything that has come before in sections 2 and 3. In this sense, the penultimate chapter is really the only important chapter in the second half of the book. If a reader wanted to take everything I have to say on faith, he or she need read only that one chapter. All the chapters that come before in sections 2 and 3 simply serve to make the case that the penultimate chapter effectively summarizes most of what we know about human choosers at a neuroeconomic level. The last chapter provides a more semantic summary of the book as well as providing a summary of what I consider to be the four most important accomplishments of the discipline to date. That chapter also lists what I consider to be the six most pressing unanswered questions in neuroeconomics today.

I want to point out here, though, that navigating this material may be unexpectedly complicated for many readers who are unused to reading technical material from outside their own disciplines. To aid readers in moving through the material, I have begun each chapter with a précis. This should help readers identify the central goal of each chapter as they move through the book. The précis both describes the goals of the chapter and identifies the types of readers for whom the chapter was primarily intended. Economists, for example, may choose to skip the chapter on the objects of neoclassical thought; this is a chapter intended primarily for psychologists and neuroscientists. Psychologists may find the chapter on psychophysical theory unnecessary. Neurobiologists may skip the review of basic neuroscience concepts. In general, however, I would urge most readers to tackle all of the chapters in the order in which they are presented, simply skimming chapters that contain material with which they are already familiar. As mentioned above, the penultimate chapter summarizes, in fairly mathematical form, the insights I have tried to provide throughout the book. I want to forewarn readers without any mathematical background that this chapter may be a bit intimidating. I believe that for these readers this chapter can simply be skipped or skimmed.

The only readers for whom I might suggest an alternative route are neoclassical economic theorists. These readers might proceed immediately to the next to last chapter for an overview of the nuts and bolts of the standard theory I present here. That chapter can then serve as a kind of technical appendix for sections 2 and 3 for these readers. My hope is that this last chapter will reassure my more skeptical economist colleagues that going through all of this psychology and neuroscience really does lead one to the Canaan of obviously economic territory.

As this introduction has doubtless made clear, this is a book directed primarily at scholars working on (or interested in) the study of human or animal decision making, whatever their academic or philosophical affiliations. I have tried to make the work complete enough that any serious scholar—whether a graduate student in psychology, a post-doctoral fellow in neuroscience, or a professor of economics—will find the exposition complete. The book provides what I believe to be the emerging standard neuroeconomic model of human choice. For scholars who have publicly doubted that such a model is possible (or desirable) my plea is simply this: Read this book.

Section 1

The Challenge of Neuroeconomics

I

Standing at the Threshold

What guides human choice? Can we predict the behavioral decisions made by individuals or groups? What are the origins of our preferences; how and why do they change? Why do people behave the ways that they do? These are a few of the persistent core questions that scholars and laypeople alike have asked since the Enlightenment. Economists, psychologists, and biologists, among others, have developed partial answers to these questions, but what is striking, if one takes a global view, is how partial and unconnected our answers to these questions remain. The incompleteness of our answers to these questions is even more striking because our answers to so many other ageless questions have become startlingly global, or *conscilient*, during the past century.

The question of where we come from is another one of these kinds of questions. At the turn of the 20th century that was also a question to which we had many partial answers, but no clear view of how those partial answers interconnected. A chemist working at that time might have argued that we are the product of well-regulated chemical reactions that build us from molecules common in the local environment. A biologist might have said that we are the product of our heredity; the features of our parents are passed to us, from generation to generation, and it is these inherited features that define who we are and who we will be.

Both the early-20th-century chemist and the early-20th-century biologist are answering the same question, but answering it in unconnected ways. Each has a fairly complete theory of our physical origins, but there is almost no overlap in their explanations; there is not even an overlap in the objects of the theories they use to answer what is obviously a single common question. The chemist speaks of molecules and the biologist of hereditable traits. Both knew that there must be some material relationship between their answers, but their answers were so different that there were not even grounds for common discourse in their theories. Were an early-20th-century chemist to propose a detailed theory of how large aggregates of molecules became self-replicating, his biological colleague might well insist that this theory was, in principle, of no interest to him.

James Watson and Francis Crick (1953) changed all of that when they discovered that the chemical compound deoxyribonucleic acid was the physical agent by which traits are inherited. Today when biologists speak of traits, genes, and DNA, they use these words as virtual synonyms. Today we have a global and quite complete theory of our physical origins. We can view that same theory through the lens of paleontology, chemistry, biology, or even neuroscience. Indeed, while there are still paleontologists, chemists, and biologists asking pressing questions, those disciplines are unified around a single global understanding of our origins.

Our understanding of how we choose, of what behaviors we decide to produce, lacks this unity. Like our 20th-century scholarly counterparts, early 21st-century economists, psychologists, and biologists all strive to answer a common question, but answer it in unconnected ways. Social scientists and natural scientists define the sources of our actions in such different ways that many insist the theories and insights of the other groups are, in principle, of no interest. To make this incredibly important point clear, consider a simple example. Let us examine a pair of humans making a single set of real choices and try to understand those choices using the tools first of economics, then of psychology, and then of biology. What we want to do is to ask how the same behavior would be understood by these three groups of early-21st-century scholars. To do that, of course, we need to select a behavior for which all three groups of scholars have well-developed conceptual frameworks. To include the biologists, this means that the behavior we examine will have to include decisions related to reproduction—to sex.

Understanding Behavior

Two adults walk into a hotel bar: a man and a woman from different cities, both attending a professional conference. We observe that they encounter each other for the first time, begin talking, and become more animated in their discussions as time passes. From prior inquiry we have learned that both adults have serious, valuable (and explicitly monogamous) sexual relationships at home, but as they interact it becomes clear that they have discovered a strong mutual physical attraction. Were we to interview the woman at this point, she might tell us, "If I sleep with him, I will regret it tomorrow." Were we to interview the man he might report, "If that woman and I were to spend the night together, I would never be able to face my partner at home." Eight hours later we learn that they have, in fact, spent the night together. Seventy-two hours later we find that they are both at home with their partners, miserable, wracked by guilt, and clearly unhappy. Interviews after two weeks reveal that they have both concluded that sleeping together was an enormous mistake that did not maximize their happiness, and of course this is an outcome they each precisely anticipated. Why did they do it? In what sense was it a mistake? How do we understand this behavior?

The common goal of biology, psychology, and economics is to answer these kinds of questions. Inasmuch as all three sciences take human choices as a logical object of study, these three disciplines all seek to answer such questions as "Why did these two people choose to sleep together?"

An Economist Answers

For a very traditional neoclassical economist, the goal of theory is to explain *observed* choice. Things in the outside world that we can measure and that have an impact on the actions of others are the "choices" that a traditional economist seeks to explain. Critical to the esthetic of the modern economic approach is a desire to accomplish this explanation with the absolute minimum number of theoretical constructs and intermediate variables. The goal of a traditional economist trying to understand why the man and the woman slept together is simply to generate the most parsimonious theory that can explain the observed choice of these two individuals with a minimal number of assumptions.

To accomplish that goal, the traditional (neoclassical) economist begins by rigorously categorizing the choices that each individual faces.[1]

---

1. I assume, for the purposes of this exposition to non-economists, that the subjects behave "consistently" in the technical economic sense of that word. Let me note for

If we take it as a given that both the man and the woman have an accurate knowledge of both the sexual experience that they might have and the objective external risks that they will face at home next week if they sleep together, then we can describe them as choosing between (1) a sexual experience in the near term and a small later risk of discovery that may cost them their permanent relationships, or (2) no sexual experience in the near term and no risk of losing their permanent relationships.[2] What we observed is that they slept together, so we *have* (as economists) to conclude that they *preferred* a near-term sexual experience to safety in their long-term relationships. As Paul Samuelson taught all economists in the 1930s, the key feature of *choice* for an economist is that it "reveals" a subject's underlying preferences. Preferences, to Samuelson, were simply the shadow of choice: We *know* what the man and the woman preferred because we *know* what they chose. It is that almost circular relationship that lends unequalled clarity and simplicity to the economic approach.

We also know, however, that the man and the woman later report verbally that the choice that they made was a "mistake" in some general way. Could a neoclassical economist agree with this conclusion drawn by the man and the woman? Probably not. The fact that these individuals keep saying to themselves that they are miserable, or that they wish they had made another choice, is simply not an element of the neoclassical story *unless it has an impact on what they do.* Imagine that they meet the next year at the same professional conference and decide not to sleep

---

economists that my slightly unusual (if orthodox) focus on preferences rather than on consistency is driven by the requirements of the theory that follows.

2. I need to point out that I have taken a *very* traditional neoclassical economic approach here. I have not allowed such feelings as "guilt" or "regret" to enter into the economic explanation. This is because the path-blazing economists of the first half of the 20th century, people like Milton Friedman and Paul Samuelson, wanted to condition economic theories only on things that could be observed in the external world. How do we measure these "feelings," Friedman and Samuelson might have asked if we had proposed adding them to an economic explanation. If we include these "unobservables" as things to be explained in our theories, we are needlessly complicating the job of prediction, they might have argued. In more recent times, however, economists have drawn from psychology the notion that to explain some classes of choices with minimal complexity, "feelings" sometimes do need to be postulated as the outcomes of choices. This is a point to which we will turn in the pages that follow.

together a second time, under identical circumstances. Then an economist might be willing to entertain the possibility that their first decision was a mistake. If they slept together again, regardless of how that later made them feel, then no reasonable economist could present a model that both predicted their choices and described those choices as a mistake. Adding the word "mistake" would add nothing to the model of choice behavior. Why would an economist concerned only with choice add that word? The fact that they keep asserting that they made a "mistake" is simply talk.

The critical point here is that economics seeks to explain choices with the simplest possible theory. Subjects reveal what they prefer by their actions. Economists use observed choices to infer preferences. If we observe enough choices and make a few simple assumptions about the nature of our subjects, we can do a fairly complete job of inferring the global structure of these hidden preferences, and we can even use these "revealed preferences" to accurately predict future behavior. As economists, we make no commitment to the idea that these preferences are physical events or mental states. They are simply compact variables, related *only* to observed choices, useful for predicting future choices. Preferences are the stuff of economic theories, and these preferences are the simplest possible tools for explaining choice. Thus economic theories (at least in their original form) must neglect anything we cannot observe directly and must be silent about whether our subjects have things such as goals, hopes, or desires. We have to content ourselves with the subjects having only preferences, and even those in the most limited of senses.

A Psychologist Answers

For most psychologists, the story of the man and the woman is more complicated than it was for economists. The choice that these two individuals face is not simply between sexual intercourse and a risk of discovery, but rather a choice between mental states and a choice about happiness. For a typical psychologist these two people are choosing between the feelings they will have during sex and the miseries they will (or may) face at home later. The experience of these choices and consequences is mediated by *mental states*. The psychologist thus typically begins by assuming in advance what these two individuals want to accomplish with their choices: They want to maximize their "happiness." Psychology knows what the two individuals are trying to do, what the goal of their choices is—a critical difference between it and economics. Indeed, it even allows us to define mistakes in a new way. A year after these two people have slept together we interview them and simply ask whether overall they are happier having slept together or whether they would have been happier if they had not slept together. We simply ask them to tell us whether or not sleeping together was a mistake.

Suppose as psychologists we conduct this interview and the subjects tell us that, exactly as they expected, they were miserable for 2 months. They tell us that the experience of sleeping together was not worth the price they paid. A typical rigorous contemporary psychological explanation for the behavior might then go this way: The first thing that we have to explain about the choice is how the two subjects came to make this mistake. Clearly this was a mistake (the subjects told us that), and daily measurements of their happiness confirm that the choice they made did not make them on average happier for a week, let alone for a year. We might postulate that the choice they faced was really a kind of internal conflict between two inner selves. The first is an impulsive inner self that can see only as far as the attractive person on the next stool at the bar. The other is a more patient rational self that can see the long-term mental costs of the affair. If we accept this theoretical framework, then the observation that the two subjects slept together is evidence that the impulsive self triumphed over the patient self. That the two subjects are unhappy later is evidence that the impulsive self should not have triumphed, and indicates that the decision was a flawed one.

Let me note that in generating this kind of explanation as psychologists, we lean heavily on our own personal (introspective) experiences of mental life. We (correctly, I think) see joys, sorrows, and regret as the products of the subjects' choices. We also see those choices as reflecting a conflict between two or more internal "selves" that compete for control of behavior. In this, we borrow a truly ancient classical tradition familiar to most of us in the form of Freudian theory. It is Freud's competition between *id* and *ego* (Freud, 1923) that mirrors the conflict our explanatory theory hypothesizes in the minds of the subjects.

There are thus two key features that the psychological explanation incorporates: (1) the notion of mental states as outcomes, choices trading not between traditional economic observables—sex, money, marriages—but between feelings that shape our daily internal lives and mediate the impact of these external variables on our actions, and (2) the notion of a goal, the idea that human choices seek to maximize happiness, or perhaps fulfillment, or some other set of mental states that we try to capture with the word *happiness*. Economics has no such object. In economics we infer preferences, an approach that precludes statements about goals or judgments about mistakes. It keeps the theory compact and well focused, but at the cost of appearing to miss something that seems powerfully important, if admittedly ill defined.

To put this last distinction more formally, the economic tradition answers the question of why the subjects did it by invoking their preferences. These two subjects slept together because they preferred the immediate sex to guaranteed future stability. Another pair of subjects might have acted differently, revealing a different set of preferences. In economics, the preferences of the subjects serve in theory as what one might call the *proximal causes* of their behavior.[3] In the psychological tradition we take a different route. We begin to ask *why* at a deeper level. If we start with the assumption that the goal of the two adults is to maximize their own long-term happiness, then can we really identify their decision as a mistake? In psychology, we can identify maximizing long-term happiness, or some related set of mental processes, as the larger goal of behavior—as the *ultimate cause* of their behavior in general. This is, of course, both a strength and a weakness of the approach. We can define the ultimate cause of behavior using this approach, but often we observe behavior that fails to be closely related to this cause. We then have to label the discrepancy between what we imagine to be the ultimate cause of behavior and the behavior we actually observe as "mistakes." In the case of the man and the woman described here, this does seem to capture something the economic explanation lacks, but at the risk of introducing a new kind of theoretical subjectivity to the analysis.

---

3. Although Samuelson himself might have argued that one would do better to see preferences as caused by choices rather than the reverse.

A Biologist Answers

For most biologists, the starting point for understanding the behavior of the man and the woman is the starting point for much natural scientific explanation: Darwin's theory of evolution. In this regard, the natural scientists differ markedly from the social scientists. Biologists view all behavior as the product of evolution, so it becomes natural for a biologist to ask this same question in yet another way that does not arise in either the economic or the psychological traditions: How is this behavior related to reproduction, or more specifically to the "inclusive fitness"[4] of the two subjects?

Consider the following anecdote from a primatologist friend of mine. A mated pair of Siamangs (a monogamous ape from the gibbon family) live together defending a territory. The male goes out foraging and while away, a solitary intruder male enters the pair's territory and produces courting behavior directed towards the female. After a brief period of courtship, the female consents and the two apes begin to mate. As they finish mating, the resident male returns and makes a number of distress vocalizations. He makes aggressive gestures towards both the intruder male and towards his mate. After a few minutes of this behavior, the intruder male retreats. The resident male then settles into a high branch of a nearby tree and curls up. He does not look at the resident female. After another few minutes the resident female climbs the tree and begins to groom her mate, who intermittently pushes her away. What is going on here?

For a biologist this is easy. All animals work to maximize the number of their genes that occur in future generations. Or, to put that more precisely, the animals that survive are those whose behavior maximizes the number of their genes in future generations. The goal of behavior is

---

4. "Fitness" in the technical biological sense is the relative probability that the hereditary characteristics of the decision-maker will be reproduced in future generations. "Inclusive fitness" is the relative probability that the hereditary characteristics of the decision-maker will be reproduced in future generations regardless of whether those characteristics descend from the decision-maker himself or from other individuals who share those hereditary characteristics with the decision-maker. For a clear formal presentation of this material, the reader is referred to Futuyma's (1998) *Evolutionary Biology*.

to maximize fitness.[5] Starting from that point we can understand why, in the sense of a biological *ultimate cause*, the female Siamang decided to mate with the intruder male. We know that female primates who have permanent partners incur both costs and benefits from the partnership. They successfully defend larger resource-containing territories, a benefit. They share the task of defending their progeny from predators, which reduces infant mortality, another benefit. They also, however, produce offspring who are very similar genetically. This is a clear drawback because it means that when the environment presents risks to one of the female's offspring it usually presents that same risk to all of her offspring. For example, if her mate and hence her offspring have light-colored skin, then changes in the color of the foliage could present a risk to all of her children. In other words, by having one mate she has, so to speak, put all of her eggs in one basket.

So, having a permanent mate has both advantages and disadvantages for the female from the point of view of evolution. Viewed through that lens, the behavior of the female Siamang then makes perfect sense. The ultimate goal of the female's behavior was to maximize the genetic fitness of her progeny. She attempted to accomplish this by *covertly* mating with a novel male. How did she feel afterwards? Did she regret her decision? To be honest, an evolutionary biologist (much like an economist) would

---

5. I have to admit that I have atrociously simplified Darwin here. First, one needs to acknowledge that Darwin argued that two things shape the behavior of animals in the absence of human breeding programs: both *natural selection* and *sexual selection*. In this discussion I am making it look like only natural selection is important, which is simply not the case. Second, from here on in I will be assuming that the pressures of evolution yield animals that largely succeed in maximizing their "inclusive genetic fitness." While most biologists are comfortable with this conclusion from empirical studies of animal behavior, some are not. While all biologists agree that evolution pushes animal behavior towards the goal of maximizing fitness, some argue that real behavior does not often achieve or approximate that goal. My own reading of the literature as a working biologist is that real animal behavior, except in very dynamic environments where the rate of evolution has trouble keeping up, almost always comes close to maximizing fitness. There is no real doubt that almost every behavioral measurement of efficiency that we have available to us indicates that if a species is in a stable environment for many generations, its behavior largely achieves this single well-stated goal. My previous monograph, *Decisions, Uncertainty and the Brain*, dealt with this issue in detail. For the purposes of this discussion, we begin from the assumption that animal behavior in stable natural environments approximately maximizes genetic fitness.

consider these questions largely irrelevant. It was an effort to increase the genetic diversity of her progeny. What the evolutionary biological story points out is the ultimate cause of the Siamang's behavior in an objective biological sense. Her behavior maximized her fitness. This is a central concept in the biological approach, and a feature that will be critical in relating the social and natural sciences in the pages that follow.[6]

At a much more proximal level, however, the biologist can also begin to ask questions about how this behavior was accomplished. What neural circuits became active when the female Siamang saw the intruder male? How did the play of synaptic activity through her cortex and basal ganglia lead to activation of her hypothalamus and later to the activation of the motor control circuits for mating behavior? How were her estrogen levels related to the excitability of these circuits?

Thus for the biologist, like the psychologist, two levels of explanation arise: the proximal and the ultimate. The proximal level is one of neural circuits and computational algorithms. The ultimate level is one of evolution and fitness in stable environments.

So how then would a biologist understand the behavior of the man and the woman at the professional conference? Much in the same way that he or she understood the behavior of the Siamangs. At the level of an ultimate causation lies evolution. From an evolutionary perspective, the decision to have sex was a rational one that would have maximized the inclusive fitness of both individuals.[7] At a proximal level the behavior of the man and woman was shaped by interacting neural systems.

If I ask my graduate students why people have sex, their answer is, "because people like having sex." This is the definition of a *proximal cause*.

---

6. Again, let me admit to simplification for the purposes of exposition. Of course what the female Siamang risks when she copulates with the other male is defection by her partner. Formally, that means that she is engaged in a kind of evolutionary game. This is a fact of which biologists are well aware. The classic work on the subject is J. Maynard Smith's (1982) *Evolution and the Theory of Games*.

7. One should point out here that the human subjects may well have chosen to use contraceptives, which would render the mating fruitless. Does that render the ultimate causal explanation false? The very important answer, to which we will return several times in these pages, is no. Evolution achieves efficient behavior in stable environments. Contraceptives are a very recent change in the environment. Many humans now use contraceptives, though evolution could now be selecting for humans who hate contraceptives.

It is a statement about mental states (or perhaps about preferences). But *why*, a biologist asks back, do people like having sex? Even the most hesitant reader has to acknowledge that people evolved to like sex *because* having sex leads to reproduction. This is the definition of an *ultimate cause* in the biological sense.

If, as biologists, we acknowledge that the physical attractiveness of the man and the woman played a role in their mating, then we can even, as biologists, try to understand this at both the proximal and the ultimate level. At the proximal level we could search for the neural circuits that identify attractiveness, and indeed many of these circuits have been identified (e.g., Aharon et al., 2001; Winston et al., 2007). Activation of these circuits is something humans and animals will expend effort to achieve (e.g., Deaner, Khera, and Platt, 2005; Klein, Deaner, and Platt, 2008). Humans and animals reveal to us by their actions that they prefer these attractiveness circuits to be active. At a more ultimate level we can hypothesize that attractiveness is a marker for certain genetic characteristics in a mate. Indeed, a group of studies seems to suggest that the more attractive a person is, the more closely he or she approximates a particular set of desirable genetic traits (Etcoff, 1999; Penton-Voak et al., 1999; Perrett et al., 1998).

The most puzzling problem for the biologist, then, is the discovery that after two months the subjects tell their psychologists that they are unhappy about having slept together. They both feel that this was a mistake and they both regret it. If they were really maximizing their genetic fitness, and their behavior really was the product of a unified behavioral strategy, then why are they unhappy?

The truth is that for a biologist this isn't really puzzling at all. Brains are complicated and highly modular—a point to which we shall return. Dozens of actions we take every day are completed without any conscious awareness. Many of these actions help us to survive and reproduce even if the parts of our brains that produce the conscious verbal narrative we share with others remain unaware of these events. To put it in a more mechanistic way, our verbal narrative reflects the actions of Broca's area (among other areas), a part of the brain also known as Brodmann's areas 44 and 45. These brain areas are connected with some, but not all, of the behavior-generating areas of our brains. When we ask the subjects why they did something, we ask their Brodmann's areas 44 and 45 to use what resources those areas have to answer that question. Our current evidence suggests that these areas have little direct access to, for example, the activity patterns in the hypothalamus. Inasmuch as hypothalamic activity governs behavior, asking Brodmann's area 44 and 45 to tell us why the behavior occurred may simply be asking the wrong part of the person. If Brodmann's area 44 and 45 tell us that sleeping together was a mistake, they are giving us a limited assessment of behavior provided by a small portion of the *neuraxis*. They are not telling us much about the overall community of brain mechanisms that make up each of the conference-attending subjects.

To put that another way, the ultimate cause of behavior is not an effort to maximize happiness or pleasure as reported verbally or by introspection. Happiness and pleasure are two of many proximal mechanisms by which the nervous system achieves its ultimate goal of fitness maximization. Obviously we did not evolve to be happy; if we had, then people would be as good at being happy as they are at having sex. That is an important point that any synthesis of the social and natural sciences will have to acknowledge.

Are We Standing at the Threshold?

Economists, psychologists, and biologists can all offer local explanations for the behavior of the two subjects we have examined in this chapter, but what is striking is the unrelatedness of their explanations. Other disciplines, such as sociology or biochemistry, may even offer explanations that are more unrelated.

Another striking feature is that these explanations are extremely local. Each of these explanatory frameworks allows us to make only very limited predictions about how these subjects will behave in the future, and each explanation makes those predictions under different conditions. The economic explanation may make predictions about behavior during future sexual encounters by these subjects. The psychological description may make predictions about future impulsivity in these subjects. The biological explanation may make predictions about future choices bearing on gene frequencies. What we lack is a global theory that can unite these disciplines and their explanations for human and animal behavior.

Could such a theory exist? If it did, what would it look like? How could we link these three explanatory traditions? If we accomplished such a linkage, what would it buy us?

2

Epistemological Constraints on Consilience

Précis

Fundamental conceptual tools available in the physical and natural sciences, such as Darwin's theory of evolution and Schrödinger's wave equations, have at least partially succeeded in linking the many independent explanations for physical and biological phenomena produced by the many independent disciplines of these sciences. These linkages have both broadened our understanding of physical phenomena and improved and extended our ability to predict those phenomena. Can similar linkages be forged between economic, psychological, and neuroscientific explanations of human behavior? If so, how certain can we be that the explanatory systems that anchor these three disciplines to one another will prove useful?

In this chapter, we explore the metaphysical constraints that the "Theory of Knowledge" places on efforts to link any two or more independent explanatory systems. We review the role of the *logical positivist* philosophers in describing how the reductive synthesis of two disciplines typically occurs, and we explore the well-described and explicit philosophical constraints on those synthetic approaches. This discussion serves as an essential prelude to any effort to build a neuroeconomic approach to human decision making because it tells us what we can—and cannot—expect to accomplish. For readers familiar with reductive syntheses and logical positivism (both its strengths and weaknesses), this material will be a review. Such a reader might well skip ahead to Chapter 3. For those unfamiliar with this line of philosophical inquiry, or even for those who suspect (I think erroneously) that reductive linkages between the sciences must always succeed, this chapter will be an important next step towards understanding how a single comprehensive theory with shared logical elements can serve to both link and extend modern studies of human behavior.

Metaphysical Constraints on any Future Neuroeconomics

To begin to better understand linkages between independent disciplines, consider first the physical sciences. Contemporary physics provides us with a standard "theory of matter." This theory describes how fundamental, or elemental, particles such as electrons, protons, and neutrons interact. Electrons, for example, interact in spin pairs and fill orbitals around atomic nuclei according to physical "laws." These are abstractions at (or near to) the lowest level of physical reality.

Contemporary chemistry provides us with a description of a different set of logical primitives,[1] the elements of the periodic table. These fundamental particles cluster into groups and interact according to chemical "laws."

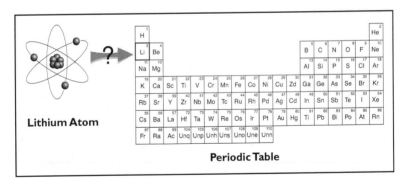

FIGURE 2.1   A lithium atom and the periodic table.

---

1. *Logical primitives* are the irreducible building blocks upon which a given theory stands. Objects such as neurons are logical primitives for neuroscientific theories as are objects like choice and utility for economic theories.

How are these two sets of abstractions related? Can we, for example, completely reduce the higher-level "laws" of chemistry to the lower-level "laws" of physics? Can we rephrase any arbitrary statement about a group of atoms to an equally accurate statement about electrons, protons, and neutrons? Interestingly, the answer to this particular question seems to be yes. We can, for example, predict the structure of the periodic table and define the elements it contains from an understanding of the basic physics of matter. This is one of the greatest accomplishments of the 20th century, but it raises the specter of an even larger reconciliation that has dominated discussions of the philosophy of science for decades: Can this kind of explanatory relationship between levels of physical description, the reduction of chemistry to physics, be extended throughout the sciences?

The Origins of Modern Reductionism

At the time that it was becoming clear that insights from physics were shaping chemistry and vice versa, the Viennese philosophers Rudolph Carnap and Moritz Schlick were struggling to understand how different kinds of knowledge about the universe were related. The notion that the many different branches of science might share a common foundation began to be clearly developed in the 1920s within a school of European philosophers and scientists that developed around the physicist, psychologist, and physiologist Ernst Mach in Vienna and Berlin (Mach, 1886). Following Mach, philosopher-scientists such as Carnap and Schlick (Schlick, 1918; Carnap, Hahn, and Neurath, 1929) came to the conclusion (originally proposed by Mach) that all classes of knowledge were related by the fact that all of our insights about the world descend from sensory experience. The critical idea for these *logical positivists* was that since all we know about the world, whether about the movements of masses or the decisions of the masses, comes from a common sensory source, all of these kinds of knowledge must be "reduce-able" to a common language or starting point.

Their argument, which was really explored most deeply by the American philosopher Ernest Nagel (1961), went this way: Imagine that we were to consider the sciences as a series of "levels of explanation." At the lowest level we would encounter the physics of sub-atomic particles.

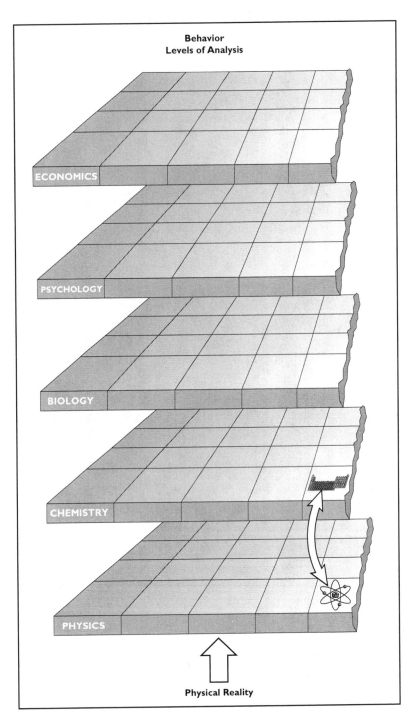

FIGURE 2.2   Levels of explanation.

At the next level we would encounter chemistry, the systems of laws and equations that describe the elements and molecules from which physical reality is built. Above that we can imagine the biological sciences, which describe the aggregate properties of huge conglomerates of molecules that we call organisms. Above that we can describe the psychological sciences that relate mental life and mental constructs to the actions of humans and animals. Above that we can describe the economic sciences as laws and principles that relate features of the environment to the actions of individuals and large groups of humans. This is the level at which, for example, the Marshallian "laws of supply and demand" emerge. The logical positivists pondered how these different levels of description are related.

At a purely logical level, they can be related only if they share common logical objects. Without any common elements in the two sets of theories, no two levels of abstraction could ever hope to be related. This seems obvious, and it is one of the well-taken points presented by Faruk Gul and Wolfgang Pesendorfer in their widely read essay "The Case for Mindless Economics" (Gul and Pesendorfer, 2008). They point out that the goal of economics is to predict choice, not brain states; thus, they argue, economic and neuroscientific levels of analysis are independent and must remain independent as long as the body of economic theory contains no biological objects of any kind.

In the 1920s a similar critique was advanced by C.D. Broad (1925), who argued that chemistry and physics were independent levels of analysis that could not be related. There is nothing, Broad said, about the nature of hydrogen and oxygen (conceptual objects he identified with physics) that would allow one to predict the properties of water (an object he tied to chemistry). One could not predict from physics, for example, the fact that water is transparent, because physics lacks the concept of transparency. Broad was right, albeit in a very local sense. The theory of physics available at the turn of the 20th century was not able to predict the properties of water; chemical concepts such as optical transparency were not objects in the then-extant theory of physics. Importantly, though, Broad's argument did not mean that such linkages are impossible, simply that they did not exist. In fact, we now can predict the transparency of water from the physical properties of atoms. This is because our modern theory of physics includes such objects as photons, and we can link chemical objects such as transparency with the movements of these photons. Chemistry and physics are now related because the theories now share at least some objects, and this makes it possible for us to map at least some ideas and insights from one theory to another.

Reduction: How Low Can We Go?

Can the many levels of analysis and scholarship that range from neuro-science to economics be related, at least at a metaphysical or conceptual level, in the same way that physics and chemistry are related? Chemistry can, one might suppose, be used to completely describe biological processes; biological processes can, one might hypothesize, be used to completely describe mental processes—and so on to the level of socio-logical analysis. One can imagine such reductions, but is this degree of inter-theoretic linkage really possible?

This notion that (at least in principle) all knowledge rests on a common foundation and thus all knowledge is (again, at least in principle) reducible to the language of physics is referred to by philosophers as *ontological reductionism*. Figuring out whether we accept ontological reductionism seems an important step towards understanding whether, like Gul and Pesendorfer, we reject interactions between neuroscience and economics in principle, or whether we can consider embracing them. So the first question that any effort to unite the social and natural sciences must engage (although not necessarily affirm) becomes: Is all knowledge reducible to a common physical language?

The data that began to emerge in the physical and natural sciences during the middle part of the 20th century seemed to suggest that the answer to this question was going to be yes. The development of the wave equations in the 1920s was among the key insights that led to the strong interactions between chemistry and physics mentioned above. These were insights that gave birth to a field now called *physical chemistry* (or perhaps more precisely *theoretical chemistry*, which is a sub-discipline of physical chemistry).

In the 1940s and 1950s, scholars using the methodologies of chemistry began to study biological molecules; in 1953 Watson and Crick famously used this approach to describe the structure of DNA. That was a huge reductive watershed. After that discovery, the techniques of chemistry could be used to describe (admittedly with some modification) the biological laws of heredity. The field now called *biochemistry* was born.

During this same period, biologists and mathematicians also began to take aim at psychology in yet another reductive step. In perhaps the first (and arguably the most famous) example of this, in the 1940s the mathematical biologists McCullough and Pitts (1943) tried to use models of idealized neurons to account for fundamental properties of human thought and behavior in their famous paper "A Logical Calculus of Ideas Immanent in Nervous Tissue." It was studies such as this one that gave birth to the field we now call *neuroscience*.

These empirical insights suggested to many that the *reductionist program* of the logical positivists was inescapable. All of scientific knowledge would someday be unified, and the appeal of this unification

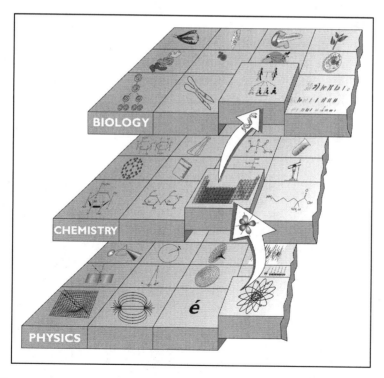

FIGURE 2.3

seemed to push aside the fears of many scholars. (It particularly seemed to embolden those working at lower, or reduced, levels of analysis, who began to take a conquering imperialist view of higher-level sciences.) But Nagel and like-minded philosophers recognized that the existence of fields such as biochemistry was certainly not proof that all of scientific knowledge was soon to be subsumed by physical descriptions of subatomic particles and Schrodinger's wave equations. Imagine, Nagel and others like him pointed out, that we were to seriously try to describe an entire biological organism using the physical laws of elementary particles. Even if such a reductive description were possible in principle, could any human really profit from its existence? Could we humans gain meaningful insight from describing, say, human behavior at the level of sub-atomic law? Regardless of the progress of the reductionist program, the answer to this question is almost certainly no. There are almost certainly practical limits to how far we can take the reductionist program even if we concede that an ontological reductionism is possible.

This line of reasoning suggests that we can identify two fundamental challenges to reductionism: *ontological* and *empirical*. Ontological antireductionism is the claim that—in principle—a reductionist approach to (for example) the social sciences is not possible. Empirical antireductionism is the claim that although such a reduction is possible in principle, in practice this reduction would be useless or impossible given the limitations of human minds and real human-gathered data, or even that in practice it simply will not occur (e.g., Kitchener, 1986).

As an aside from this point, it may be interesting to note that when a world-famous economist says something like "While neurobiologists may someday know enough to impose constraints on economics, everything that neurobiologists have learned up to this point is far too limited to be relevant to the practice of economics," he is making only a very, very limited critique of the reductionist program. The statement seems to explicitly accept that an ontological reduction of economics to neuroscience is possible; it even seems to accept that an empirical reduction is possible—it simply asserts that such a reduction is not *yet* possible. It is frustrating that such a claim by any highly visible scholar implies that, after a careful and deep study of all of modern neuroscience, the speaker has concluded that relationships between the brain and economic behavior simply cannot be forged today—frustrating because many of the scholars making these well-publicized statements often know less about modern neuroscience than a third-year undergraduate. We all have to acknowledge that this is not a very compelling criticism. But good criticisms are possible, and these are the criticisms we need to consider here.

Before moving on, however, let me pause to reveal my own convictions about the limits of reductionism, convictions that some readers may find surprising. For reasons we will turn to next, I would describe my own stance as an *ontological* opposition to complete reductionism. Unlike the economist quoted above, I do not believe that all of economics can be reduced to neuroscience. This is actually a very important point, and it is why my own scholarly career has been devoted to the study of economics, psychology, and neuroscience. To understand why I came to this ontological position, we turn next to the fundamental challenges to reductionism raised in the 1970s.

Emergent Properties and Anti-Reductionism

What, really, are the alternatives to reductionism? Perhaps the most obvious alternative to reductionism is to argue that the properties of the world we humans observe at the level of the social sciences (like the preferences of some people for chocolate over vanilla) are simply not governed by (or the product of) physical law. This is an essentially anti-materialist stance held by many people outside the academic community. These critiques reduce to the statement "People are guided in their choices by phenomena that lie entirely outside the province of the material word, and thus any effort to use physical law to describe the behavior of people (the central domain of the social sciences) must fail."

Without being intentionally disrespectful, I am going to have to say that this kind of magical thinking should be dismissed out of hand for two reasons—first, because it is a call to abandon the search for knowledge of human behavior before one even begins, and second, because there is no evidence whatsoever that materialism will fail to describe human behavior.

If we accept, as a starting point, that the goal of science (social or natural) is to describe the world around us as the product of material phenomena, then are there alternatives to ontological reductionism? The answer is a resounding yes. To quote Thomas Nagel:

> How could the following two propositions be true?
> (1) Every *event* that happens in the physical world has a fundamental description and a fundamental physical explanation.
> (2) Some *facts* about the world do not have a fundamental physical explanation, but do have a higher-level explanation. (Nagel, 1998, italics mine.)

The answer to this question is that whether both propositions can be true depends on how we define facts—or, more precisely, how we group together ideas into what philosophers often call "natural kinds."

To understand this criticism of the reductionist program, let us return to the stacked "levels" of the sciences, here focusing on the relationship between chemistry and biology. In Figure 2.3, one can conceive of each of the squares in the "mesh" I have labeled "biology" as being core ideas. In the front row, for example, we can see the "idea" of heredity and within that idea lies the mathematical concept of an inheritable "gene" first proposed by the 19th-century monk Gregor Mendel (1866). These objects, heredity and genes, are central explanatory ideas from which biology is built. For a philosopher, these bundles of ideas and concepts are called "natural kinds." Importantly, biology, as a set of explanatory concepts that relate and explain observations in the living world, is composed of many such "kinds." The definition of the pancreas (in the second row) is yet another example of a biological kind. Figure 2.4 shows an expanded view of just a few of these relationships.

The question that we have to ask is how these "kinds" that occur at the level of biology relate to "kinds" that occur at the level of chemistry. The first example I have chosen (heredity and genes) is one where this relationship turns out to be very clear. At the level of chemistry we can find another group of "kinds" called nucleic acids. As is widely known today, a sub-group of the nucleic acids are the deoxyribonucleic acids, DNA. Watson and Crick revealed in their famous study that the chemical "kind" of DNA when it is found in cells corresponds almost precisely to the biological "kind" of a gene. Genes, at least in a general sense, could be thought of as *being* DNA. Indeed, it turned out that biological theories describing how genes must be duplicated and passed from parent to

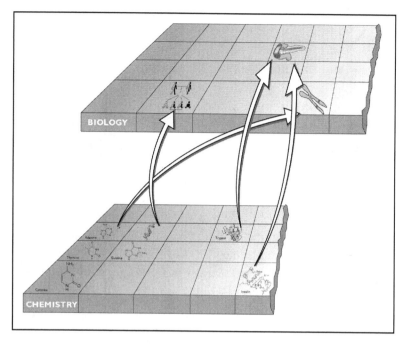

FIGURE 2.4

offspring could (with only minor modifications) also be reduced to statements about the replication of strands of DNA. The reductive relationship between biology and chemistry in this area seems nearly perfect (or can be amended to be so), and it is observations like these that led the reductive revolution.

The concept of the pancreas, however, provides a different example. Since antiquity, the pancreas has been a unitary conceptual object in biology. It is a yellowish-red organ attached to the digestive tract by a small duct, or tube. Damage to this duct produces deficits in digestion. The classical concept of the pancreas in biology is a single logical object. Chemical and microscopic studies of this same physical object during the 20th century, however, revealed that at the level of chemistry the pancreas could not be viewed as a single logical object. At a chemical level the pancreas has to be viewed as involving two separate and unrelated logical objects: an insulin-producing system and a digestive-enzyme–producing system. Biochemistry relates these pre-existing logical categories when it re-categorizes the biological entity of the pancreas into one group of cells that secretes insulin into the bloodstream in response to blood glucose levels and a second independent group of cells that secretes digestive enzymes into the duodenum of the stomach in response to gastric loads.

In other words, what we see here historically is a mismatch between two levels of description—a failure of reduction. To chemists, insulin and digestive enzymes are fundamentally unrelated logical concepts. To biologists, the pancreas is a unitary object. Biochemistry related these two sets of kinds by altering the biological-level concept of the pancreas. The concept of "the pancreas" in biological theory was replaced by two logical objects: "the acinar cells of the pancreas" and the "islets of Langerhans in the pancreas." This modified theory, it is important to note, then makes enhanced predictions (for example about disease) at the biological level. The result was that a reductively driven re-definition of a biological kind resulted in a strengthened higher-level (in this case biological) science. What is interesting and instructive about this example is that it begins as an apparent failure of reduction but ends with a modification of the biological kind to more precisely approximate the two bodies of knowledge. The end product is a strengthening of the predictive power of both disciplines.

Must these kinds of "reductive" linkages *necessarily* occur? Is it possible that there are some important natural kinds discovered by biologists that cannot ever be mapped (or redefined and mapped) into single kinds at the level of chemistry? Consider the biological concept of an "ecosystem." What is the relationship between that concept and the ideas that form the natural kinds of chemistry? It may be that many different pieces of chemistry contribute to the idea of ecosystem, but perhaps not in a simple way that permits a direct reductive mapping. It is possible that the concept of "ecosystem" *emerges* only at the level of biology. It is possible that, unlike the modified theory of the pancreas that emerges from biochemical study of the thorax, the concept of an ecosystem is fundamentally *non-predictable* from the study of chemistry and physics.[2]

---

2. Non-predictability is the critical issue here. Recall that it was Broad's claim that the transparency of water could not, in principle, be predicted from the physical properties of atoms.

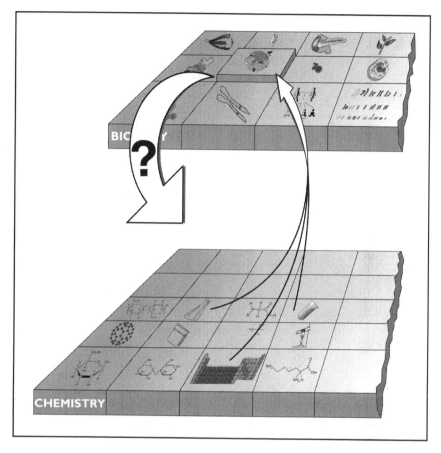

FIGURE 2.5

What we have are two basic possibilities. The first is that there are clear reductive linkages possible between the sciences. Formally, we call these "homomorphisms": The mapping of one mathematically defined set onto another such that any operation performed on the first set corresponds to a specific operation that can be performed on the second with identical results. One possibility is that all concepts in biology are (or after modification could be) homomorphic to concepts in chemistry. The second is the possibility that there are some concepts in biology that could not ever be meaningfully mapped into chemistry. Such concepts would be said to be "emergent." They are philosophical kinds that emerge only at the level of analysis undertaken by biologists.

The critical questions that face any reductionist approach to linking the social and natural sciences are thus:

- Are all concepts at the level of economics homomorphic to concepts at the neurobiological level?
- Are all concepts at the level of economics emergent, or is it the case that some concepts are reducible (as is, or after modification) while others are emergent?

I have to stress here that at a metaphysical level we simply do not know the answer to this question. We cannot say with absolute certainty that even part of biology will turn out, in the far distant future, to be reducible to chemistry. The apparent reduction of genes to DNA may later turn out to have been an error. On the other hand, it may be that everything will be reducible. The apparent failure to reduce "ecosystem" to a set of concepts from chemistry may reflect an incomplete knowledge of chemistry, or at some future date we may abandon the notion of ecosystem and choose to replace it with some much better concept. Either of these is possible, so how are we to proceed?

My answer to this is simple, mostly pragmatic, and probably shaped by my own experience as a young psychologist in the 1980s. At that time, the argument I just outlined (which is actually quite old) had been presented to the psychological community by the American philosopher and psychologist Jerry Fodor (1974). Fodor was interested in classical psychology: concepts such as grammar, emotion, and attention. At that time, reductionism was in its heyday and many young psychologists believed that all of psychology was on the verge of being reduced to biology by neuroscience. Fodor pointed out that reduction would not necessarily succeed with psychology because homomorphisms between the natural kinds of psychology and the natural kinds of neuroscience might simply not exist. In fact, Fodor went a good deal further, arguing that all of the core ideas of psychology would likely resist reduction—that psychology was at its heart an emergent science. His prediction was that the effort to reduce psychology to neurobiology would largely fail because there would be no natural mapping between neurobiological kinds and such psychological concepts as attention, emotion, and grammar. We know today that Fodor's extreme view was wrong, at least at the empirical level where psychologists operate now. There is hardly a psychology department in the world today that does not own, or at least employ, a brain scanner. Attention seems to be mapping well to brain states, and contemporary theories of psychology and neuroscience now share many logical objects and reductive links. But it is also important to point out that so far, Fodor also appears to have been at least partially right. The mapping between brain areas and emotion has proven far more difficult than at first suspected (although huge progress has been made on this front[3]), and I think it would be fair to say that the key concepts from the study of grammar, although under active investigation at the neurobiological level, have so far entirely escaped reduction.

This history, then, tells us something fairly clear that can guide us as we try to relate neurobiology, psychology, and economics. At an empirical level there almost certainly will be regularities that homomorphically map some economic kinds to neurobiological kinds. (Indeed, the bulk of this book will be a precise description of the mappings of this kind that have already been discovered or postulated.) It also seems very likely that there will be emergent concepts in economics that resist reduction. What I am saying here is that the reductive relationship between neurobiology and economics (largely via psychology) will be incomplete—but only a real extremist could argue today that no such mappings of any kind will ever be found to exist. So far, every scientific discipline that has ever faced a reductive challenge (whether it be chemistry, biology, psychology, or anything else) has demonstrated at least a partial set of linkages to the more reduced disciplines. These partial reductions have also been influential; they have reshaped the logical kinds of the higher-level discipline. There is no reason to believe that economics will be different. Indeed, the data that I will present in the pages that follow will, I believe, make this case incontrovertibly.

So What Are the Obstacles to, and Benefits of, Synthesis?

To summarize, the very concept of building an interdisciplinary synthesis like the one neuroeconomics offers faces two key challenges. The first is

---

3. For an overview of the strengths and weaknesses of this particular reduction, see Phelps (2002) and Phelps (2006).

whether the synthesis of disciplines as different as economics, psychology, and neuroscience is possible. The second is whether such a synthesis, even if possible, would prove valuable to the parent disciplines. What I hope this historical and philosophical chapter has conveyed is that the answer to the first of these questions is that it is possible to link (at least partially) these three disciplines. I hope it has conveyed, with regard to the second question, that such a linkage will almost certainly improve the predictive and descriptive powers of all three parent disciplines.

Why should we believe that linkages between the disciplines are, in principle, possible? Consider the alternative. Consider the possibility that, in principle, no reductive linkages of any kind between the explanatory levels of economics, psychology, and neuroscience are possible. This is exactly the same as saying that *all* of the features of the psychological explanation of behavior are emergent properties at the level of psychological analysis and that *all* of the features of the economic explanation of behavior are emergent properties at the level of economic analysis. For reductive linkages between the disciplines to be impossible, all of economics and all of psychology must be non-predictable from lower-level theories *in principle*. While we cannot rule out this possibility, it is important to understand how extreme a set of assumptions is required for this to turn out to be true. It is also critical to understand that in the history of scientific inquiry, such an extreme degree of non-predictability has never before been observed. It seems almost inescapable that some kind of meaningful reductive synthesis between these disciplines must be possible. The goal of this volume is to present exactly such a synthesis, but we have to begin here by taking the ontological stance that such a synthesis, or at least a partial one, is in principle possible.

Given that such a synthesis is possible, the question of whether synthesis will yield real benefits to its parent disciplines of course remains. This is a question that has troubled economists in particular during the past decade. If one could create a neuroeconomic framework, would it be of any interest to economics *cum* economics? To understand the answer to this question, we have to understand that neuroeconomics would not be simply the linkage of three existing bodies of theory: neuroeconomics would be a revision of three existing bodies of theory into a more powerful linkable form. This is a subtle point, but one that is terribly important. If we assume that there exist, in the real physical universe, reductive linkages between neurobiologically, psychologically, and economically observable phenomena (the point made in the preceding paragraph), then we assume that an ideal theory of economics, for example, would come ready-made for maximal linkage to, say, psychology. Put another way, if we believe such linkages are a feature of physical reality, then theories perfectly aligned with that reality (perfectly predictive theories) would be linkable without modification. In such a world, linkages between economics, psychology, and neuroscience would have no impact on any of the disciplines—but we do not live in such a world. Our existing theoretical frameworks in all three disciplines are imperfect. That means that searching for alterations to each of those frameworks that allow linkages allows us to improve each of those sets of theories. If we believe partial reduction is possible in an ontological sense, then that means we can use knowledge gained in one field to constrain the structure of knowledge in the other fields. It means that knowing how the brain works, for example, will help us to constrain economic theory.

Not only can we draw this conclusion at a philosophical level, we have every reason to believe that we can draw this conclusion empirically, based on the experiences of other disciplines. There is no doubt that the theories of physics have been changed by physical chemistry, that the theories of biology have been changed by biochemistry. In short, there is every reason to believe that the theories of economics, psychology, and neuroscience will be changed by neuroeconomics.

An Example of Interdisciplinary Modification and Reduction

In the real practice of science, this kind of interdisciplinary reduction happens all the time, and it has even begun to happen in economics and psychology. What I have pointed out in this chapter are the philosophical foundations of this process so as to lay bare my ontological goal. To take perhaps the most famous example of this process, consider the following.

In the 1980s, the economist and psychologist George Loewenstein recognized (like many before him) that there are a number of circumstances in which economic theory makes very poor predictions. The situation that interested him most at that time was one he described in a famous study of humans making hypothetical choices that formed the core of his doctoral dissertation (Loewenstein, 1987). Loewenstein found in that study that if Yale undergraduates were asked to place a monetary value on the opportunity to kiss the celebrity of their choice 1, 2, 3, 4, or 5 days in the future, they placed the highest value on a kiss in 3 days. This result defied prediction with the standard economic models available at the time used to understand intertemporal choices, the choices we make between gains at different times. Loewenstein hypothesized in that paper, at a psychological level, that subjects chose 3 days because they wanted to enjoy anticipating the upcoming kiss. Interestingly, however, he explained the behavior at an economic level by expanding pre-existing models of intertemporal choice. What I think this revealed was a fundamental mismatch between the class of explanatory objects available to him as an economist and the class of explanatory objects available to him as a psychologist. It seems clear that mapping "the pleasures of anticipation" to "the curvature of a positive discount function" will yield at best only a partial homology.

It was about a decade later that this fundamental tension was resolved for many economists and psychologists when Andrew Caplin and John Leahy published their landmark paper "Psychological expected utility theory and anticipatory feelings" (Caplin and Leahy, 2001), wherein they laid out the notion that an "anticipatory feeling" could be explicitly considered a logical object within the framework of traditional economic theory. In essence, they looked at the mismatch between the psychological and economic theories and then suggested modifications to the "kinds" in both domains so as to better align the two sets of explanations. What they produced was a modified form of neoclassical economics with better explanatory power, although admittedly a form with a higher degree of complexity.

Crossing the Threshold

There has been a huge amount of debate in the past few years swirling around the effort of a few determined scholars to go beyond Caplin and Leahy (2001) in their efforts to link the social and natural sciences.

The most visible of these scholarly groups have been the neuroeconomists who have sought to relate economics, psychology, and neuroscience. While this effort to describe the neurobiological basis of human decision making has been immensely popular with the lay press, neuroeconomics has received intense criticism from many established scholars in each of its parent disciplines.

Many of these critiques arise from a misunderstanding of the theory of knowledge on the part of both the supporters and detractors of neuroeconomics. If we are trying to build principled linkages between these fields that will have real theoretical traction, we must do so in a serious manner. The critical idea here is that our goal must be to modify the theories of each of the parent disciplines so that they align toward a common endpoint and share as many reducible logical kinds as possible. We have to do this in the same way that notions of genetics were successfully related to the biochemistry of DNA, or insulin and digestive enzymes were related to the two-part concept of the pancreas. This will require a group of scholars who can move freely in all of the areas of theory employed by the parent disciplines. The empirical claims of hostile economists about the limits of a neurobiological theory they do not know are of no more importance to this project than the claims of neurobiologists who lack a theory of choice.

With this in mind, what follows next is an effort to describe the critical elements of existing economic, psychological and neuroscientific theory. My goal is to give readers just enough of the tools and esthetics of each of the parent disciplines to allow them to see how reductive linkages can be forged, and to convince them that such reductive linkages are worth forging.

3

Economic Kinds: Understanding the
Abstractions and Esthetics of
Economic Thought

Précis

One of the core ideas of Chapter 2 was that in order to link economic,
psychological, and neurobiological models of human choice behavior,
one must understand and appreciate the disciplinary frameworks that
one is attempting to link. All too often during the past decade, neurobiologists working as neuroeconomists have published papers about
choice that at best are irrelevant to, or at worst fundamentally incompatible with, economic thought. If neurobiologists and psychologists want
to seriously engage economists, not only must they learn the language of
economics, but they also must appreciate what economists strive to
accomplish. They must understand the esthetics of economics, particularly
as those esthetics apply to the logical objects economists call "preferences."

This chapter is an effort to provide readers whose primary training
is in neuroscience or psychology with an overview of the key ideas—the
logical primitives—that make up much of microeconomic theory. Doing
this in a single chapter requires a heavily selective presentation. Most
economists will find this material superficially treated and of limited
value to them; I urge them to skip ahead to Chapter 4.

For readers who do choose to work through this chapter, I want
to offer the following guidance. There are a wide range of views in
economics, as in all fields. Not all economists would agree that all of the

selections from the corpus of economic thought that I have made were the right selections. Some might, for example, argue that I have placed too much emphasis on preferences and not enough on the critical notion of consistency. I must stress that I am not trying to present non-economist readers with the single true center of the worldview of economists, but rather to present a worldview that all economists would recognize as economic. What I hope to do most of all is to convey to non-economists how economists think and what economists value. To do that, of course, we will encounter all of the most important logical primitives of choice theory. The ones to which I devote the most time are those that I believe will best serve neuroeconomics.

The Decision Models of Classical Economics

All economic theories of decision making have their roots in the insights of the Enlightenment mathematician Blaise Pascal. These insights gave rise to classical economics and defined the tradition against which modern neoclassical economics, and the esthetic that guides it, rebelled. If one is to really understand neoclassical economics, one has to have a deep appreciation for what was wrong, and of course right, with classical economics.

Pascal was the first Western thinker to ask how people should, in a normative sense, choose between uncertain alternatives. Should an individual prefer to buy a lottery ticket that yields a 50% chance of winning 100 gold florins at a price of 45 florins, or should he pass up the ticket and keep his 45 florins? For Pascal the basic technique for answering this question was simple: one multiplied the *probability of winning* by *the amount to be won*, which yielded an average, or expected, value for the action. One then selected the option having the larger of the two *expected values*.

Importantly, Pascal did not see this as an approach limited in application to the analysis of monetary choices. He argued that a similar approach could be used in situations as complicated as deciding whether or not to believe in God.

From the point of view of later economists (and insurance companies for that matter), Pascal's approach had three very important features.

	Probability x	Value =	Expected Value
#1	0.5	100	50
#2	1.0	45	45

FIGURE 3.1   Expected value.

First, it identified two variables that were important for guiding choice behavior: the size of the gain or loss associated with an option, and the probability of realizing that gain or loss. Magnitude and probability of gain (or loss) are key concepts that recur throughout the history of economics as core primitives. Pascal identified these concepts as critical.

Second, Pascal provided a clear algorithm for normative choice. One multiplies magnitude by probability to yield a single decision value, *expected value*, and then chooses the option having the largest expected value. So Pascal provides a model of human behavior in a way that will be familiar to many biologists and psychologists. He starts with a set of assumptions about what kinds of things choosers *should* care about, proposes that humans can extract and encode these properties of the outside world, hypothesizes that a particular mathematical operation should be performed in the brains of human choosers, and then finally proposes that the result of these mathematical operations performed on each element of the current choice set are compared and the highest value option selected. That is Pascal's detailed model of how choice should be accomplished.

Third, and perhaps most importantly, Pascal's theory tells us what it means for a choice to be correct or incorrect. If a human chooser selects an option that is not the element with the highest expected value on his menu of choices, he has made an error. Pascal even shows how to correct that man's error. Take a famous example that interested him (and his colleagues Antoine Arnauld and Pierre Nicole [1662]). A woman is frightened of death by lightning but not frightened of death by disease. We know that a death by lightning is of lower probability than a death by disease; thus she makes an error by having this fear, and we can help her by convincing her that it is illogical to fear death by lightning and not death by disease. What Pascal purports to show us, in the language of modern economics, is how to maximize the *welfare* of people by guiding their choices.

In what is perhaps Pascal's most famous piece of writing, a passage from his *Pensées* (1670) known as *The Wager*, he develops this argument clearly with regard to the belief in God. One must choose, he argues, between believing in God and not believing in God. To understand how to choose, we start with gains, losses, and probabilities.

If God exists and we believe in him, we gain eternal happiness in heaven. If he exists and we do not believe in him, we gain eternal misery in hell: infinite happiness versus infinite misery (or more formally, infinite negative happiness). If we conclude that the probability that God exists is a number greater than zero (however small), the algorithm requires that we multiply this small probability by the value of salvation (in this case valued at infinity). The result of this multiplication is, of course, infinity—a quantity Pascal defines as the expected value of believing in God. To compute the expected value of not believing in God, we multiply negative infinity by any non-zero number and we get negative infinity—the expected value of not believing in God. We must, Pascal concludes, choose to believe in God. Anyone who does not believe in God makes a formal error in decision, and most importantly (and perhaps perniciously), we know from this logic that we help that person if we force him to believe in God using any means possible. Importantly, *this is true regardless of whether or not God turns out to exist*; it is true as long as the

Pascal's Wager				
	If God Exists	If God Doesn't Exist		
	(Prob × Value)	+ (Prob × Value)	=	Exp. Value
Believe in God	>0 × ∞	+ ≥0 × 0	=	∞
Do not Believe in God	>0 × −∞	+ ≥0 × 0	=	−∞

FIGURE 3.2   Pascal's Wager.

existence of God is uncertain and we have correctly defined the costs and benefits of belief.

What stands out about Pascal's contribution are thus three factors. He provides us with a statement of what variables should influence choice. He provides us with a clear model of how the mathematical algorithm of choice should operate. He argues that anyone who deviates from this algorithm is behaving incorrectly and that we can help this person by correcting his or her choices.

Bernoulli's Contribution

It soon became obvious, however, that the choices of many humans seemed to violate the predictions of Pascal's algorithm. In the example of the lottery/gold florins choice discussed above, Pascal tells us that we must choose the 50% chance of winning 100 florins over the guaranteed 45 florins. In real life, however, most people choose the sure thing (the 45 florins) over the risky lottery. And a second issue that arose at the same time was that philosophers and economists began to challenge Pascal's idea that people who chose the 45 guaranteed florins were doing something wrong that should be necessarily corrected.

The person who most clearly stated these challenges to Pascal's theory was the Swiss mathematician Daniel Bernoulli. Bernoulli urges us, in a famous paper published in St. Petersburg in 1738, to consider a beggar on the street who has only a single penny in his pocket. Walking along he discovers a lottery ticket lying on the ground that offers a 50% chance of winning 20,000 florins. He now owns an object with an expected value of 10,000 florins. A wealthy man walks up to him and offers 7,000 florins for the ticket. Should he take it? Pascal's answer is no, he should not. But can we be so sure that the beggar has made a mistake if he accepts the rich man's offer? He is choosing between being certain that he will have enough money to pay for food and lodging for years to come or facing a 50-50 chance of either continuing in poverty or being roughly three times as wealthy as if he accepts the rich man's offer. Surely there would be nothing illogical about accepting the 7,000-florin offer under these conditions. Bernoulli leads us to question the notion that we, as decision scientists (or politicians—remember always that economics is at least as much about social policy as it is about scholarly inquiry), know for sure what is best for the beggar.

So how did Bernoulli resolve this problem with the expected value theory of Pascal? His answer was to take a route often traveled by natural scientists today: he made Pascal's model just a little bit more complicated. Bernoulli's idea was, in essence, to add two additional parameters to Pascal's model. The first idea was to build the overall wealth of the chooser (a variable we could, at least in principle, measure) into the model. The second was to replace the measurable external world variable "value" with a mathematically transformed version of value hidden inside the chooser that could account for the observed aversion of humans to risks. This is a hidden variable that came to be called *utility*.

Bernoulli proposed that the algorithm of choice works the following way. First, rather than assessing the desirability of an option by multi-plying value and probability directly, instead we take the logarithm of value (after correcting for wealth) to produce a hidden variable called utility and then we multiply utility by probability to yield our decision variable. To make this clear, consider the beggar who has an initial wealth of a single penny, which we will treat colloquially as a wealth of zero.[1]

For that man, the utility of the 20,000-florin ticket is simply the logarithm of 20,000, or 4.3 utils. Multiplying 4.3 by 0.50 (50%) we get 2.15 as the expected (or average) utility of the ticket to the beggar. Now consider the offer he receives of 7,000 guaranteed florins from the rich man. That has a utility of 3.8 utils multiplied by 1 (since the gain is certain) and hence an expected utility of 3.8. Obviously the beggar should take the 7,000 florins. To put this slightly differently, the logarithmic compression of value means that even though the lottery ticket offers almost three times the objective value of the 7,000-florin payoff, it offers far less than twice the *subjective value*. Given that the higher payoff is only half as likely as the lower payoff, it is the lower payoff that has the higher expected utility. The key idea here is that for the beggar, the decrease in probability associated with the 20,000-florin ticket is not adequately compensated for by the increase in subjective value offered

---

1. Putting a penny in the beggar's pocket is intended to save us from the mathematical indignity of having to take the logarithm of zero.

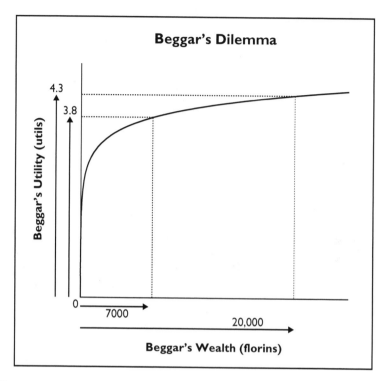

Beggar's Dilemma

FIGURE 3.3

by 20,000 florins, making it undesirable. *That is why Bernoulli's beggar is averse to taking a risk on the lottery ticket.*

How, though, can we explain that the rich man prefers the lottery ticket to the 7,000 florins? This is where Bernoulli's inclusion of wealth into the model comes into the picture. As was the case for the beggar, for the rich man the issue he must address is how many utils each of the two options will add to his total life stock of utility. For the beggar this was easy because he had no utils to start with,[2] but for the rich man who has a non-zero starting wealth we perform a slightly different computation.

Let us imagine that the rich man has a starting wealth of 1,000,000 florins (6 utils). If he pays 7,000 florins for the ticket and it wins, he adds

---

2. I assume here that money is his only source of utility. I do that just to make the math simpler. As will become clear, one could easily extend this problem to include even the most abstract or personal forms of non-monetary wealth.

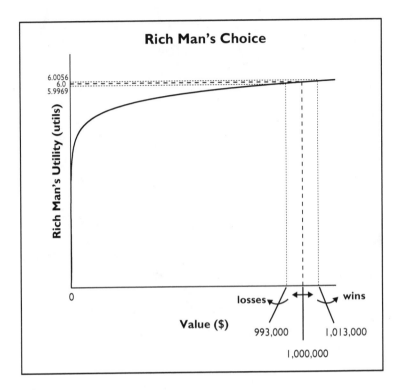

FIGURE 3.4

13,000 florins (20,000 florins less the 7,000 florins he paid) to his overall wealth. If it loses, he subtracts 7,000 florins from his wealth. The lottery ticket thus has a 50% chance of yielding 1,013,000 florins total wealth (6.0056 utils) or a 50% chance of yielding 993,000 florins total wealth (5.9969 utils). Thus the expected utility of the ticket is simply the sum of those two calculations:

$$EU = (0.5 \times 6.0056) + (0.5 \times 5.9969) = 6.00125$$

Thus the subjective value of buying the lottery ticket for the rich man is 6.00125 utils, and of course the value of not buying the ticket is his previous wealth level of 6.00000 utils. Obviously the rich man should buy the ticket.

The Bernoulli model is interesting for two reasons. First, it predicts choices in circumstances like these where Pascal's model failed to predict choice accurately. Second, it introduces the almost psychological notion that the value of money, or goods, is a subjective property hidden inside the chooser and that this subjective value is influenced by wealth. (Although as we will see, the very need to postulate such an unobservable variable, something that can never in principle be measured, is something that modern economists often find disturbing, for very good reasons.) To accomplish this, however, Bernoulli has added quite a few complicating factors to our model of choice. Now we have a model in which we assume that: (1) People compute and represent probability objectively, (2) People represent the quantity utility (a thing that we cannot observe or measure directly) and that this representation includes total wealth and a logarithmic transformation, (3) People take the product of each of these representations, and (4) People select the option from their set of alternatives that has the highest product of these values.

What is the evidence that this is a better model than Pascal's? The answer is that the model fits the data better; it accounts for human choices more accurately than does Pascal's. Indeed, it accounts for choice behavior *much* better than does Pascal's model.

Interestingly, though, Bernoulli's model allows us to preserve the notion of right and wrong choices. If we agree that utility is the logarithm of value, then as was the case for Pascal's model, we can identify the course of action for each of our citizens that maximizes his or her individual utility if we know his or her total wealth. Further, we can help them if they are about to make a mistake by making a better choice for them.[3]

The Problem of Parameters

During the two centuries of economic thought that followed Bernoulli's famous paper, models of choice grew steadily more complicated, included more and more hidden variables, and began to more accurately

---

3. I need to add here that Bernoulli and the scholars who used this theory after him were not overly committed to the logarithmic function as the only possible way to translate between objective value in florins and subjective value in utility. The economists of the 18th and 19th centuries explored many classes of utility functions.

predict choice. Most of these models explored different mathematical ways to compute utility from objective, real-world values such as dollars and cents. They examined the choice predictions of utility functions represented by power laws, natural logarithms, and ratio scales, among others. And as these additional models were explored, they were related systematically to such ideas as happiness and fulfillment, compelling abstractions that were not subject to direct measurement.

This is exactly the same way that most modeling in the natural sciences has progressed over the past century: One harvests an intuition about how some behavior or process might be generated, then uses that intuition to write down a formal mathematical model, preferably one with not *too* many parameters and not *too* many unobservable properties. The free parameters that are included in the model are then adjusted (in the language of the empirical sciences, they are *fit*) so that observable behavior or neural activity is "predicted" by one or more elements in the model. The resulting model is generally declared a "good fit" if it outperforms some other specific model with which it is in competition in a rigorous statistical sense. Failures to achieve a good fit lead to the search for other related models that can better approximate the subject of study, whether it be behavior or neural activity.

In the history of economics, however, two factors arose with regard to this standard approach that began to trouble a group of extremely rigorous Lausanne-based economic scholars in the late 1800s. This group of scholars was worried about how arbitrary and unstructured models of economic choice had become, and how these arbitrary models filled with immeasurable variables were being used to decide what was best for people. Consider a version of Bernoulli's model in which we begin with the *a priori* hypothesis that humans want to maximize expected utility. Next we assume that expected utility is the product of an accurate representation of probability, an accurate representation of value in dollars, a transformation of dollars to hidden utils via a power function (as opposed to a logarithmic transform) with an adjustable exponent and a multiplication.

For each subject, our goal is to fit the model to his or her behavior by determining the exponent for the power-utility function that best accounts for his or her behavior. To do that, we observe our subject making 20 choices and simply select the exponent with which the model

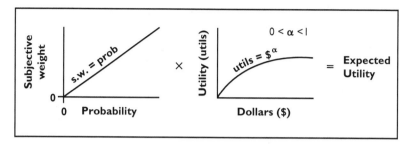

FIGURE 3.5   A classical choice model.

most accurately predicts these 20 choices. Armed with our four assumptions about what is represented and our data-fit derived exponent, we can draw conclusions about what utility might look like inside this person—even for situations we have never explored directly. Then we can use this hidden variable and our assumptions to begin to make out-of-sample predictions about the behavior of our subject. We can even begin to identify choices that are mistakes: choices not predicted by the model.

We can furthermore compare the "utilities" induced in our citizens by government policies. With just one more assumption we can even make these comparisons *across* individuals. Imagine we were to consider, as policy-makers, outlawing sexual interactions among attendees of professional conferences, and we had agreed that our social goal was to maximize the aggregate utility of our society.[4] With a well-fitting model that yielded exact numerical estimates of utility, we might be able to determine how many utils this law would add to the lives of the partners of conference attendees. We could then ask whether the loss in utility to the attendees of conferences was numerically outweighed by the gain in utility by their partners. In other words, with these numerical models in hand we could set about a choice-by-choice optimization of the cumulated welfare of all of humanity.

---

4. I assume here that we have agreed on maximizing aggregate utility as the goal of our social policy. Of course the argument that follows holds for many broad classes of social welfare functions. I select this one only for ease of exposition.

What was troubling about this approach to the economists of the Lausanne school, scholars such as Leon Walras and Vilfredo Pareto, should be obvious. First, the model rests on utility—the model is uniquely *about* utility—even though *there is no independent evidence that utility exists and no way to measure utility*. What one observes and measures is choice; from this one infers what utility *might* be like. Second, the model is terribly *ad hoc* in nature. How do we know that another Bernoulli-type function will not come along tomorrow and suggest an entirely new and better formulation for computing utility and that this new formulation would lead to a different conclusion? We do not. Many sciences face the problem that theories evolve in unexpected ways, but in economics this problem seems particularly pernicious because we want to use the outputs of these models to say what is best for people and to guide the policies of governments. Third, and key to understanding the philosophical positions of these scholars and nearly all modern economists, it can be demonstrated that even the basic assumption that utilities are unique numerical quantities that we can compare across individuals represents a technical mathematical error that the classical economists had made.

The Neoclassical Revolution: Defining the Tools and Esthetics of Modern Economic Thought

A mathematically inclined economist working at the end of the 19th and the beginning of the 20th centuries, Vilfredo Pareto was very aware of the arbitrary and *ad hoc* quality economics had taken on in the preceding century or two. He worried that the models being developed in his day contained too many assumptions and that these assumptions posed real philosophical challenges. He worried particularly about the issue of inter-individual comparisons of utility that arise from the classical notion of what a mathematician would call a *cardinal* scale. This is a critical point that anyone who wants to appreciate the logical primitives of modern economic theory must understand, so it is essential that we engage it.

By the end of the 19th century, many economists had begun to use choices to fit models of utility. This yielded unique numerical estimates of utility for goods and policies. What was beginning to happen was that economists were starting to use these numerical estimates of utility to compare "goods" and "bads" within and across individuals. If an action by the government increased the overall utility of one individual more than it decreased the overall utility of another, then a classical economist who hoped to maximize aggregate social utility might conclude that it was a justifiable policy. This troubled Pareto because this conclusion is based on the assumption that utilities could be represented by *unique* numerical values, and he recognized that this assumption is wrong.

To make Pareto's point clear, consider two subjects: Milton and Oskar. We observe that Milton chooses apples over oranges over grapes. Let us assign (based on our model) a utility of 3 to an apple, 2 to an orange, and 1 to a bunch of grapes. Those are utilities that perfectly predict Milton's preferences among these three fruits. Next we observe that Oskar chooses apples over grapes over oranges. We therefore assign the utilities: Apple = 3, Grapes = 2, Oranges = 1 for Oskar.

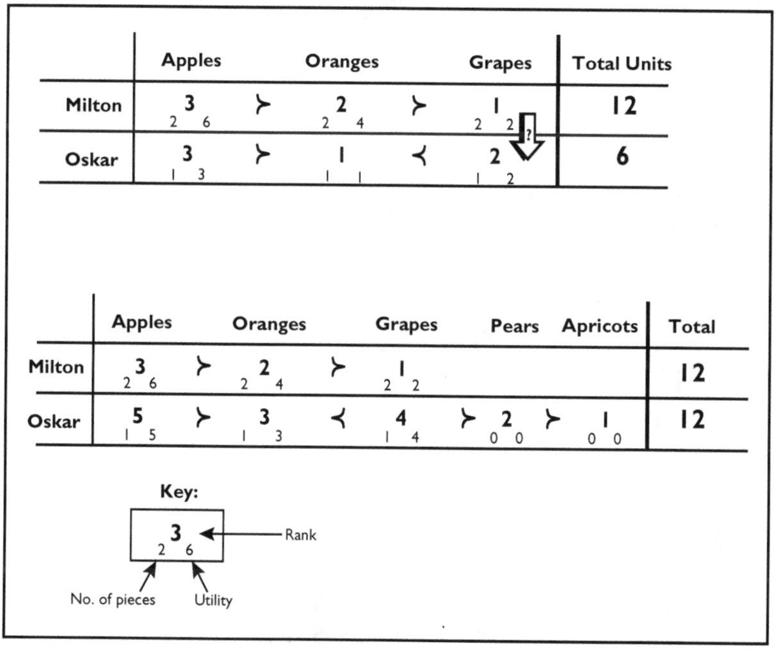

FIGURE 3.6   Preferences and assets table for Milton and Oskar.

Now consider a situation in which Milton is found to have two of each piece of fruit and Oskar to have only one of each piece of fruit. We conclude that Milton has a total utility of 12 and Oskar has a total utility of 6. As a benevolent despot, what should we do to maximize their joint utility? If we were to take Milton's grapes away from him and give them to Oskar, we would reduce Milton's utility by 2 but we would increase Oskar's utility by 4. Clearly this yields a net increase in aggregate utility for the pair, so it seems an entirely justifiable action for someone committed to maximizing aggregate utility. But this conclusion is based on a mathematical error in our understanding of utility, a fact that was clear to Pareto and to few others at that time (Pareto, 1906). The error rests on our belief that we have identified in some unique way the actual numerical utility experienced internally by Milton and Oskar based on observations of their choices. To make that error clear, consider what happens if we now ask Oskar (the one who seemed to start with fewer utils) to tell us his preferences again, this time including pears and apricots in our survey. This time we find that his preferences order as: Apples ≻ Grapes ≻ Oranges ≻ Pears ≻ Apricots. Now that we have two new fruits in the set, we should really reassign Oskar's utilities as: Apple = 5, Grapes = 4, Orange = 3, Pear = 2, and Apricot = 1. Using this assignment of utilities (an assignment just as well supported by our data as the first assignment) we conclude that the initial redistribution of fruit made above was actually fairer than it had appeared at first. Now we conclude that Oskar has 12 utils in hand, and we reach this new conclusion that utils have been equally distributed *simply because we included pears and apricots in our initial survey* of Oskar's preferences. Of course, surveying Oskar's utilities in this way also leads us to conclude that if we were to take all of Milton's fruit away and give it to Oskar, we would be maximizing aggregate utility.

This example only scratches the surface of the problem that Pareto uncovered. Choice data, he pointed out, tell us how subjects rank the objects of choice (usually called *goods* in economics) in terms of desirability. We can talk about utilities as ways to describe this ranking, but we must always remember that utilities are only really good for *ordering* things. Treating utilities as numbers that can be exchanged across subjects (or even used in cardinal computations with regard to a single subject) goes way, way beyond the data we have.

Pareto reacted to all of this by turning away from the models of his time, which rested on complicated, unprovable, and often false assumptions about utility. Instead, he argued, economists should strip down their models to include a minimum number of assumptions and a minimum number of parameters. A "good" model, he argued as a political economist, is one that assumes almost nothing, and what it assumes must be either testable or infallibly true. Of course the drawback that this esthetic imposes is that it means that the power of economic models is going to be necessarily limited. Pareto recognized this and tried to explore the kinds of minimally complicated statements that an economist could safely make. He concluded, for example, that one could sometimes define one distribution of goods among individuals as better than another. Consider a world in which either:

Oskar has 2 apples and 2 oranges; Milton has 0 apples and 0 oranges.
or
Oskar has 2 apples and 2 oranges; Milton has 1 apple and 0 oranges.

Obviously the second case is better largely irrespective of one's assumptions.[5] What Pareto went on to stress is that utility functions are only about ordering, not about discrete numerical values. Mathematicians refer to numerical scales that provide information only about ordering as *ordinal scales*; what Pareto argued was that any numbers associated with utilities must be viewed as representing only an *ordinal relationship*. If one good is concluded to have a utility of 4 and another good is concluded to have a utility of 2 (for a given chooser) then we know that the first good is better for that chooser, *but we do not really know how much better*. This stands in contrast to numerical systems, in which 4 really is twice the size of 2. These systems, where numbers represent unique mathematical

---

5. To be precise, the second case is better only if we assume "(increasing) weakly monotonic utility functions." This was a point Pareto developed in detail and because he was comfortable with the simplifying assumption of increasing monotonicity (the idea that a subject's utility curves never go down as the number of pieces of fruit a subject has goes up). He would have concluded that the second world is a better world than the first because both Oskar and Milton are better off in that world. Stated more formally: **Pareto optimality** is the assertion that the resources of a society are not optimally allocated as long as it is possible to make at least one individual better off while keeping all others at least as well off as before.

quantities rather than simply representing orderings, are referred to as *cardinal*. Pareto proved that existing utility theories were ordinal even though they were often erroneously employed in cardinal calculations.

Paul Samuelson

The result of Pareto's work was that a growing number of mathematically sophisticated economists began to distrust most existing economic models. They asked whether models that made really detailed predictions were ever possible, and they began to search for new mathematical approaches to modeling economic behavior. In particular, this group became very skeptical of models with hidden and immeasurable parameters that were adjusted to achieve maximal "goodness of fit." Models of this kind can be rated as better or worse than one another, but it has often been argued in the history of science that there is no way to objectively falsify models of this kind, a problem faced today by much of modern biology and psychology.

What this new group of economists wanted was to develop a new way of modeling that included strict criteria for falsifiability that rested on empirical tests of observable phenomena only, that made a minimal number of testable assumptions, and that respected the true ordinal nature of utility. The group found that new approach in the work of the American economist Paul Samuelson when he published the paper, "A note on the pure theory of consumer's behaviour" (Samuelson, 1938).

To understand Samuelson's approach and the modern economic esthetic it embodies, one has to begin by recalling that what troubled Pareto most about Bernoulli-style models was the assumption that utilities are unique numerical values, fully cardinal objects. What troubled Samuelson even more was that utilities cannot—in principle—be directly measured. Imagine that we begin with a set of hypotheses about utility and a model of how utility influences choice. Put more formally, we describe a rule that takes us uniquely from utility to choice. If we hypothesize that utility is a specific power function of magnitude, then in any situation we can predict exactly what choice we will observe. *What troubled Samuelson is that the reverse is not also true.* If we observe a choice of a particular kind, it does not uniquely make any particularly interesting predictions about utility. Specific utility theories may make unique predictions about choice, but that relationship is not invertible. And it is choices, not utilities, that are real events in the real world. If we observe a particular choice being made, that observation is compatible with many possible utility representations, as demonstrated by the example of Milton, Oskar, and their fruit. This is essentially Pareto's point but seen in the other direction, as seen from a focus on the only thing we can actually measure: choice. Choice and utility are linked in traditional utility theories but, Samuelson suggested, they are linked in only one direction (from utility to choice) *and at best that is the wrong direction*. What one wanted, Samuelson argued, was a theoretical approach that either avoided utility entirely, or at most made linkages in the other direction. What one wanted was to use choice to say something directly about choice, or at most about utility, but not ever to use utility to say something about choice.

In his 1938 paper, Samuelson thus asked what might seem a slightly odd question to a natural scientist: What is the simplest model of human choice behavior that still makes positive predictions about consumer decisions, and how might such a model constrain the nature of utility? Samuelson answered that question by proposing a "model" of human behavior that assumes that if we *observe* that a person consistently chooses (for example) [4 apples and 2 oranges] over [2 apples and 4 oranges], then this means that we can *assume* that the person *does not also* consistently prefer [2 apples and 4 oranges] to [4 apples and 2 oranges].

In other words, Samuelson's "model" proposes that if a subject is observed to prefer A to B, then we can assume that he cannot also prefer B to A. To a pre-Pareto classical economist, of course, this would have seemed an insanely small thing to assume and not the stuff from which a model could be built. When one reads Samuelson's paper one has the sense that he presents this almost playfully. Indeed, one's intuition is that such a model makes almost no predictions of any kind about utility. What makes Samuelson's work special, however, is that he was able to show that even this simple statement (or model) allows us to make quite surprisingly useful predictions about choice and to constrain statements about utility.

Consider, Samuelson urges, a subject who we are convinced strongly prefers apples to oranges and strongly prefers oranges to pears. If one is convinced of that, then all theories, *literally all possible theories*, of ordinal utility require that this chooser must prefer apples to pears even though we have no prior information about that preference. Can we though, to pursue the esthetic of simplification even further, simplify even this approach to preferences? Yes: we can simply eliminate oranges from the story. If we do that, we can boil down our observation and theory even farther. If we are convinced that a subject strongly prefers apples to pears, then we cannot also be convinced that he strongly prefers pears to apples and still preserve any ordinal notion of utility. Samuelson could have stopped there and he would have accomplished something significant. He would have made a statement about choices that placed a unique constraint on utility—or would he have?

In fact, what Samuelson recognized was that even this statement goes too far. (If one can come to appreciate this fact, one can go far towards understanding the esthetic of modern economics.) What we observe are choices, not strong preferences or weak preferences, but choices. The theory described above states that we observe a subject who strongly prefers apples to pears, but in fact we could never observe anything of the kind. We observe that he chooses an apple over a pear. Does that mean he really prefers apples over pears? Not necessarily. It might mean that he finds apples and pears exactly equal in desirability. We simply have no way of knowing. That is a crippling fact, but Samuelson's genius was in realizing that it was not *completely* crippling. If we observe him to pick an apple over a pear we do not know that he prefers apples to pears, but we do know that *he cannot prefer pears over apples*. (At worst he can only view them as equivalently desirable.)

This logic is the reason that Samuelson constructed his theory the way that he did. If a subject is observed to **choose** A over B, then we can assume that he cannot **prefer** B to A. So what then, if anything, does this tell us about utility and choice? First, Samuelson went on to prove irrefutably using mathematical tools that anyone who showed choice behavior that followed this admittedly weak rule could be treated as if he had a coherent utility representation. If one observes that a subject chooses A over B and at the same time never can be shown to prefer B over A, then that subject can be described as behaving exactly as if he had a utility-like representation guiding his choice behavior.[6] Second, he was

---

6. Importantly, the reverse is not necessarily true. If we see a violation of Samuelson's rule it does not necessarily mean that no utility-like representation is possible.

able to demonstrate that this conclusion has some profound implications for predicting his future choice behavior. This relationship is now widely known as the Weak Axiom of Revealed Preference (WARP) and is almost universally considered the starting point for modern neoclassical economics.

So to recap, WARP has two features that are critical. First, Samuelson has created a theory (for the first time) that points in the right direction by using statements about choice to constrain utility, not the other way around. Second, the theory is either beautifully elegant and simple or annoyingly weak, depending on your point of view. For people trained as economists it is almost always viewed as beautifully elegant and simple.

Why? What does WARP mean? What does it do? Consider thinking about the behavior of a human chooser using WARP as our starting point. WARP's single axiomatic statement is that "if one observes that a subject chooses A over B, one can predict (in the sense that any model makes predictions) that she can never be shown to prefer B over A." If one adds to this only the notion that "more is better than less"[7] then one can begin to make quite specific statements about what choices tell us about utility; one can make quite specific predictions about future choice; one can even develop unexpected ways to test whether WARP's assumption, the model of human behavior it captures, is correct.

To understand this, consider a man who has $6 to spend on pieces of fruit (either apples or oranges) that cost $1 each. Effectively, he is asked to select a point from the shaded portion of the graph in Figure 3.7, which describes all of the combinations of apples and oranges he can afford. The dark line describes his budget constraint: this is the most fruit he can afford to buy.[8] If we observe that the subject chooses the point

---

7. One can incorporate this idea into WARP in a number of ways. Perhaps the simplest and oldest is Walras' rule, which assumes that we study only circumstances in which subjects spend all of their money. That behavior implies that subjects prefer having more to less under the circumstances we are studying.

8. In a real analysis we would obviously need to include all of the other things on which that subject might choose to spend his money. One can accomplish this either by adding additional dimensions to the graph or by labeling one of the axes "all other stuff one could buy." Samuelson demonstrated that both techniques work and that the two approaches are logically/mathematically identical. In any case, we will assume away this subtlety by placing our subject in a world of only apples and oranges where the explanation is easy to follow.

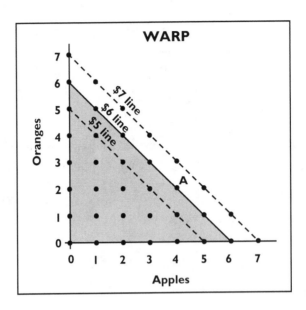

FIGURE 3.7

marked A (four apples and two oranges), then *what WARP says is that we can conclude that no point along the dark line can be better than A for our subject* or he would have picked it (of course these points could be equally good). We can even go one step farther if we assume that in this limited world more fruit is better than less fruit (which is implied by the fact that our chooser spent all of his money). Recall that we are assuming, from WARP, that (1) every other point along the dark line (those points marked with Bs) is at least as good as A for our subject. From the fact that he spent all of his money we can conclude that (2) every point inside the triangle is strictly worse than at least one point on the dark line because it results in his having fewer pieces of fruit than the points on the line, none of which can be better than A. From these two facts we can conclude that our subject prefers A to every point inside the triangle, and A is at least as good as every point on the dark line, for our subject.

Simply by observing that a subject chooses A over B (in this case that he chooses A over all of the possible Bs), and by taking WARP as our core model of his behavior, then we can infer something very tangible about the preferences of our subject. We can conclude that he behaves as if the utility of A is greater than the utility of all of the points inside the triangle.

If we then observe what he prefers to purchase when he has $5 and later $7 in hand, we can actually build a quite complete ordinal ranking of utilities *from only his budgetary choices and the WARP model*. We can build this ordinal ranking from a model that rests on only two basic ideas:

1. If you choose A over B you cannot also prefer B to A.
2. More of a good thing is better than less of a good thing.

At its inception WARP defined a minimalist esthetic that dominates economics to this day. How little can you assume in your model and how much can it prove? These are the questions economists ask every day in their models.

GARP

What followed the publication of Samuelson's WARP paper were a series of papers by important economists that extended his approach. We turn now to one of those modifications, principally so we can better understand the process and esthetic of modern economic inquiry. WARP is probably all of the logical foundation we need for neuroeconomics, but I want to show how an economist would explore the kinds of models offered by WARP-like approaches.

In the 1940s Hendrik Houthakker (1950) developed a model in the style of WARP that could make stronger predictions about choice, the theorem we know today as the generalized axiom of revealed preference (GARP). GARP states explicitly as an assumption that choosers can never be satiated. Imagine that we observe A is chosen over B, B over C, and C over D. We can think of these as choices among groups of budget sets as we imagined them in Figure 3.7. To see how GARP handles this graphically, look at Figure 3.8 and consider our previous budget problem.

In this example we consider a situation in which each apple costs $1 and each orange costs $1. Under these conditions we observed that our chooser picks fruit bundle A. Now we double the price of oranges and halve the price of apples. When that happens, what the subject can afford changes; what he can now afford is shown by the dotted line. Can we make any predictions based on our previous budgetary observation? Houthakker assumes in his model that we can. If we know that A is at least as good as everything on the solid line, and better than everything inside the shaded triangle (which is the essence of GARP's single axiom), then if we offer our chooser everything on the dashed line he cannot chose anything to the left of the point A because we can assume that his previous choices revealed that these were not preferred to A.

So what GARP proposes is that we can use observations like "A is chosen over some set of alternatives B" to infer some of the choices subjects would make when asked to choose among a new set of alternatives. This is the model at the level of choices. Of course, the most interesting question is, What would such a model tell us about utility? Samuelson's WARP assumes something very simple about choices, and Samuelson proved that if you accept this assumption then you can use choices to construct an ordinal scale of utilities. But what GARP tells us turns out to be something much more. Houthakker proved that saying a subject's observed behavior obeys the assumptions of GARP is exactly the same as saying that he has the monotonic utility function Pareto was after.

To put that in another, and slightly more rigorous, way, GARP proved that any subject who shows no circularity in her choices (who does not choose inside the shaded region when presented with the second budget in Fig. 3.8) behaves exactly as if she were really trying to maximize a weakly monotonic utility function.[9] Her behavior does not tell us much about the shape of that utility function, but it does tell us that for her, a utility function (or more accurately, a family of equally valid utility functions) could be described that fully accounts for her behavior.

---

9. A monotonic utility function in this sense is one that goes up as the quantity goes up. It is a utility function that captures the idea "more is better." To be more precise, monotonic utility functions come in two flavors: weakly monotonic and strictly monotonic. Weakly monotonic functions go up or stay flat; "more is never worse." Strongly monotonic functions always go up. Modern theory recognizes that this is never really the case. At some point one must have so many apples that more apples really would be worse. These are called satiating utility functions, and it is this class of utility functions that GARP assumes away. But in a general way, it should be obvious that most of the time more (of a good thing) really is at least as good as less and it is these most generally applicable circumstances that we focus on in this brief introduction.

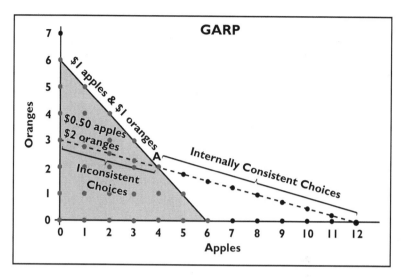

FIGURE 3.8

This was an amazing accomplishment: it resurrected the utility function in some sense, but now on more rigorous and for the first time entirely testable grounds that come from observed choice and not the other way around. Now one could ask: Is this subject's behavior describable *in principle* with some kind of utility function? If her behavior obeys the rules described in the GARP model, we never observe her to make choices like those inside the shaded region of Figure 3.8, then the answer is yes. If, on the other hand, she does make these kinds of choices, then the GARP model is falsified for her. In a very real sense GARP reconciles the kinds of minimalist arguments that Samuelson introduced with the reduced ordinal notion of utility with which Pareto was comfortable. What WARP and GARP did, in essence, was to introduce a new kind of model-chooser: the *Rational Actor*.

Understanding Economic "Rationality"

One key element for understanding neoclassical economics is seeing that models such as WARP and GARP are really just compact descriptions of choice behavior that internally consistent. In fact, some economist readers of this chapter may even have found my focus up to this point unusual. The chapter has presented the mathematical logic of choices and preferences but, they might argue, missed the point. All of these models are really designed only to describe minimal conditions for calling any behavior internally consistent.

To understand this point, imagine a chooser who had the following strict preferences (recall that a strict preference rules out indifference) and who considers a penny an infinitesimally small amount of money:

apples $\succ$ oranges

oranges $\succ$ pears

But oddly also: pears $\succ$ apples

How would such a chooser behave in the real world? Imagine that this person had a pear and $6 and I offered to sell her an orange for her pear plus 1 cent. She accepts because she prefers oranges to pears. I then offer her an apple for the orange I just sold her plus one more cent. She accepts because she prefers apples to oranges. Then I offer to sell her back her original pear for the apple plus one cent. *She accepts because she also prefers pears to apples.* Notice that at the end of these trades she has lost 3 cents, has her original pear in hand, and considers each trade she has made a good trade.

After an hour of this she still has her original pear, but I have her $6. Still, she considers herself well treated. This is a chooser who violates the GARP model because her behavior is internally inconsistent; for her the model is falsified. But because obeying the GARP model also means that you behave as if you were maximizing a utility function, we therefore know that this subject's behavior cannot be described as an effort to maximize a monotonic utility function.

For an economist, such a person's behavior is *irrational*, where the word irrational has a very precise technical meaning. Irrationality here means that the subject has inconsistent preferences—that she violates GARP or WARP.[10] This is a very important point, and one that has generated no end of confusion in the interactions of economists with

---

10. For the very technically minded, let me concede it could be taken to mean that her preferences were either inconsistent or what is formally called *incomplete*.

normal people. If our chooser tells you that she loves apples over all other fruits, there is nothing irrational about this in the economic sense. If she reveals that she prefers a piece of fruit to a million dollars, nothing irrational is implied. If a person is rational in the economic sense, it simply implies that one cannot pump money, or fruit, out of her as in the above example. It implies that her preferences are internally consistent— *and thus by GARP it implies her behavior can be described with a utility function.* It places no constraints on what she likes, how she feels about those likes or dislikes, or even whether the things she likes include things we are convinced it is dumb to like. Rationality is consistency and nothing more, a point to which we will return again and again.

Axioms: The World According to GARP

For someone trying to build a model of natural world phenomena, models such as GARP are both interesting and frustrating. GARP is a theory about representation. Put even more precisely, GARP is a theory about theories of representation. GARP says that if a set of observed choices obeys some very minimal constraints, then the chooser is behaving exactly as if he had internal utility functions that were monotonic. What is frustrating to a natural scientist about this is that GARP does not tell us much about what those utility functions look like. It is not a theory that tells us, This chooser has a utility function of the form

$$Utility = \# \, of \, Apples^{0.5}$$

or

$$Utility = \frac{1 - \exp(-\alpha(\# \, of Apples)^{1-r})}{\alpha}$$

Instead, what it tells us is something that is at the same time weaker *and* more powerful. It is weaker in the sense that it is a theory about the representation of value that places very few constraints on that representation. It is, however, much more powerful when one thinks of it with regard to the standard logic of scientific inquiry, a logic (Popper, 1959) that says that our goal is not to prove theories but rather to falsify them.

If we observe that a subject's choices violate GARP, then we can conclude that *there is no model of any kind that rests on a monotonic utility function that can describe this behavior.* It is in this sense that the economic approach is most powerful, and it is in this sense that the axiomatic approach embodied by GARP differs from all other approaches used in scientific inquiry.

To make this distinction clear, consider two scientists studying the same choice behavior. The first tries to account for the observed choices of a subject by fitting the data with a power utility function. The best fit he obtains is:

$$Utility\,(apples) = \#\,of\,apples^{0.43256}$$

But he also observes that the variance accounted for by this model is only 20% of the total variance in the dataset, so this looks like a bad model. What he does next is to try another utility function and repeats the process, perhaps indefinitely. Now consider a scientist who looks at the raw choice data and asks if he can see direct violations of GARP. That scientist observes that about half of the choices made by our subject violate the axiomatic basis for understanding utility functions that GARP provides. What is interesting is that this second scientist knows something that the first does not *and his insight is not subject to future reinterpretation.* The second scientist knows that no one will ever succeed in finding a monotonic utility function for describing this subject's behavior because GARP proves that no such function exists.[11] GARP thus allows us to ask a first-order question in a very global way: Is there at least one member of the class of all possible monotonic utility functions that can account for the observed data?

The Limits of Tools such as GARP and WARP

Of course, tools such as GARP are also quite limited. There are many utility functions compatible with GARP-like functions. If, for example, we know that a chooser obeys GARP, we know quite a bit about her

---

11. For economists following along here, let me reassure you that I will pick up the thread of Random Utility Models in the next chapter.

budgetary choices. We also know that a utility function exists that can account for her behavior. In fact, we know that a related family of functions exists that can account for her behavior. The most important limitation that we must keep in mind, however, is that not only are we ignorant of the "right" functions, but we also know that *in principle* there is no unique "right" function, only a family of "right" functions—all in the family being equally valid. This was Pareto's point when he developed the notion of ordinal utility, and it is a point that holds true for—indeed, is a key feature of—models such as WARP and GARP.

I want to focus on this point because understanding this is important for understanding economic theory, and it is something that very few psychologists and neurobiologists appreciate. Imagine that I demonstrate that a particular chooser obeys GARP in her choices among fruits. Then imagine that I find (perhaps by fitting some function to her choice data) a utility representation that predicts her choices among all the fruits or bundles of fruits I have ever examined directly, or could imagine drawing conclusions about using graphs such as the one in Figure 3.8. The utility in this function of an apple might be equal to 3, an orange = 2, a pear = 1. Great. I actually do know something, but it is critical to remember that even with GARP, the numbers I am using are basically made up. Their order is constrained by the data, but the actual magnitude of these numbers is not very much constrained, which was Pareto's point. I know from observed choice that an apple is better than a pear, but in no sense do I know that an apple is exactly 3 times better than a pear. That is simply going beyond my data—a fact that the GARP approach makes clear because of the very weakness of the constraints it imposes. If I squared all of the values in my utility list so that Apple = 9, Orange = 4, and Pear = 1, my function would have exactly the same predictive power as it did before. Any increasing monotonic transform of these utility numbers will preserve choice ordering and preserve compliance with GARP. (I also know that I cannot take the reciprocal of each of these numbers. This is a non-monotonic transform that GARP tells me cannot work with these data.[12])

---

12. Taking the reciprocal also fails to preserve the ordinal structure of these particular objects. For more complex functions, one can generate cases where a transformation preserves ordering locally while failing to maintain global monotonicity. This is a class of

To summarize, what the neoclassical approach provides are very minimalist models. These models are built out of logical statements about choice called axioms. A good model of this type has (for our purposes here) three important features. First, the statements are concise, they are easy to understand, and they seem likely to be true. Second, an underlying mathematical proof relates choices that obey these axioms to a clear theory of value or utility (not the other way around). Third, the theory of value described by the axioms cogently defines a large class of important sub-models (as GARP defines classes of utility functions) and this means that falsifying an axiomatic model, finding choice behavior at variance with the axiomatic statement, unambiguously *falsifies this entire class of models for all time*. That is the core of this approach.

Adding Axioms: Moving Towards a Richer Theory with Expected Utility

What the preceding section should have made clear is that one can use choices to understand or describe utility, and one can even determine whether the theories of subjective value embodied by the class of monotonic utility functions (a class often called "Bernoullis" in economics) applies to a particular chooser. There are, however, clearly things missing from GARP that we would like to be able to study. GARP does not, for example, tell us how the utility of a pile of apples grows as the number of apples in the pile increases. Is having 1,000 apples 1,000 times better than having 1 apple, or only 50 times better? GARP can tell us only that it is better. Is there an extension of these original models that places stronger constraints on the shape of the utility function—that places more explicit restrictions on choice—that can be built from this basic approach? The standard answer to that question is yes, and the axiom group typically used to generate that answer forms the core of *Expected Utility Theory*.

Expected Utility Theory was developed by John von Neumann and Oskar Morgenstern (1944) specifically to describe a more explicit theory

---

functions specifically incompatible with GARP in the way I have described but detailing those functions here would unnecessarily sidetrack this presentation.

of value (somewhat like the one Bernoulli had proposed) but using the more rigorous neoclassical economic approach. One major discrepancy between the objects of study in classical and neoclassical economics was uncertain or probabilistic events. Pascal had invented the original theory of valuation, the theory of expected value, to describe choices among uncertain events. In the cases Samuelson studied, subjects were choosing between objects such as apples and oranges. In principle one could extend this to choices among things such as lottery tickets. Which does a chooser prefer: a 50% chance of winning an apple or a 28% chance of winning a pear? But it is important to note that neither WARP nor GARP treats a 28% chance of winning a pear and a 29% chance of winning a pear as being similar in any way. None of these super-compact theories of choice gives us the tools to treat similar probabilistic outcomes as having related utilities.

Having come this far, it now probably seems obvious that using a neoclassical approach to describe choice under uncertainty became a natural goal for the neoclassical movement. To achieve that goal, von Neumann and Morgenstern started with essentially the same axiom that forms the core of theories such as GARP, but they added three additional pieces (von Neumann and Morgenstern, 1944).

1. Defining the Objects of Choice: Probabilistic Outcomes

Von Neumann and Morgenstern's first step was to define the kinds of objects people would be asked to choose between in their formulation in such a way that uncertain events could be studied and related. They did this by describing an "object of choice" that they called a "lottery." This is an object of choice defined by two numbers: a probability and a value. So, for example, one might choose between a 50% chance of gaining a pear and a 25% chance of gaining an apple within the context of their theory. Both of these are referred to formally as "lotteries," and are composed of the thing you might get, often called a "prize," and a probability that you will get that prize.

It is natural to think of these choice objects as being like the lottery tickets sold at casinos or newsstands, and indeed one often sees that description used, but it is important to stress that von Neumann and Morgenstern meant this to be a general way of talking about almost anything you could imagine. How, as economists, do you think about the value of asking a fellow conference attendee to sleep with you? You place some value on the event and some probability on his or her saying yes. Lotteries are meant to be a general-purpose tool for describing any certain or uncertain "prize" in mathematical terms.

2. First Axiom: Continuity

Given this new way of talking about the objects of choice as probabilistic events, what we next need is to develop an axiom that represents the fact that a 10% chance of an apple and an 11% chance of an apple are similar in a way that apples and oranges are not. Our goal as economists is to communicate this idea as a testable minimalist rule that will contribute to our overall theory of value in a useful way. To achieve this goal, von Neumann and Morgenstern settled on the "continuity axiom." Imagine that we establish that you prefer apples to oranges to pears. The continuity axiom simply says that if you prefer a 100% chance of winning an apple to a 100% chance of an orange, then even if you add a tiny, tiny, tiny probability of also winning a pear to the certain orange, your preferences should not change. Put somewhat more formally, the axiom states that there is some probability of winning a pear, usually denoted ε (epsilon), that is so small that adding it to either of the other prizes has no effect on the subject's choice. In essence, this amounts to a minimalist assertion that probabilities are special—that probabilities describe a continuous axis in prize space, which things such as apples and oranges need not necessarily do.

This may seem like an incredibly weak statement. Surely von Neumann and Morgenstern should have included an axiom along the lines of "Double the probability and you double the subjective value of a choice." The problem with a rule like that, however, is that it is circular. We have no way of measuring the subjective values our subjects place on prizes directly. Instead what we are trying to do is create rules (axioms) about choices that will let us later say something about subjective values, or utilities. And as we will see in a moment, the truth is that this very minimalist statement is going to be enough, coupled with the other axioms, to yield conclusions about underlying utility representations very much like "Double the probability and you double the subjective value of a choice."

3. Second Axiom: Independence

One of the other disappointing features of such theories as WARP and GARP is that they were silent about the fact that "prizes" could actually be made up of bundles of separate things, and that how these bundles were composed mattered. The independence axiom states, in essence, that if you prefer an apple over an orange, then you must also prefer an apple plus a tiny, tiny bit of a second apple over an orange plus that same tiny, tiny bit of the second apple. Put more generally, the axiom says that if you add a common prize to each side of a choice relation, it should not change the subject's preferences. If a subject prefers a 50% chance of winning $100 over a 25% chance of winning $200, he should also prefer a 50% chance of winning $100 and a 5% chance of winning $10 over a 25% chance of winning $200 and a 5% chance of winning $10. This is, in essence, the independence axiom.[13]

The Expected Utility Theorem

So what does all this mean with regard to a theory of value? If we say that we have a chooser who obeys in her choices the axioms of GARP, that turned out to be the same as saying that we have a chooser who behaves as if she had a monotonic utility function. Von Neumann and Morgenstern proved that if we have a chooser who obeys GARP plus the continuity and independence axioms, it is the same as saying that she has some monotone utility function (as in GARP) and she computes the desirability of any lottery by multiplying the probability of the gains or losses presented in the lottery by the utility of those gains or losses.

---

13. My more technical readers may have noticed that these lotteries do not, in actual fact, provide a *mathematically precise* example of the axiom's requirement. To generate a mathematically precise version, one does better to use a three-prize lottery of the form used by Allais (1953). I present such an example in Chapter 5. I have avoided it here to achieve clarity about what the axiom means for a non-economic audience.

To put that another way, an expected utility-compliant chooser behaves as if she chooses by multiplying probability by utility. It should be immediately obvious that von Neumann and Morgenstern have gotten us almost back to where Bernoulli left us—but in a much more powerful way. Bernoulli gave us a bunch of assumptions about the form of the human utility function, what was encoded, what was represented, and how those variables interacted. From these he specified how actual humans would choose. But he never gave us those rules in a way that allowed us to examine the choice behavior of subjects in a meaningful way. What von Neumann and Morgenstern did was to give us a few simple rules that describe choice behavior. If you can prove that a chooser obeys those axioms in his or her choices, you know quite a bit about how he or she constructs and represents subjective values, at least in a theoretical sense. If you can prove that the chooser did not obey those choice rules, then you have falsified the theory, at least with regard to that chooser and that set of choice objects.

A second feature of expected utility theory is that it very much strengthens (but does not completely recover) the cardinality of our original notion of utility. If we observe a subject whose choices obey the axioms of expected utility, and we observe that she finds a 50% probability of winning an apple exactly the same as a 100% probability of winning an orange, then we can say that *she values an apple exactly twice as much as she values an orange*. One cannot stress enough what a huge advance this is for our theory of value. Von Neumann and Morgenstern essentially showed how to use probability as a yardstick to measure the relationships between the values of different prizes *for subjects who obey their axioms*. Using the von Neumann and Morgenstern approach, we can get past the ordinal bottleneck Pareto identified to some degree. Let me stress, however, that this advance does not get us to a unique number that we can assign as the utility of an object. Utilities are still only measurable *relative* to other objects (this means that if we choose to say that an apple has a utility of 4 and a pear has a utility of 2, we can also just as accurately say that an apple has a utility of 40 and a pear has a utility of 20), but our notion of utility certainly has more bite than it did under GARP, and we know how to determine when this additional bite is warranted by testing the axioms of the theory on behavior.

Conclusions

I hope that this chapter, though admittedly a tough chapter, accomplished two goals. First, I hope it familiarized non-economists with the kinds of objects that arise in economic theories. If we are really to set about linking the objects of study in economics to the objects of study in psychology and neuroscience, we have to be very clear about what these objects look like. Economics is largely made up of axioms on choice and the theories of value that these axioms describe. The theories of value, which incorporate objects such as expected utility, are conceptual objects. To economists, they are mathematical tools for predicting choice and nothing more. They are not real physical events or things that can be measured directly. But what we will begin to ask in the pages that follow is whether theoretical constructs such as utility, or the axioms themselves, can be related directly to the philosophical objects that populate neuroscience and psychology.

Second, I hope it communicated to non-economists some of the esthetics of economics. I hope it communicated why von Neumann and Morgenstern's Theory of Expected Utility is fundamentally different from, and more testable than, Bernoulli's notion of utility. This is a difference that is enormously important to economists and that I have found non-economists often mistakenly believe to be small. It is a difference in method, in falsifiability, and in philosophy. Anyone who wants to seriously do neuroeconomics simply must appreciate this point.

To move forward in laying the foundations for neuroeconomics, the objects introduced in this chapter that we need to keep most careful track of right now are those related to expected utility theory: That we can treat choosers who obey the axioms of expected utility as if they:

1. Construct monotonic utility functions for things such as apples and oranges
2. Multiply the utility of each object by the probability of obtaining that object to yield an expected utility for each option in their choice set
3. Select the option having the highest expected utility.

Before closing this chapter, though, we also need to acknowledge several problems with expected utility theory in particular and with the neoclassical approach in general. The greatest power of these simple and compact theories is that they are falsifiable. Their greatest weakness is that we can therefore prove that most of these theories are false under at least some conditions. When the probabilities of an outcome are small, for example, we know that most humans violate the independence axiom (Allais, 1953; Wu and Gonzalez, 1998). When children are younger than about 8 years old, we know that they violate GARP more seriously than adults (e.g., Harbaugh et. al, 2001). These are real problems that have generated no end of tension in the economic community. As we will see in the pages that follow, these problems with the neoclassical approach have led psychologists and economists to take two different approaches to choice in recent years. One group of economists has responded to this challenge by revising the axioms so that they better align with observed choice behavior. A second group of economists and psychologists has argued that these data suggest that the logical primitives of economics, these axiomatic approaches, should be entirely abandoned in favor of the data-fitting approaches common in the natural sciences.

In this book I argue for a middle road. First, I suggest that one group of the revised sets of axioms will turn out to be very closely aligned with existing psychological and neurobiological kinds. Second, I argue that the imperfections in the alignment of these logical "kinds" offer opportunity—an opportunity to, for example, use data from neuroscience and psychology to subtly alter the structure of existing economic theory in a way that preserves its compact, choice-focused nature but makes it much more predictive. The next chapter provides our first example of such a formal linkage and realignment as we explore the relationship between the neurobiology of sensory encoding, the psychology of sensory perception (often called *psychophysics*), and a class of utility-based models (often called *random utility models*). What we will see is that the neural machinery for encoding properties such the sweetness of a sugar solution, the psychological description of how we discriminate the sweetness of the foods we encounter, and the economic description of how we choose among sweet objects already all share an almost identical logical structure—a pre-existing structure close enough to permit the kind of philosophical reduction I proposed in the preceding chapter.

4

Using Psychology to See the Brain in Economics

Précis

In this chapter I hope to develop the first of several linkages between economics, psychology, and neuroscience. In the preceding chapters I have laid the conceptual foundations for such linkages; here I hope to give a first example of exactly what it means to say that a concept from economics can be mapped to a concept in psychology and thence to neuroscience.

I propose to accomplish that goal in several steps. First, I have to provide non-psychologist readers with an overview of classical psychophysics. This is a heavily mathematical sub-discipline of perceptual psychology concerned with understanding how physical stimuli in the external world give rise to a hidden subjective experience called a *percept*. It employs a class of mathematical models for describing this process, usually called signal detection theory.

Second, I have to demonstrate that the mathematically described relationship between stimulus and percept can be mapped fairly directly to neurobiological models of sensory transduction. Reductive linkages of the kind described in Chapter 1, linkages between psychological models of perception and neurobiological models of stimulus transduction and encoding by the nervous system, have already been well developed. This chapter provides examples of these pre-existing conceptual reductions between psychology and neuroscience.

Finally, I have to demonstrate that one of these fully linked neurobiology-to-psychology concept groups can be relevant to economics.

In light of the previous chapter, it should come as no surprise that I will argue that a key neurobiology–psychology concept group can be directly and obviously linked to economic notions of utility. That linkage is mediated by a class of models from economics called Random Utility Models (RUMs), which were developed by Daniel McFadden, a leading economist who was attempting to incorporate psychophysical tools for the study of stochasticity into economics (McFadden, 1974, 2000).

The chapter will thus end with the explicit claim that economic models of the random utility of directly consumable rewards are, in their present form, reducible to psychological models of percept and thence to neurobiological models of biochemical transduction. Let me stress that this first reductive link between the parent disciplines intentionally offers few new insights. While many readers may find it amazing to discover the biochemical mechanism of preference encoding for one class of consumable rewards, this is not an insight that will change economics, nor is it supposed to be. It is simply meant to serve as a compelling existence proof, a demonstration that clear reductive linkages between these three sciences are unarguably possible.

To make this case in the pages that follow, I present a fairly detailed history of the models employed in sensory psychophysics. Beginning with the work of Weber, I trace that history through Fechner and Stevens to Green and Swets and beyond. For trained psychologists this will be a review; I ask that these readers skim these sections but still take the time to read the overall chapter. The last section of the chapter, in particular, presents information critical to the discourse that follows. With that précis in hand, we turn next to a psychophysical parable meant to communicate some of the logical kinds of psychology.

Searching in the Dark: A Parable

Imagine a man moving through a dimly illuminated nightclub constructed of three sequentially arranged rooms. The first room is lit only with blue light, a second only with green light, and a third only with red. The club owners have made sure that each room is illuminated with equal intensity; each contains an equal number of photons. The man is searching for a particular woman, perhaps one he met at a professional conference.

The likelihood that she will recognize him, it turns out, depends on the room in which she sits. We know for certain that she is much more likely to see him if she sits in the green room than in either of the other two rooms.

This may seem odd because in all three rooms the man reflects an equal number of photons,[1] although the reflected photons have the different wavelengths associated with each of the rooms. Most physical properties of the three environments are identical, but her actions are not. How do we, as psychologists, understand this?

To understand this behavior, a classical sensory psychologist postulates the existence of a hidden variable inside the mind of the woman called a *perception*, or a *perceptual experience*, that links the sensory stimuli in the outside world and the actions of the observer. The action, in this case, is the probability that she will detect the man.

As psychologists we can indirectly access that variable, the perceptual experience, in a number of different ways. The simplest possible way would be to ask the subject if she saw anyone she recognized. More complicated techniques might be employed. Regardless of the precise method, though, our goal would be to describe a mathematical function that relates properties of stimuli in the outside world, in this case wavelength, to an underlying perceptual experience that the woman uses to guide her behavior.

Taking This Example Seriously: The Psychophysics of Scotopic Vision

Since at least the mid-1800s, perceptual psychologists have tried to understand the functions that relate stimuli to percept in rigorous ways. In no field is this clearer than in the study of the simplest kind of vision, the perception of light intensity as a function of wavelength described in the preceding example.

To understand that area in the study of perception, one must begin with the early observation that mammalian vision operates in two distinct modes: *scotopic* and *photopic*. Scotopic vision is what we use under conditions of very dim illumination, and its most marked feature is that

---

1. In fairness, this would make him unusually monochromatic.

humans operating under scotopic conditions cannot discriminate colors. A number of other discontinuous functional features separate scotopic and photopic vision (see Wandell, 1995, for more on these issues). Under conditions of dim illumination when only the scotopic system is active, subjects can make judgments about the relative intensity of lights but not about their color. Under photopic conditions, in contrast, humans behave as if they use a three-color perceptual system to discriminate the properties of light as colors ranging from red to green to blue.

This initial qualitative observation led a number of researchers working in the early 20th century to hypothesize that such behaviors as the woman's inability to perceive the man searching for her in the red and blue rooms might be easily and rigorously characterized at a mathematical level. To achieve that characterization, psychologists turned to a set of techniques known collectively as psychophysics. To better understand the strengths and weaknesses of psychophysics, we review the study of scotopic perceptual brightness.

Scotopic Percepts

The stimuli (the physical events) in the red and green rooms described above can be characterized by the number of photons they emit and the wavelengths of each those photons. While it is true that we humans can report the existence of photons having a wavelength of 650 nm by saying that we see a red light, it is important to remember that there is nothing intrinsically "red" about those photons. Indeed, there are many combinations of photons having different wavelengths that all give rise to an indistinguishable perception of "red" (e.g., Wandell, 1995). Radiance (number of photons) and spectral (wavelength) distribution are properties of the outside world. What we experience mentally is a percept, and it is the mapping from stimulus to percept that psychophysicists seek to characterize. In the case of light intensity it is a mapping from *radiance* to *brightness*, where brightness is the psychophysical name given to the perceptual experiences associated with changes in radiance.

In the real world around us most light sources—for example, an electric light—give off photons having a broad distribution of wavelengths. Figure 4.1 gives an example of this, showing the spectral distribution of a typical incandescent bulb.

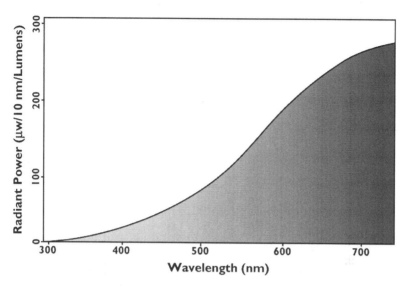

FIGURE 4.1   Spectrum of lightbulb.

How can we hope to characterize the scotopic perceptual experience, the internal subjective variable, associated with viewing that particular incandescent bulb? To do that, we take the following standard experimental approach (Wandell, 1995). First we seat the subject in a dimly illuminated room (so that her vision remains in the scotopic mode) facing a circular display (see Figure 4.2). Onto the left half of that display the incandescent light we hope to characterize is projected at an intensity (an objective radiance) controlled by the experimenter. On the right side of the patch a special light source that emits photons at a single wavelength, a *monochromatic light*, has been prearranged. The subject is then provided with a simple instruction: Turn a knob that adjusts the intensity of the monochromatic light until it appears to be exactly equal in intensity to light from the incandescent bulb we are trying to characterize. Adjust the magnitude of the monochromatic light, we tell her, until your brightness judgments are "indifferent" or subjectively equal.

Once the subject reports that she perceives the two lights as having exactly equal perceptual intensity, the number of photons per second emitted by each light source is determined and plotted on a graph. Next, the intensity of the incandescent light source is incremented, the new

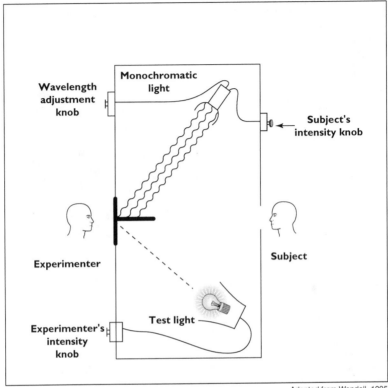

Adapted from Wandell, 1995

FIGURE 4.2   Wavelength sensitivity experiment.

point of subjective equality is established, and the process is repeated several more times. What results is a graph of the intensity pairs (the intensities in the two lights) that yield identical *percepts* of brightness. Perhaps surprisingly, when this experiment is done, one always observes that when the *wavelength* of the monochromatic light is held fixed, these pairs of points all fall along a straight line that passes through the origin of the graph.

Next, the entire experiment is repeated, but this time after shifting the wavelength of the monochromatic test light. Again we plot the intensity pairs, which again fall along a straight line passing through the origin but this time with a different slope. This may seem complicated, but it has a simple logic. We are asking the subjects to perform a kind of

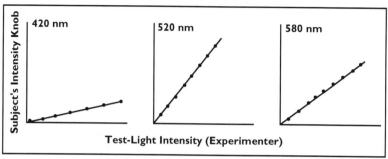

FIGURE 4.3   Subjective intensity matches.

substitution experiment—how many photons at a particular wavelength do we have to add to match the addition of any given number of photons to the incandescent test stimulus?

In the last step of this psychophysical experiment, we can quantify how effectively *photons of different wavelengths* substitute for increases in the test stimulus by simply plotting the slopes of the many graphs we obtained as a function of wavelength. The result is often called a *spectral sensitivity curve*; it describes, for this subject, the relationship between the percept of brightness and the wavelengths of the photons that give rise to that percept of brightness. Figure 4.4 plots that curve for a typical human subject (Wald and Brown, 1956; Wandell, 1995). What we can see is that for this typical human, photons having a wavelength of 550 nm produce a much bigger increment in the perception of brightness (the hidden internal value) than do photons having wavelengths of 650 nm or 425 nm. This has been found to be true for all humans with normal vision.

This observation explains why the woman in the parable at the beginning of the chapter would have failed to notice her partner if she had been sitting in the red or blue rooms. In our example the red and blue rooms were illuminated, respectively, with 650-nm and 425-nm photons. At a psychological level of analysis, these are photons that give rise to weaker intensity percepts than do the 550-nm photons used to illuminate the green room. In the green room the perceptual experience was simply stronger.

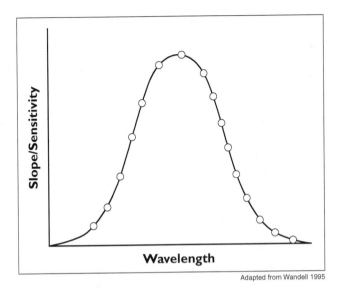

Adapted from Wandell 1995

FIGURE 4.4   Scotopic sensitivity.

The interesting thing about this explanation is its similarity, in many ways, to a classical economic study. While the judgment the subject is making is very simple (and perhaps economically uninteresting), we can understand that decision in terms of a hidden process, in this case a mental process that we relate with a specified function to observable variables in the outside world. The subject is not incentivized monetarily for the decision in a typical psychophysical experiment as he would be in an economic experiment, but the results speak for themselves. The repeatable linearity of the measured functions across individuals clearly indicates the existence of an important regularity.

What makes this particular example crucial, however, is its relationship to neuroscience.

Reduction: Percept to Rhodopsin

About 10 years after the psychophysical story detailed above appeared in the scientific literature, a number of biochemists began to make serious headway in understanding the mechanisms by which photons were captured by molecules in the retina and used to produce neural action potentials, a process called *phototransduction* (Wandell, 1995). Their studies suggested that under scotopic conditions, each molecule of a compound called *rhodopsin* was transformed in structure when it interacted with a single photon of light. When many photons entered the retina, many molecules of rhodopsin were transformed; when only a few photons entered the eye, only a few molecules were transformed. This naturally led these biochemists to ask whether the efficiency with which photons are absorbed by rhodopsin, the rate at which light transforms individual rhodopsin molecules, varies as a function of wavelength. Do rhodopsin molecules more easily capture photons of some wavelengths than others?

To answer that question, Wald and Brown (1956, 1958) developed a simple apparatus to measure the fraction of photons captured by a sheet of rhodopsin. They coated a sheet of glass with a layer of rhodopsin and then examined the fraction of photons chemically absorbed by the sheet as they varied the wavelength of light bombarding the rhodopsin film. They found that rhodopsin did a rather poor job of absorbing photons at wavelengths including 425 and 650 nm but a rather good job of absorbing photons at wavelengths such as 550 nm. More quantitatively, they were able to generate *absorption spectra* for the chemical rhodopsin much like the wavelength sensitivity spectra that behaviorally measured the percept of light intensity in the experiment above.

What was most amazing about this process was the close match between the perceptually measured curve and the biochemically measured curve. If we correct the biochemical curve to allow for the wavelength-specific absorption spectra of the parts of the eyeball that are interposed between the lights we were using in the behavioral experiment and the retina, the curves that measure biochemical absorption and the curves that measure verbally reported mental experience were identical. You can see this in Figure 4.5: the black dots plot the spectral sensitivity of the brightness percept and the white dots plot the absorption spectra of rhodopsin.

So what does this mean? It almost certainly means that the absorption spectra of rhodopsin and the optical elements of the eyeball account entirely for the psychological function that relates wavelength to percept. In fairness, many of my economist friends and colleagues scoff at such a claim of perfect mental to physical reduction. Sure the match is perfect,

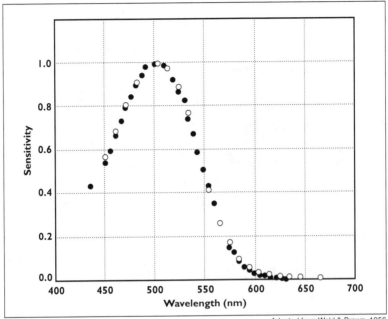

Adapted from Wald & Brown, 1956

FIGURE 4.5   Behavioral and biochemical sensitivity curves.

but perhaps that is just chance. I think a further observation disproves that hypothesis: human subjects who do not have rhodopsin (either from an experimental manipulation called photobleaching or through a genetic defect) have no scotopic vision. Rhodopsin is required for scotopic vision *and* the absorption spectra of rhodopsin accounts for the perceptual curve (Baylor et al., 1987).

This also, of course, implies two other even more amazing facts, that perceptual experience is a quite direct function of rhodopsin absorption and that human verbal reports of brightness equivalence are essentially perfect indicators of the underlying perceptual experience.

To me this is a simply astounding observation, and one clearly relevant to the issue of whether neurobiology and economics are likely to be relatable to one another in a reductive sense. But to explore that issue in greater detail and to examine what it means for such concepts as utility, we turn next to the history of psychophysics.

Ernst Weber and the Birth of Modern Psychophysics

The modern notion that perceptual experience could be studied as a mental phenomenon distinct from external physical measurements has its origins in the work of the 19th-century German physiologist Ernst Weber. He was interested in understanding the limits and properties of human sensory judgments (Weber, 1834). He made a number of discoveries in this regard but is most widely known for a set of experiments on the accuracy of human perceptual judgments about touch.

Imagine that we give a subject a sack of sand weighing 1 kilogram that we refer to as the "reference" stimulus. We then hand him a second, or "test," sack of sand and ask him if this second sack is lighter or heavier than the reference. As we vary the weight of the test sack, we find that the likelihood he will call the test sack heavier increases slowly (as the weight of the test sack increases), a finding shown in Figure 4.6.

The first thing this reveals is that human perceptual judgments are imperfect; as the weights of the two sacks become close, human observers have trouble distinguishing them. In fact, their judgments become quite probabilistic as the two sacks approach the same weight. The second thing that it reveals is that human perceptual judgments, although probabilistic, are quite lawful. As the weight of the test sack increases, the likelihood that the subject will say that this is the heavier sack grows slowly and steadily. Even more important than this, however, was Weber's study of the way in which this kind of judgment changes as the weight of the reference stimulus changes. Weber found that if one repeats this experiment with a 10-kilogram sack, the range of weights over which the subject makes errors grows significantly *but stays a fixed fraction of the reference stimulus magnitude*. Thus, if a subject has trouble distinguishing the difference between a 0.95-kilogram and a 1.0-kilogram sack, then Weber found that the subject would also have trouble distinguishing between a 9.5-kilogram sack and a 10-kilogram sack. In fact, he found that this was a consistent feature of sensory judgments at many weight levels. In other words, Weber found that the *just noticeable difference* in weight is, across a very broad dynamic range, a fixed fraction of stimulus weight (or *intensity*, in the generalized language of psychophysics). If the minimum increment in weight a subject can detect reliably (say with 75% accuracy) is 0.5 kilograms at a base weight of 10 kilograms, then the

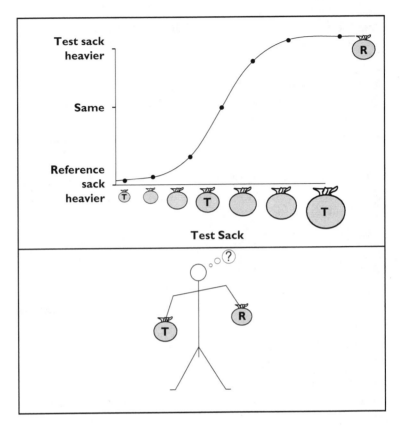

FIGURE 4.6   Weber's experiment.

just noticeable difference in weight for this person will be 5% at essentially all weights.[2]

In subsequent experiments, Weber's observation was made in a variety of sensory systems, and the notion that the accuracy (or more

---

2. It should be acknowledged that this regularity breaks down as the stimulus approaches the subject's detection threshold. In this example, that means that as the weight of the reference sack approaches the minimal weight that a subject can actually detect (something less than a gram), the just noticeable difference ceases to be a constant fraction of the reference weight.

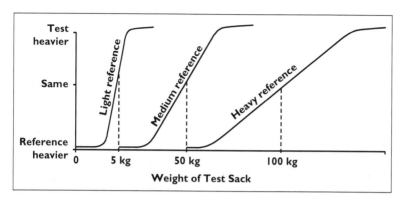

FIGURE 4.7

precisely the confusability) of perceptual judgments scales as a constant fraction of stimulus intensity became codified as a psychological law.

Gustav Fechner

Starting from these discoveries of Weber's, the German physicist Gustav Fechner set about both mathematizing and extending Weber's work (Fechner, 1860). He began by reanalyzing Weber's work from a more quantitative perspective, focusing on the fact that this constant fractional accuracy had some interesting implications. If we replot Weber's data on a logarithmic axis, as in Figure 4.8, one sees immediately that the slopes of the discrimination curves—the sizes of the just noticeable differences as a function of stimulus intensity—are constant. Whence do these slopes arise?

If one considers perceptual experience as an imperfect representation of the external world, then understanding Weber's data becomes quite simple. Imagine that each time a 5-kilogram weight is placed in a subject's hand this gives rise to a percept, but each time it is a slightly different percept because of the imperfection of the representation. To keep things simple, let us imagine that Figure 4.9 plots the distribution of perceptual experiences that are produced by a 5-kilogram weight. This is a Gaussian

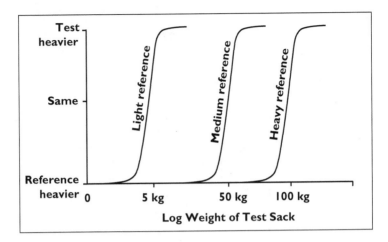

FIGURE 4.8

distribution, centered here arbitrarily on a perceptual intensity of
1 "exper."[3]

One way that we can think about this is that each time our subject
picks up a 5-kilogram sack he "draws" a perceptual experience at random
from a Gaussian distribution of possible perceptual experiences. The
curve in Figure 4.9 thus tells us the likelihood a particular percept will
be drawn each time he picks up the sack. If we assume that each of the
two sacks that our subject is examining is transformed into a mental
experience by a similar Gaussian distribution, then we can understand
why the judgments of our subjects change in the way that they do as the
test stimulus begins to approach the reference stimulus in weight. If we
ask our subjects to discriminate between two very similar weights, then
they will actually have perceptual experiences that may be overlapping
(see Figure 4.10). In contrast, the distributions of experience will be
quite different if we use very different weights.

---

3. Let me hasten to add that the units of perception in the literature are sensory-
system specific. *Brightness* is used for judgments about light intensity, *heaviness* for judgments
of weight, etc. Collapsing all of these units onto a single common unit, I adopt the
convention of the "exper," which I use here as the universal unit of subjective intensity.

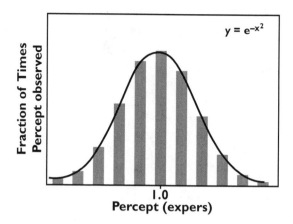

FIGURE 4.9   The distribution of perceptual experiences produced by a single stimulus intensity.

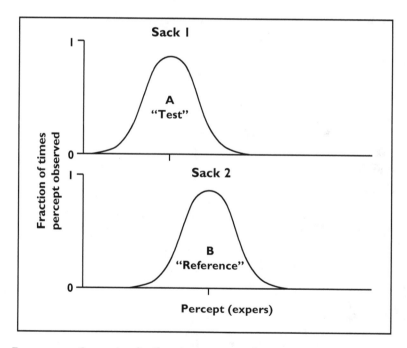

FIGURE 4.10   Comparing distributed percepts in Weber's experiment.

Weber's observation that confusability is a constant fraction of magnitude tells us that these distributions of perceptual experience have a constant width on a logarithmic axis. From this line of reasoning Fechner derived what is now called *Weber's Law*:

$$\frac{\Delta I}{I} = k$$

or, in words, the just noticeable difference (ΔI) divided by the actual weight (I) is always equal to a constant.

Fechner then took this observation a step farther, and in a very important way. Weber's studies had all been about confusability, about how subjects discriminated between two stimuli, but he really wanted to know about the intensities of the perceptions themselves. What fascinated Fechner was the relationship between mind and body, and he wanted to discover the function that related these two. Fechner thus hypothesized that the relationship between stimulus and percept and the relationship between stimulus and variability of percept were both captured by Weber's law. Percept, Fechner hypothesized, grows as the log of intensity in just the same way that Weber had shown that variance in percept grows as the log of intensity. To put this in units of expers, consider Figure 4.11.

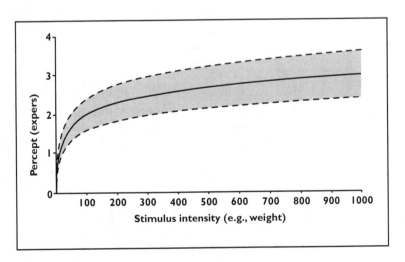

FIGURE 4.11

If I place a 10-kilogram weight in your hand, you can experience any of a number of percepts. But these percepts are distributed around 1 exper (the log of 10) and have a constant variance as a function of position along the subjective curve of expers.

What I hope will be immediately obvious to any reader is the similarity between this curve and the one Bernoulli proposed for understanding choice. Fechner proposed that as the magnitude of the stimulus increases, the subjective experience of that stimulus grows as the logarithm of that stimulus magnitude. This is an idea very similar to the one developed for choice by Bernoulli a century earlier. An important difference between these two formulations, however, is the notion of variance. In classical economics, Bernoulli did not include a concept of trial-by-trial variability, but it was from Weber's focus on measurements of trial-by-trial variability that the Fechner curve emerged.

Fechner's curve has a number of other implications that also need to be considered because they play a key role in understanding later neurobiological and psychological studies of choice. First, we should note immediately that Fechner's curve yields a largely cardinal notion of perceptual experience, but not one as explicitly cardinal as Bernoulli's. The reason for this is simple. Bernoulli imagined that one could compare the utilities of any two objects by simply asking a subject to choose between them. If we imagine a utility function for gold and a utility function from silver, we can scale those two curves to each other by asking subjects to choose between a fixed quantity of silver and a variable quantity of gold. This allows us to define an equivalence point between gold and silver that allows us to scale these two utility functions to each other. For percept, most (but admittedly not all) scholars argue that no such scaling is possible because we cannot ask our subjects to tell us when a variable sack of sand is heavier than a fixed light is bright.

The second, and probably more important, feature of Fechner's curve is that variance and magnitude are related by a constant. As magnitude grows, so does variance, and at exactly the same rate. This is a tremendously important feature of the cardinality of expers for an empirical scientist, because to fully quantify a perceptual experience one needs only to measure either the subjective magnitude of the percept or the variance of the percept. By knowing one, you reveal the other (to within a constant scaling factor). This may seem a trivial point, but much of neurobiological choice theory rests (erroneously, I believe) on this assumption.

To summarize, psychophysics began with an effort to rigorously quantify one facet of perceptual experience. Ernst Weber measured the confusability of stimulus judgments, focusing on tactile sensations. He found that confusability (a property called the *just noticeable difference*) scales as a constant fraction of variance. From this observation and the axiomatic assumption that the variance and magnitude of percept are linear transformations of one another, Fechner proposed a complete description of the relationship between a hidden mental process that we call "perceptual experience" and observable stimulus intensity.

S. S. Stevens

The *Weber-Fechner Law*, as Fechner's model came to be known, stood as the central insight for understanding the relationship between stimulus, percept, and percept variance for almost a century. This was true despite the fact that the Weber-Fechner Law rested on the largely untested assumption that perceptual intensity scales with perceptual variability. Fechner had a strong conviction that measurements of perceptual variability revealed the way perceptual magnitude scaled, but he had little direct evidence to support this conclusion. In this regard, Fechner was at a significant disadvantage when compared to Bernoulli and his studies of utility. Bernoulli could begin to measure the shape of the utility function by using probabilistic lotteries. His idea was that if one halved the probability of winning a lottery, one also halved the utility of that lottery (an assumption related to the independence and continuity axioms of von Neumann and Morgenstern). Fechner had no such technique for halving the number of expers in a percept.

In the 1940s and 1950s the Harvard psychologist Stanley Smith "Smitty" Stevens began to approach this problem by trying to develop a direct method for measuring percept. Stevens' idea was, in reality, quite simple. He would present a subject with two stimuli and ask the subject to adjust a third stimulus until it was "midway between the two test stimuli in intensity," a technique he called the *bisection method*.

In one experiment, Stevens performed this procedure using lights of differing intensity in an effort to map the relationship between stimulus and percept for brightness. He found in that case that the function that best predicted these bisection judgments was indeed something like a logarithmic transformation, as Fechner had imagined. When he performed these same experiments on other perceptual stimuli, however, Stevens obtained a very different result. The scaling between stimulus and percept, he discovered, is very stimulus-type dependent. The apparent length of a line, for example, is a perfectly linear function of objective length. The subjective intensity of an electric shock, in contrast, grows faster than its objective value (Stevens, 1961).

Stevens performed literally dozens of these kinds of measurements and obtained data that related these perceptual bisections to stimulus intensity for everything from the sense of sweetness to the heaviness of weights. His many datasets led him to conclude that the magnitude of percepts grows *as a power function of objective stimulus intensity*, with the size of the exponent of the power function being a different number for each sensory system. Warmth, for example, he found to be well described by the equation

Perceived warmth of a large patch of skin $= (Temp \ of \ that \ skin)^{0.7}$

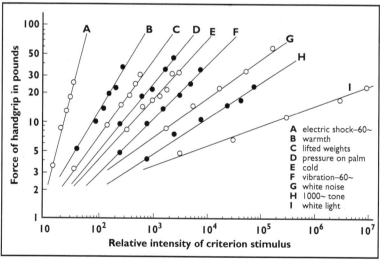

After Stevens, 1961

FIGURE 4.12

In contrast, he found that:

Perceived intensity of an electrical shock = *(Electrical current)*$^{3.5}$

Stevens' findings came to be broadly accepted, and the Stevens Power Law has now largely replaced the Weber-Fechner Law as the standard model for understanding the mapping between stimulus and percept. That advance meant that perceptual variance and perceptual intensity could once again be considered independent properties. As we will see later, that has huge implications for understanding important decision-related neuroscientific work such as Newsome and colleagues' studies of perceptual decision-making.[4]

Signal Detection Theory

While the Stevens Power Law is widely accepted among the cognoscenti of the psychophysical community, there remains a certain level of discomfort about the bisection method used to derive these functions. What does it mean, a rigorous scientist might ask, for a subject to say that one stimulus is "halfway between" two others? That seems a reasonable concern. The Stevens Power Law measurements describe something repeatable—but what? Stevens called the thing they describe "percept," but how we relate that hidden variable to the actions of humans doing other things than turning an intensity knob has always been difficult. One result of this difficulty is that, since Stevens, psychophysics has tended to return to the studies of confusability that Weber pioneered.

As a result, the study of judgment about confusability has come a long way, mathematically, since Weber's time. Today, the core techniques for understanding confusability judgments are referred to collectively as signal-detection theory and take a form familiar and comfortable to

---

4. This is important for understanding the Newsome experiments because that work is specifically about the confusability of two stimuli. Because confusability in their experiments is primarily determined by perceptual variance, their experiments tell us very little about the perceptual experience of their subjects. This is a point about which there has been no end of confusion in the scientific literature despite the best efforts of Newsome and his colleagues to make this clear.

neuroscientists, psychologists, and economists. Signal detection theory, largely developed by David Green and John Swets (1966), begins with a tractable set of assumptions that are meant to correlate stimulus properties directly with judgments about confusability. The key assumptions of signal detection theory (in its most basic form) are that real-world stimuli give rise to percepts through a random process like the draw from a Gaussian distribution described above. More specifically, their approach assumes that if we perceive two objects that we are trying to compare, both objects produce a mean perceptual intensity plus or minus a symmetrical variance term, and the magnitude of the variance term for the two percepts (typically in the log domain) is identical.[5]

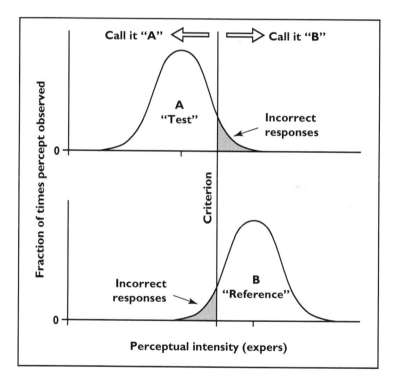

FIGURE 4.13   Choosing amongst distributed percepts.

5. Let me hasten to add that modern theories and tools allow one to relax almost all of these assumptions. I present classical signal detection theory for ease of exposition. The interested reader is referred to MacMillan and Creelman (2005) and Jean-Claude Falmagne's (1985) book *Elements of Psychophysical Theory*.

To make the implications of this assumption clear, consider lifting two sacks of sand each having slightly different weights and then being asked to tell an experimenter which is heavier. As shown in Figure 4.13, the two percepts are assumed to be drawn from two Gaussian distributions of equal variance and then to be compared. Because the distributions are overlapping, sometimes just by chance the lighter object will give rise to a heavier percept and the subject will make a "mistake." Of course, to the subject, no mistake has been made. She is making a correct judgment about her perceptual experience, but that perceptual experience is not accurately reporting which of the sacks weighs more.

This is the core approach to perceptual decision making in signal detection theory, but the overall theory does go much farther. If, for example, we were to instruct a subject to tell us which is heavier, A or B,

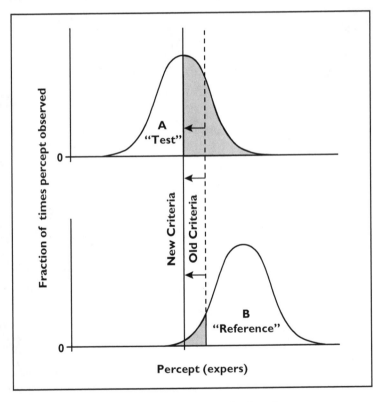

FIGURE 4.14   Choosing asymmetrically amongst distributed percepts.

but we were also to tell her that we would pay her $1 on correct "A" trials and $2 on correct "B" trials, we might expect this to change her decision process. Signal detection theory models this by assuming that subjects operating under these conditions effectively shift their criterion (see Figure 4.14) for saying that "B" was heavier. They shift into a mode in which they require more evidence to say "A" than "B" because saying "B is heavier" is more profitable. Green, Swets, and their followers showed mathematically how such a weighting of percept should occur normatively. They explained how an ideal decision-maker would operate when comparing percepts under a range of conditions.

For us, however, the most important thing about signal detection theory is how it treats "mistakes." Consider the circumstance in which a subject is asked, for a reward of $10 each time she is correct, to identify the heavier of two sacks. The first sack weighs 9.8 kilograms and the second weighs 10.0 kilograms. According to the assumptions of signal detection theory, these two sacks give rise to percepts that vary probabilistically, and then the subject, aware of this variation but unable to do anything about it, simply reports accurately which sack is perceptually heavier. Although the subject may not earn $10, in no sense can we call any of her judgments a mistake under this framework. She is accurately reporting what she perceived.

Random Utility Models

For a psychologist, this notion that subjects have variable internal experiences from the same stimulus will be quite intuitive, but for neoclassical economists such as von Neumann and Morgenstern this notion may not have been quite so natural. There is nothing variable or stochastic about the utility curve of Expected Utility Theory. This is an infinitely thin mathematical abstraction that relates the objective value of a good to the subjective value of that good (Figure 4.15).

That means that if a chooser is asked to select between any two options in standard utility theory, either she says one is better than the other or she says they are identical in subjective value. This makes the neoclassical economics of the middle of the 20th century and perceptual psychology quite different. When a subject makes a perceptual judgment,

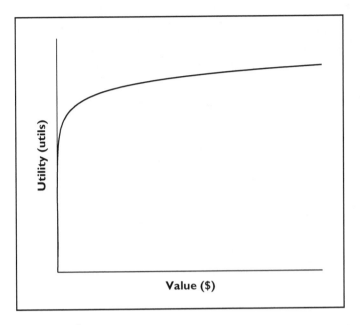

FIGURE 4.15   A utility curve.

she experiences a stochastic percept and makes a stochastic judgment. That is a core feature of both theory and empirical measurement in psychology. In all of the core theories of economics I have presented so far, this feature is neglected.

To highlight this point, imagine that we ask a subject which of two sacks filled with silver she prefers to possess. As the amounts of silver in the two sacks grow similar, the choices of the subject become more and more variable. What we observe in this case (and in basically all cases that have ever been studied) is that the choice function (shown in Fig. 4.16) transitions smoothly from a preference for sack A to a preference for sack B. So how should we think about this process? In theories such as WARP and Expected Utility, we really have only one option: we have to think of these curves as representing errors by our subject. That is an interesting philosophical stance but one that is at variance with the psychological notion that our subject is experiencing a stochastic percept of the weight of these two sacks.

To make this issue even clearer, consider a subject choosing between 10 oranges and a variable number of apples. Early neoclassical-style

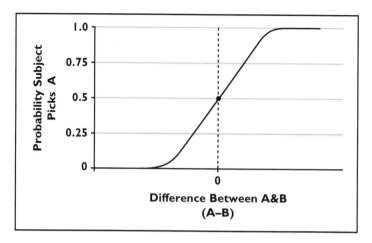

FIGURE 4.16   Choices amongst bags of silver.

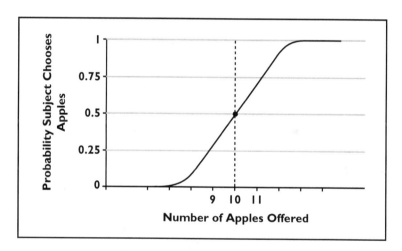

FIGURE 4.17   Choices between apples and oranges.

models predict an abrupt transition in such curves, but if one actually performs this as an experiment, we see, as we did in the silver experiment above, a smooth (and hence stochastic) transition between choosing the apples and choosing the oranges. For us to understand this process from the philosophical position of a model such as GARP, what we have to conclude is that the subject behaves as if each quantity of apples has a fixed utility, but the decision process itself includes some "error." This has obviously important policy implications. If we know the subject's average response to a given choice situation, we can tell her which option to choose on a given trial and can thus reduce her error, whether she is choosing over fruit or sacks of silver.

In the 1970s, the economist Daniel McFadden found himself struck by this logic and how it differed from the kinds of logic being used in signal detection theory (McFadden, 1974). This led him to a ground-breaking proposal that today draws psychological and economic descriptions much more closely together. McFadden proposed that like the percept curves of psychophysics, the utility curves of economics should be considered variable.

McFadden's idea, in a nutshell, was that the very same tools used to study confusability in perceptual judgments should be brought to bear on "errors" in choice observed under economic conditions. He proposed a class of theory now called "Random Utility Models" in which the axioms assume that the utility inferred from a subject's choices can be treated as a variable quantity in almost exactly the same way Weber treated the percept of heaviness.

This notably suggests a natural reduction between the theories of psychology and the theories of economics. The notion of "Random Utility" and the notion of "Percept" are very closely aligned. If we were

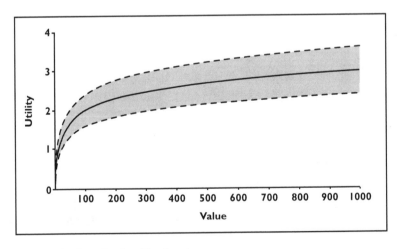

FIGURE 4.18   A stochastic utility function.

to believe, for some reason, that percept and utility were, at least on occasion, actually the same phenomena being studied at different levels of philosophical abstraction, then we would be highly tempted to perform a philosophical reduction between these two concepts. But how could we convince ourselves that this kind of inter-theoretic reduction makes sense?

The Sweet Taste of Success

Consider a little-read neurological and psychological paper from the 1960s (Borg et al., 1967). Two human neurological patients are undergoing surgery. As part of that surgery, the main nerves from the tongues of those patients will be exposed while they are awake and alert. So their surgeons ask them to participate in an experiment. The surgeons will pour sugar solutions of different concentrations on their tongues (while holding the long-term average sweetness constant) and record the activity in the nerves. The surgeons note that although variable, the mean firing rates as a function of sugar concentration increase as a power function having an exponent of about 0.6.

Next, the surgeons adopt Stevens' bisection method and ask the subjects to perform ratings that allow them to construct perceptual intensity curves. The surgeons find that the perceptual curves also describe power functions, again with an exponent of 0.6. They therefore hypothesize that the percept of these subjects is simply a linear report of activity in the nerve.[6]

Although we do not know for sure, these patients were almost certainly food restricted the night before their surgery. In an admittedly casual attempt to replicate this, I recently asked the members of my laboratory to forgo food for a few hours before coming to work one morning so that they would be sure to place positive values on food.

---

6. Although I tell this as an isolated story, Vernon Mountcastle (1998, 2005) and his colleagues spent nearly two decades demonstrating that percepts of the kind Weber studied are almost always linearly related to activity in peripheral nerves. This is also the phenomenon we observed in the visual experiment about percept described at the beginning of this chapter.

I then asked them to sample some sugar solutions of varying concentration. After they sampled these solutions I asked them to make choices between different glasses of sugar solutions offered as prizes in lotteries. What I did was perform a standard economic experiment to assess the utility functions for sugar solutions in these individuals. They then made choices and received sugar solutions to drink after their choices were complete. Importantly, these sugar solutions were all that they could consume during a one-hour period that followed their choices, so what they chose really mattered. Perhaps surprisingly, I found that these measurements yielded an estimate of the utility curve that could be well described with a power function having an exponent of roughly 0.6.

I want to be careful, now, not to over-interpret this set of trivial observations, so let me say only this: Suppose that we were studying an imaginary creature called NewMan who we knew employed a tongue transducer that encoded sugar concentration in firing rate as a power function with exponent 0.6. The simplest possible creature of this kind would directly experience that firing rate as a percept. Such a creature would make choices in a way that simply maximized the expected value of tongue firing rates. (He would be choosing so as to maximize the average number of action potentials in the nerve when he obtained his chosen sugar solution to drink.)

This imaginary creature would still be showing risk aversion over sugar solutions, but that risk aversion would arise at the level of the tongue. Evolution, as it were, would have put risk aversion there, rather than in some more complicated structure. Of course not all of the NewMan's risk-averse behavior arises in its tongue. But it is without a doubt interesting that for this creature, under at least some limited conditions, a partial reduction between the neurobiology of sucrose transduction, the psychology of signal detection, and the economics of random utility theory would be entirely plausible.

5

Behavioral Economics: Exceeding the Limits of Traditional Neoclassical Models

Précis

The preceding chapter suggested a clear path for linking economic notions of utility with both psychological notions of percept and neurobiological notions of sensory encoding. At first blush it does look like the economic primitives we call "preferences" may map fairly directly to some well-described objects in the theories of psychology and neuroscience. Were all of economics, psychology, and neuroscience to show such obvious mappings, then neuroeconomics would be a straight-forward, if un-influential, reduction.

However, we already know that reductive mappings between much of economics and psychology, let alone neuroscience, will be much more problematic than the previous chapter implied. There is a wealth of decision-related phenomena that are poorly described by the neoclassical models we have encountered so far in this exposition, and this strongly suggests that many linkages between these disciplines will call for modifications to existing theories.

In this chapter I hope to highlight several of the important decision-related phenomena that are poorly described by the early neoclassical approach, and to review the existing responses of economists and psychologists to those challenges. I will argue that until fairly recently, decision-scientists have tended to fall into one of three categories. The first of these categories of scholars I identify as "the deniers." These scholars argue that no significant phenomena at variance with the traditional neoclassical program have yet been identified. The second of these groups of scholars, "the naysayers," asserts that the discovery of phenomena poorly predicted by traditional neoclassical models deals a fatal blow to the axiomatic basis of economic thought, and hence to any effort at a reductive linkage of these models to psychology or neuroscience.[1] The third group of scholars, "the middle grounders," argue that the addition of new adjustable parameters to models originally associated with axioms will be the most valuable strategy for the future. Although these extended models have been unarguably valuable, this approach reflects, in my opinion, an effort to return to the multi-parameter fitting strategy that characterized economics before the neoclassical revolution and that characterizes much of the natural sciences today.

I am also convinced, however, that a fourth class of responses to these challenges has begun to emerge: "the revisers." The scholars making these responses have begun to argue that economics (as well as psychology and neuroscience) should stay true to the pre-existing logical "kinds" that dominate those disciplines, but should remain open to the extensive theoretical revisions required for interdisciplinary linkage. The best developed of these models are neoclassically-styled axiom sets that attempt to capture behavioral insights that have their origins in existing psychological theories. If one believes, at an ontological level, that measurements of brain properties can be related meaningfully to behavior, then one has to believe that reducible sets of models that span disciplines will be more powerful than models isolated within a single discipline. The recent successes of models that employ the tools of economics to incorporate the insights of psychology (e.g., Caplin and Leahy 2001; Gul and Pesendorfer, 2001) are proof that explicit interdisciplinary linkage will offer real value in the study of human behavior. On these grounds I base my core argument that disciplinary boundaries need to be relaxed, and that the goals of each discipline must be broadened (although without sacrificing the logical primitives of each discipline), if we are to develop models of human behavior as quickly and as accurately as possible.

---

1. This constitutes a fatal blow because if we knew for sure that real human choice could not be accurately modeled using the axiomatic approach, then we would know for sure that an accurate global theory of choice could not include axioms.

Before developing these points, however, we need to understand why the traditional neoclassical models we have already encountered are inadequate. We therefore turn next to the most famous of the challenges to the neoclassical revolution of the mid-20th century: the paradox of Maurice Allais.

The Allais Paradox

In 1952 the French economist Maurice Allais, who was to win the Nobel Prize for economics in 1988, conducted a simple survey experiment meant to test von Neumann and Morgenstern's axioms of expected utility directly (Allais, 1953). He first asked 100 subjects to choose between two options:

(1A) a 100% chance of winning $1,000,000 or
(1B) an 89% chance of winning $1,000,000, a 1% chance of winning $0, and a 10% chance of winning $5,000,000.

By standard expected utility theory, either option could be preferred by any given chooser; which option a chooser prefers simply depends on his or her degree of risk aversion.[2] The expected value of option 1A is, of course, $1,000,000. The expected value of option 1B is $1,390,000. Option 1B, however, carries a 1% risk of winning nothing, and this possible outcome drives a risk-averse chooser towards option 1A, although a risk-neutral subject would select 1B. In any case, when Allais posed this hypothetical question to his 100 subjects, nearly all of them selected option 1A; they demonstrated a reasonable degree of risk aversion.

What Allais did next was to ask the same subjects a second question: Which would you prefer:

(2A) an 89% chance of winning $0 and an 11% chance of winning $1,000,000 or
(2B) a 90% chance of winning $0 and a 10% chance of winning $5,000,000?

In response to this question, nearly all of Allais' subjects reported that they preferred the second option, the 10% chance of winning $5,000,000.

---

2. Or the degree of curvature in their utility function. As I hope Chapter 3 made clear, these are by definition equivalent statements.

What was amazing about this pair of questions is that the choices of Allais' subjects demonstrated conclusively that the axioms of expected utility theory were false. To see how these two simple questions accomplished that amazing feat, we have to return to the theory of expected utility presented in Chapter 3.

Recall that von Neumann and Morgenstern constructed the theory from four simple axioms—rules that human subjects ought to obey if they were to be internally consistent in their choices. One of these rules was the independence axiom. The independence axiom argued that if you prefer an apple over an orange, then you must also prefer an apple plus a tiny, tiny bit of apple over an orange plus a tiny, tiny bit of apple. Or stated the way I put it in Chapter 3, if you prefer a 50% chance of winning $100 and a 5% chance of winning $10 over a 25% chance of winning $200 and a 5% chance of winning $10, you should also prefer a 50% chance of winning $100 over a 25% chance of winning $200.

What Maurice Allais did was to test this assertion directly. To understand how he did that, we can simply restate his first question in the following way:

(1A) an 89% chance of winning $1,000,000 and an 11% chance of winning $1,000,000, or
(1B) an 89% chance of winning $1,000,000, a 1% chance of winning $0, and a 10% chance of winning $5,000,000.

Of course option 1A is the same whether we call it a 100% chance of winning $1,000,000 or an 89% chance of winning $1,000,000 and an 11% chance of winning $1,000,000. When we ask subjects which gamble they prefer, they still answer 1B. Simple enough. Now, imagine we simply remove the 89% chance of winning $1,000,000 from both 1A and 1B. What we get is an 11% chance of winning $1,000,000 or a 10% chance of winning $5,000,000.

These are exactly the gambles presented to Allais' subjects in question 2, so any subject who obeys the independence axiom and prefers option 1A must also prefer option 2A. Similarly, any subject who prefers option 1B and obeys expected utility theory must also prefer option 2B. What Allais found, however, was that the great majority of subjects prefer 1A and 2B—a clear and direct violation of the independence axiom that is at the very core of von Neumann and Morgenstern's theory.

Allais developed this experimental test because it was his intuition that von Neumann and Morgenstern's axioms were simply the wrong axioms. He had his doubts that human subjects represented probabilities objectively as expected utility theory hypothesizes. Instead, he favored a theory more closely tied to the work of Fechner. He advocated for a theory of cardinal utility based quite specifically in psychophysics. What he hoped was that by demonstrating this failure of von Neumann and Morgenstern's independence axiom he could drive the neoclassical economic community back towards a cardinal theory of utility rooted in his own axioms. But what actually happened was something quite different.

My reading of what happened, at a sociological level, after Allais' paradox was presented was that the three basic classes of responses I mention above began to emerge. The first of these responses was to reject Allais' observation as something too specific to trouble a very general theory of choice. This was famously the position taken by Leonard J. Savage, a co-discoverer of expected utility theory (Savage, 1954). The second response to the paradox was to conclude that the mathematical-axiomatic approach to the study of behavior and decision championed by the neoclassicists would have to be abandoned. Although this response was slower to evolve, I would argue that the contemporary "heuristics and biases" approach described below began in this way. The third of these responses was, in essence, to take a middle road, to add parameters to theories such as expected utility that did not arise from an axiomatic model, but that had the effect of improving the predictive power of the theories. I would argue that the development of prospect theory, also described below, reflects the current endpoint of this class of response.

The most important thing to keep in mind historically, however, is that before Allais' paradox was discovered, there was an almost universal conviction that axioms rooted in expected utility theory would successfully describe human choice behavior. After the paradox was discovered, that consensus began to erode and a group of alternative approaches to the study of human decision began to emerge. To understand those events, and the extent to which the traditional neoclassical models do face significant problems, we turn next to the Ellsberg paradox, the endowment effect, and risk seeking over losses.

The Ellsberg Paradox

In Ellsberg's (1961) paradox you are presented with an urn[3] and you are told that it contains 90 balls. Of these, 30 are blue, and 60 are *either* red or yellow; any proportion is possible. You are then offered a choice between two possible outcomes. Outcome 1A is a lottery ticket that pays $100 if a blue ball is drawn when you reach into the urn and pull out a ball at random (an event with a probability of 1/3). Outcome 1B is a lottery that pays $100 if a red ball is drawn. Note that the probability of both a red and yellow draw is unspecified: the choice is *ambiguous*. The probability that you will draw a red ball must range from 0 to 2/3, but you do not know the actual probability. Under these circumstances people typically choose the first lottery, which wins if a blue ball is drawn. In fact, even if you offer to pay them $200 if a red ball is drawn, they still prefer the $100 blue ball option.

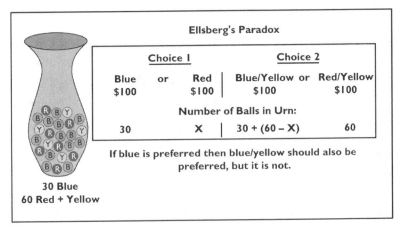

FIGURE 5.1

3. Mathematicians and economists love to use the metaphor of an "urn" to describe probabilistic events in physical terms. In this metaphor an opaque and narrow-mouthed container is filled with colored billiard balls of some known or unknown distribution and you, the reader, are asked to imagine drawing one or more balls out of the container. The metaphor probably has its origin in the writings of the French mathematician Pierre-Simone LaPlace, who used it in one of the first serious books on probability ever written (Laplace, 1814).

How can we understand this decision within the framework of expected utility theory, which postulates that humans behave as if they choose by multiplying probability and utility for each option and picking the option having the highest expected utility? Given that the payoffs in dollars are clear, according to expected utility theory the fact that our subjects pick option 1A means that they believe there were fewer than 30 red balls in the urn.

Next, before any balls are actually drawn, but with the same urn standing in front of the subject, you ask the subject to choose again, this time between lottery 2A, which pays $100 on either blue or yellow, and lottery 2B, which pays $100 on either red or yellow. Now the likelihood of winning is clear in the second case (a 2/3 probability of winning $100) but ambiguous in the first case (a probability between 1/3 and 1). People this time typically choose the second lottery, lottery 2B. The first lottery seems less attractive, because there might be *too few* yellow balls. Is there anything wrong with this behavior? If expected utility theory is correct, then there certainly is: our chooser cannot rationally think that there are too few *and* too many yellow balls in the urn at the same time.

In this very colloquial sense, then, the Ellsberg paradox demonstrated another violation of rationality—people seemed to be thinking that there were both too many and too few yellow balls, and even to a non-specialist this seems irrational. Still, the effect is very powerful and has been widely studied and documented. People behave exactly as if there are both too many and too few yellow balls.

Although not directed at a specific axiom in the same way that the Allais paradox was, the Ellsberg paradox was another example of average human subjects behaving in a way that could not possibly be described as maximizing expected utility. There is no simple utility function of the kind Samuelson envisioned that can make this kind of behavior rational.

The Endowment Effect

We begin this behavioral demonstration of the endowment effect (Kahneman et al., 1990; Thaler, 1980) by selecting two objects that have roughly equivalent market values, for example a nice pen and an inexpensive ceramic mug. Next, we invite two groups of subjects into the laboratory on two sequential days. When the first group arrives we hand each of them a free mug and stress to them that this is a gift from us, which they should put in their backpacks. Next we produce a set of pens and ask the subjects to tell us how much they would actually pay us to buy one of these pens.

Getting them to tell us how much a pen is really worth to them is not trivial. If we simply say, "How much would you pay for this pen? We will sell it to you for whatever number you pick," we are really encouraging them to say a number far below its true value. Similarly, we don't want to simply ask, "How much is this pen worth to you in the abstract?" because then their answers have no consequences. A subject who is bored could say $1,000,000 as a joke. The right way to determine how much a pen is worth to each subject is to create something like a marketplace where subjects are induced to tell us the real value that they place on the pens. One can accomplish this a number of different ways, for example by holding a pen auction, but the classic strategy in experimental economics is to employ something called a Becker, Marshack, DeGroot (or BDM) bid (1964).

To understand how the BDM process works, imagine that we place 10 possible values on the pen: $1, $2, $3, on up to $10. What we want to know from our subjects is what is the largest of these values that they still consider a good deal for the pen. So what we do is we place 10 poker chips labeled $1, $2, $3, on up to $10 in a sack (or balls in an urn if you are feeling more classical). Each subject will be asked to reach into the full bag and pull out a chip. If the chip has a number on it at or below the maximum price the subject said she was willing to pay, then she pays the price on the chip and gets the pen. If it has a number above that maximum, then the subject keeps her money and does not get the pen.

If you think about this process, what should be clear is that under these conditions the subjects are incentivized to really tell us what the pens are worth to them. Their number doesn't influence what we do in any way, so they have no incentive to bid too low, and if they do bid too low then they might find themselves unable to buy a pen that they think is worth $5 for the bargain basement price of $3. The BDM process is interesting in this way because it provides a simple way to get subjects to tell us, in a consequential manner, what stuff is really worth to them.

In any case, we use this technique to establish the average value of the pens in our group of subjects and, if this is a typical group, we get a number between $3 and $4. All of them then draw poker chips and, based upon luck and their individual valuations, many wind up buying pens.

Now comes the interesting part of the experiment. Just as the subjects are leaving the laboratory we stop them and ask them to place a BDM bid on their mugs. What we say is, "What is the minimum price you would accept for your mug?" When we do this we discover that the value the subjects place on the mugs is typically around $6. So now we know that these subjects seem to value the mugs at about twice the dollar value they place on pens. From this we can likely conclude that the average subject likes mugs more than pens.

On the next day we repeat the same experiment on a new group of subjects, but this time with one important change: we switch pens for mugs. On this day, when the subjects arrive we hand each one a pen as a gift and urge them to keep it in their backpacks. We then establish the value of mugs to this group and find that this group places an average value of about $3 on the mugs. Then as they are leaving we ask them to place a value on the pens and, like the group from the day before, they value these endowed goods at about $6. So what is happening here?

Clearly, something about the procedure of giving the subjects a pen or a mug and having them place it in their backpacks seems to have changed the value of that object to them. The objects that they get "given" as a gift generally seem to have twice the value of the same object offered in a marketplace.

At face value this seems to suggest a really profound problem with the neoclassical framework, and it was with that in mind that Richard Thaler originally drew attention to this behavior (Thaler, 1980). If we think of the BDM bids as telling us the preferences of these subjects, then we seem to have data indicating that the preferences of subjects between pens and mugs are highly mutable. This is a critical problem and, to understand why, we have to revisit Samuelson's WARP theory, which lies at the very foundation of the neoclassical revolution.[4]

---

4. Let me admit that although this "exchange asymmetry" is probably one of the most widely-cited examples of an "anti-neoclassical" behavioral result, it is also one of the

Recall that in his seminal paper on WARP (1938) Samuelson asked: "What is the simplest model of human choice behavior that still makes positive predictions about behavior?" Samuelson proposed a model that assumes that if we observe that a person *chooses* having two apples and one orange rather than having one apple and two oranges, then this means that we can assume that the person does not also consistently *prefer* one apple and two oranges to two apples and one orange. Samuelson's model proposes that if a subject is observed to choose A over B, then we can assume that he cannot also prefer B to A. Thaler's experiment seems to suggest that even this very minimal assumption is violated by real people in the real world—and violated in a big way. The endowment effect seems to lead to a doubling of valuations, suggesting that the relationship between choice and preference is unstable. If this is widely true, then one has to question even the most basic core elements of the neoclassical economic approach.

Kahneman and Tversky: Risk Seeking Over Losses

Which of the following would you prefer: (1A) a sure gain of $500 or (1B) a 50% chance of a gain of $1,000? As described in Chapter 3, most human subjects prefer 1A, and this reflects risk aversion of the kind first described by Bernoulli. In the neoclassical approach we see this as compatible with the claim that typical human subjects have concave monotonic utility functions, given that these subjects obey the axioms of expected utility theory—at least over the range of choices presented in a typical experiment. Indeed, when Daniel Kahneman and Amos Tversky (1979) asked 70 human subjects this question, 84% of them preferred 1A.

Next, answer a second question: which of the following would you prefer: (2A) a sure loss of $500 or (2B) a 50% chance of losing $1,000? When Kahneman and Tversky asked this same question of the same 70 subjects, 70% said that they preferred option 2B. Under these

---

most controversial. Charlie Plott and Kathryn Zeiler (2005, 2007) have shown that under very controlled behavioral circumstances most, if not all, of this asymmetry can be well explained with neoclassical conceptual tools.

conditions they were "risk seeking." For traditional neoclassical economics, this is another deeply troubling paradox that is very difficult to
explain or resolve. To understand why, consider the graphs in Figure 5.2.

Here we plot, in standard economic form, the relationship between
the total utility a subject has from money over his or her lifetime and the

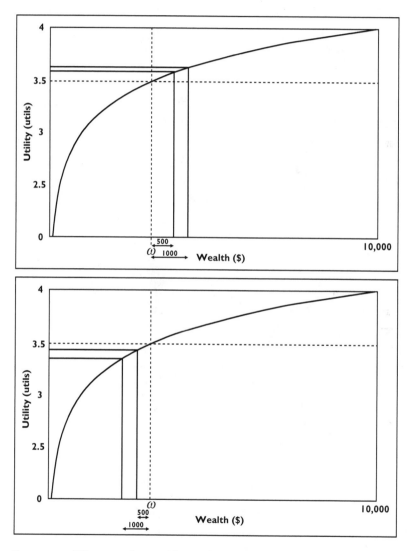

FIGURE 5.2   Wins versus losses with regard to current wealth (——).

total amount of money he or she has.[5] On the lower axis of the first panel have marked with the Greek letter omega (ω) what I imagine to be the total wealth of one of Kahneman and Tversky's subjects. Now, when we ask that subject which he prefers, $500 for sure or a 50% chance of $1000, he answers that he prefers $500 for sure because this function is concave (or compressive). He chooses the sure win because the subjective value of an additional $500 is not twice the subjective value of the original $500. So far so good, but what happens when we ask a chooser having this kind of utility function to choose between losing $500 for sure and losing $1,000 with a probability of 0.5?

The answer is shown in panel the second of Figure 5.2. The loss of $500 is less than twice the loss of $1,000, in subjective utility terms. The result? Our chooser should be risk averse over losses as well as gains. He should prefer the sure loss of $500 to the 50% risk of losing $1000, *but he does not.* How can we hope to explain this using standard economic tools? (If we use a utility function anchored to lifetime wealth, then explaining this observation is also problematic.)

Although I have presented four classic problems with expected utility in these past few pages, there are many other examples of phenomena that appear to challenge the traditional economic framework. These are just a few well-studied examples, and each of these examples is controversial in ways I have not always outlined in this brief discussion. Taken together, however, the body of data these observations are drawn from must lead us to ask how we should proceed in our study of human choice and behavior. Should we stick with this obviously erroneous approach from neoclassical economics? As I argued above, three principal responses to this question have emerged in the larger decision-making community. We turn now to each of those responses in turn.

Alternative 1: There is No Problem

While I would venture to say that the majority of people in the decision-making community acknowledge that traditional axiomatic models face

---

5. Of course, we are not constrained to make this a discussion of money. The lower axis could be about love or happiness, a point taken up in Chapter 3. Here we focus on money for simplicity.

severe challenges today, there is still a significant cohort of neoclassically trained economists who doubt that the data we have available mounts a significant challenge to models such as expected utility. When a new behavioral dataset is generated that falsifies an important model, these scholars often reply by doubting the validity of the data-gathering process or by searching for mathematically sophisticated (and to my mind unlikely) alternative explanations.

Perhaps the most famous of these kinds of critiques was produced by Milton Friedman and Leonard J. Savage (1948), who were trying to explain why the phenomenon that would later be called *risk seeking over losses* did not pose a challenge to expected utility theory. Friedman and Savage proposed that this phenomenon could be explained without abandoning or modifying any of the axioms of the existing theory if we were comfortable hypothesizing that the local curvature of the utility function is convex below a chooser's current wealth level and concave (like a normal utility function) above that current wealth level.

This is shown in Figure 5.3. If this were the shape of a subject's utility function *and* his current wealth level put him precisely at the

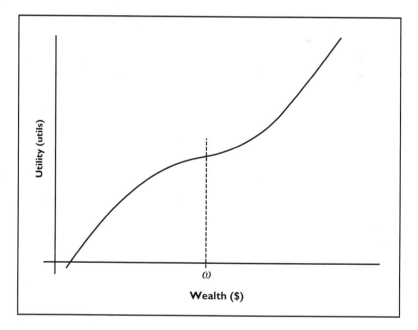

FIGURE 5.3   Friedman and Savage's utility function.

point marked ω, then the utility function would effectively be compressive for gains and expansive for losses. In other words, the decision-maker would be risk averse for gains but risk seeking for losses from his current wealth level. But a very important point is that such a decision-maker would show this pattern of risk aversion and seeking only at precisely the wealth level marked omega; at any other point he would be more consistent in his risk attitudes.

Friedman and Savage recognized that for this kind of a utility function to account for the fact that people were risk seeking over losses and risk averse over gains, then the wealth level of anyone who ever showed this pattern of behavior would have to be carefully aligned with this "kink" in their utility functions when they were showing this behavior. They attempted to resolve this issue by arguing that human decision-makers might have only one or two such inflection points in their utility functions, but that humans tended to get "stuck" for a lifetime at these particular wealth levels. They even went so far as to hypothesize that the class structure of human society might be driven by the inflection points inferred to exist in this manner.

While there can be no doubt that Friedman and Savage's proposal is both mathematically clever and entertaining, surely none of us today can consider it a compelling defense of expected utility theory. Being risk averse in gains and risk seeking in losses is a widespread feature of human decision making and is observed at all wealth levels and under a broad range of conditions. The complexity of the set of subject-specific utility functions required to account for this behavior, although mathematically possible, almost defies imagination. A utility function anchored to lifetime wealth simply cannot usefully account for these observations. Failing to acknowledge that fact—failing to acknowledge the existing data—is simply not going to strengthen economic models.

Alternative 2: Abandoning the Logical Objects of Economic Thought

Among another group of scholars the response to these observations has been to argue that human decision making should not be seen as the product of a single globally-organized strategy but rather as the product of many local strategies applied piecewise to the many choices we encounter in life. Rather than using one set of axioms, we should be looking for dozens, if not hundreds, of little local rules to describe decision making.

This approach, often called the *heuristics and biases* approach, proceeds from the assumption that the psychological mechanisms for decision making are highly modularized. What happens when we are presented with a problem is that we begin by first selecting a module, or heuristic, and then letting that heuristic control decision making for a particular problem.

Perhaps the most classic example of this comes from the work of Kahneman and Tversky on a non-economic decision-making problem known widely as the "Linda the bank teller" puzzle (1982, 1983).

> Linda is 31 years old, single, outspoken, and very bright. She majored in philosophy. As a student, she was deeply concerned with issues of discrimination and social justice, and also participated in antinuclear demonstrations. Which is more likely: that (A) Linda is a bank teller or (B) Linda is a bank teller and is active in the feminist movement?

When Kahneman and Tversky asked this question in the lab they found that the majority of subjects answered B, despite the fact that category B is obviously a subcategory of A and thus cannot be more likely. To explain this error, they hypothesized that subjects employed a "representativeness heuristic." The idea here was that when asked a question of this type, subjects simply determined whether Linda was more representative of a person in category A or a person in category B.

In a similar way, Kahneman and Tversky proposed a number of other heuristic rules that they hypothesized might account for the decisions of their subjects under a limited number of conditions. These took on names such as "the availability heuristic" (Tversky and Kahneman, 1974), "the hot hand" (Gilovich, Vallone, and Tversky, 1985), "anchoring" (Tversky and Kahneman, 1974), and "the gambler's fallacy" (Kahneman and Tversky, 1972; Tversky and Kahneman, 1974), to name a few.

Subsequent to Kahneman and Tversky's work, a number of other important psychological researchers have also argued that we can best understand decision making using a heuristics-based approach. Perhaps the most famous of these researchers today is Gerd Gigerenzer (1999). Gigerenzer has argued that while human behavior is often very efficient and approximates the kinds of maximizing solutions described in standard economic models, in fact it achieves this mechanistically with a set of heuristic rules. This is a subtle distinction and one that is fairly important. Like Kahneman and Tversky in some of their papers, Gigerenzer argues that human behavior is best described as the implementation of a series of independent decision rules. But an important difference is that Gigerenzer argues that under many conditions these rules approximate the maximization solutions that a single axiomatic system would produce.[6]

I should point out here, though, that a heuristics-based system that produced behavior indistinguishable from expected utility theory would be an ideal candidate for inter-theoretic reduction of the kind described in Chapter 2. If a complete set of heuristics were identified and did roughly as good a job of describing behavior as did expected utility theory, then the job of an interdisciplinary synthesizer would simply be to map these two theories to one another.

In practice, however, the scholars advocating heuristics-based approaches have tended to see them as very distinct from economic-type models. The focus for these scholars has been to identify simple decision-making situations and then to see whether a single rule-based model can account for that behavior. The problem with such an approach is that one risks winding up with a new heuristic for every kind of decision one studies. In the limit, this reduces to a rule for every decision—simply a restatement of the original data. Thus, inasmuch as a complete and finite set of heuristics for decision making can be developed, one has in heuristics a model of human decision making. Inasmuch as one has a heuristic named for every violation of expected utility theory ever

---

6. In fairness, I should say that Gigerenzer's point is more complicated than this. Gigerenzer takes pains to say that these heuristics yield decisions that are "superior" to the solutions of a system of the neoclassical type designed to achieve perfect utility maximization. At first blush this seems very hard to understand; after all, what could it mean to be better than perfect? What Gigerenzer means, though, is that in the real world a system designed to compute, for example, Bayes' theorem often runs into problems it cannot solve. Gigerenzer's heuristics, because they are simple and easy to compute, never have this problem. Gigerenzer's point is that heuristics outperform discrete Bayesian-style calculations in the real world when the Bayesian calculations are too difficult or too time-consuming.

uncovered in a behavioral experiment, the heuristics reflect only a list of expected utility's weaknesses.

Approach 3: Incorporating Violations as New Parameters

In the late 1970s and continuing into the 1980s, Kahneman and Tversky sought to develop a mathematically complete theory of decision making that could serve as an alternative to traditional expected utility theory (Kahneman and Tversky, 1979; Tversky and Kahneman, 1992; for a review see Fox and Poldrack, 2009).[7] Their goal was to develop a mathematical model that could describe choice behavior in situations including the Allais paradox, the endowment effect, and risk seeking under conditions of loss. The key features they hoped to incorporate into their new theory were essentially four-fold. First, they wanted to capture the fact that, under conditions like those explored in the Allais paradox, subjects tend to violate the independence axiom specifically when the probability of winning or losing in lotteries is either very high or very low. Second, they hoped to capture in their model the fact that subjects seem to make decisions from some kind of reference point or, as Thaler originally put it, with regard to the "status quo." Third, they wanted to capture the fact that subjects seem (at least under some conditions) to be risk seeking when considering possible losses from the "reference point" and risk averse when considering gains from the "reference point" (although as we shall see, exactly defining the "reference point" can be difficult). Fourth, they hoped to capture the fact that subjects appear, again under some but not all conditions, to see losses as worse than they see equivalent gains as good. The goal of prospect theory was, in essence, to develop an alternative formulation for something like utility that characterizes the subjective value of an outcome for human subjects in a way that predicts choice.

To account for the Allais paradox and other anomalies like it, prospect theory proposes that humans do not make choices based on actual probabilities, as von Neumann and Morgenstern had proposed, but

---

7. I should note that prospect theory is not the only example of theories of this type.

instead on a subjectivized form of probability—an idea first put forward axiomatically by Savage (1954). The idea here is that just as a utility function relates value to a subjective object called utility, a second function could exist that relates probability to a subjective property they called a "weight." This function, called the probability weighting function, thus plays a role similar to the utility function.

In contemporary forms of prospect theory, the probability weighting function is a curvilinear equation often described by two parameters: one that controls the degree of curvature of the function and a second that controls the point at which the function crosses the identity line for probability. The most commonly used form today was developed by Drazen Prelec (1998) and is shown in Figure 5.4, where the two free parameters gamma (γ), which controls curvature, and delta (δ), which controls where the function crosses the identity line, are fit to the observed behavioral data.

$$w(p) = \exp[-\delta(-\ln p)^{\gamma}],$$

where $\delta, \gamma > 0$

Next, to capture the reference point notion, they proposed that all computations of the utility (or subjective value) of any option were made with regard to a "reference point." Importantly, they stressed that the reference point is *not* just current total wealth, but something more complicated. Indeed, they concluded that the data they had did not permit a clear specification of what the reference point was at any given time, but they did provide a number of general rules for how the reference point ought to behave in their model.

To capture risk seeking for losses and risk aversion for gains, they cleverly used the notion of the reference point to modify the idea of the utility curve. Rather than having a single monotonic function, they proposed that the new utility curve (which they called the "value function") would have distinct shapes above and below the reference point. Specifically, they proposed that the curvature of the value function going upwards from the reference point (the domain of gains) would be concave (as was a standard Bernoulli function) but would be convex in the domain of losses.

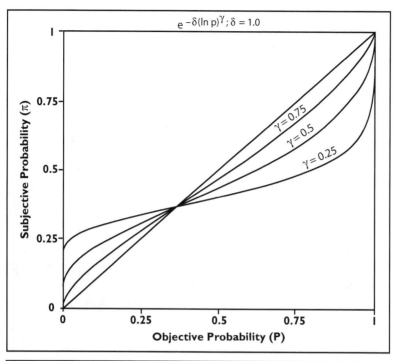

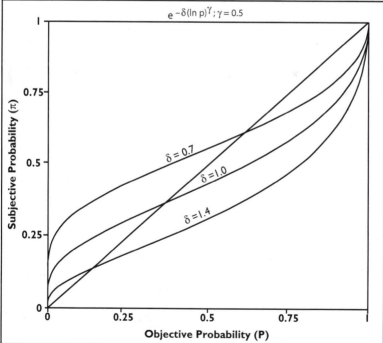

FIGURE 5.4   Probability weighting functions.

In their standard formulation of the value function the relationship between subjective values and gains is specified as

$$Subjective\,Value = Gains^\alpha$$

where Gains is the amount gained by the outcome over the reference and α is basically a power utility function fit to the observed choice data. For losses the function takes the form

$$Subjective\,Value = -Losses^\beta$$

where β is again fit to the observed behavioral data. Together, these functions yield a utility-like curve of the type shown in Figure 5.5.

Finally, to account for the observed asymmetry in losses and gains observed under many conditions, Kahneman and Tversky proposed that the magnitude of the loss-associated side of the value function was

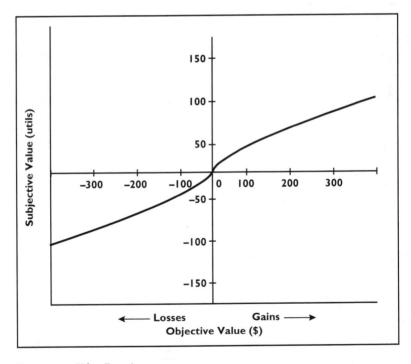

FIGURE 5.5   Value Function.

steeper than the gains-associated side of the value function. To achieve this they weighted the loss side by an additional parameter:

$$\textit{Subjective Value of Losses} = \lambda \times \textit{Losses}^{\beta}$$

where λ, the loss aversion coefficient, captures the additional sensitivity of choosers to losses over gains. Thus a chooser who viewed a $200 loss as equivalent to a $100 gain would have a lambda of 2 (see Fig. 5.6).

The full version of prospect theory thus has five free parameters. This means that to predict the behavior of a particular chooser, one has to select values for these parameters.

In fairness, one absolutely has to say that this is an enormous practical accomplishment. Prospect theory can predict behavior like the Allais paradox, the endowment effect, and risk seeking in the domain of loss. It is an incredibly powerful and widely-used theory. But it is also very important to keep in mind prospect theory's limitations, which are of two types, empirical and theoretical.

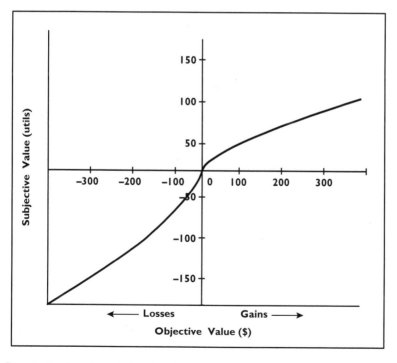

FIGURE 5.6   Loss Averse Value Function.

The Empirical Limitations of Prospect Theory

There are two key empirical limitations to prospect theory. The first is that it simply has too many interacting parameters to make it a truly falsifiable theory. To understand why this is so, consider an experiment in which one hoped to pin down the five free parameters of prospect theory for a group of individuals. In practice one would need hundreds of carefully designed questions to robustly estimate, for each individual, each of the five parameters. And this estimation is complicated by the fact that many classes of behavior that violate the predictions of expected utility theory can be accounted for with more than one parameter. So, for example, one can account for the Allais paradox either by adjusting the curvature of the probability weighting function or by adjusting the curvature of the value function and the magnitude of the reference point. Either of these two strategies works, and it is often problematic to decide which of these two strategies to employ. Indeed, automated approaches to this problem, such as maximum likelihood fitting, often yield highly unpredictable results for this reason. (For more on this see Fox and Poldrack, 2009).

To address this problem, most users of prospect theory try to use a simplified version of the approach that relies on only three free parameters. This vastly simplifies the parameter estimation problem, often with little loss of predictive power. In this reduced form the curvature of the value function for losses is taken to be the negative of the curvature of the value function for gains, and the probability weighting function is taken to cross the main diagonal of the graph (to have its prosing point fixed) at the value $1/e$.

The second major empirical limitation to the theory arises from its use of an incompletely specified theory of the reference point. Although I personally think that there is overwhelming evidence for the existence of a reference point both behaviorally and neurally (a point to which we will return in Section 2), prospect theory is almost entirely silent about how the reference point is determined and how it changes from choice to choice. This is a huge problem for users of the theory and is very rarely dealt with explicitly. In many experiments or circumstances it is enough to assume that the reference point is a constant over the course of a set of observations, but that is not always the case, and the absence of a clear specification for the reference point remains a central problem in prospect theory, even in three-parameter versions.

Theoretical Limitations of Prospect Theory

The most important thing to understand about prospect theory, however, is that it is simply not a traditional economic theory in any meaningful sense. This is not necessarily a bad thing, but it is a very important thing for someone considering inter-theoretic reductions.

Consider expected utility theory. Expected utility is a list of four axiomatic statements about consistent human behavior. Each axiom can be formally tested, and indeed experiments such as Allais' are clear tests and falsifications of these axioms under well-specified conditions. Under conditions in which all four axioms are obeyed by human choosers, we know with certainty that the observed behavior looks exactly as if the choosers were multiplying probability by a monotone utility function. There are no free parameters, simply four testable statements and an identity proof. That is the core notion of an economic kind in the philosophical sense.

In contrast, prospect theory provides a list of functions and free parameters that can be fitted and then used to predict choice—it is and was explicitly meant as a descriptive model. There is no deep logical identity here.[8] One cannot, for example, say that a subject who shows a λ of 2.0 and an α of 0.8 is the same as a subject who obeys some particular axiom or who employs some particular class of underlying representation. In this sense, prospect theory is much more a traditional model of the kind employed by psychologists and neuroscientists than it is an economic theory. Further, and this often frustrates economists very badly, it does

---

8. In fairness to prospect theory, I must note that Kahneman and Tversky's famous 1979 paper does provide an axiomatic description of a portion of their theory. These however, axioms say little about the all-important reference point and are widely acknowledged to be more a nod towards the economic method than a statement of testable axioms or logical identities.

not include a specification of the reference point, which is one of the most powerful and important elements of the theory. It is for these reasons that traditional neoclassical economists often dismiss prospect theory as uninteresting.

Let me hasten, to add however, that prospect theory "works" in a way that expected utility theory does not. With a large dataset and careful analysis, three-parameter or five-parameter prospect theory can be highly predictive of human choice behavior. Prospect theory is beyond a doubt useful. Some of this usefulness stems from its having free parameters that are adjustable and some stems from a very judicious selection of the functions into which those parameters are embedded. That prospect theory works and is useful is simply beyond dispute at this point. It is always important to remember, however, that prospect theory is not an economic theory in the sense we use that description here. It is a model fit to behavior using the traditional tools of psychology and the natural sciences. This is very important and must be kept in mind if we are to build a neuroeconomic science that explicitly seeks to link economic, psychological, and neurobiological approaches reductively.

Towards Interdisciplinary Synthesis and Constraint: The Fourth Way

I have argued that the demonstration of behaviors that are at variance with the predictions of the neoclassical models of the 1950s and 1960s led to the rise of three key schools of thought among decision scientists. The first school, made up largely of older neoclassical economists, argued that these violations were not significant enough to call for abandonment of the existing theories. A second school, made up mostly of psychologists, argued that these violations were so significant that they called for the complete abandonment of the logical primitives that defined economic thought. A third school, epitomized I think by Kahneman and Tversky's prospect theory, argued that the sophisticated model-fitting techniques of the natural sciences could be combined with insights from pre-existing axiomatic approaches to yield an empirically driven class of models for understanding human behavior.

There is, however, a fourth alternative. Perhaps without realizing it, this approach proceeds along the lines of a very traditional inter-theoretic reduction of the kind described in Chapter 2. Within economics, this approach begins by acknowledging both that phenomena exist that are poorly modeled by existing axiomatic tools, and that models in lower-level disciplines such as psychology already capture these phenomena. The approach then proceeds to ask whether the logical kinds of economics can be intentionally adjusted to achieve an inter-theoretic reduction.

Perhaps the most famous example of this is the story of *Anticipatory Utility* discussed in Chapter 2. Recall that in the 1980s the psychologist George Loewenstein (1987) had demonstrated a class of behavior that could not be reconciled with existing economic models. He found that if normal human subjects were asked to choose between a desirable event today and that same desirable event in three days, they chose to wait three days. They wanted, Loewenstein argued, to be able to enjoy anticipating the event for a few days.

What the economists Andrew Caplin and John Leahy (2001) recognized was that the failure of traditional neoclassical economics to be able to account for this behavior reflected the absence, in economics, of a logical kind that could be related to this psychological notion of anticipation. What they did was to axiomatically construct a logical kind specifically designed to capture this psychological-level construct. I am arguing here that in doing so they performed an inter-theoretic reduction of exactly the kind we desire. What is most exciting, however, is that Caplin and Leahy are not alone in this achievement. David Kreps and Evan Porteus, for example, have axiomatized the "utility of knowing" (1978, 1979). Graham Loomes and Robert Sugden have axiomatized the notion of "regret" (Loomes and Sugden, 1982; Sugden, 1993). Botond Kőszegi and Matthew Rabin (2007, 2009) have begun to develop an axiomatic model of the reference point. Perhaps ironically, Faruk Gul and Wolfgang Pesendorfer, although they insist that inter-theoretic linkage is of no value, have axiomatized "the cost of self-control" (Gul and Pesendorfer, 2001). These are all clear examples of modifications to the standard economic corpus in ways that better align it with the corpus of psychological thought, but accomplish this goal without abandoning the key logical primitives of economics. And most economists agree that these insights have improved the predictive power of economics. Can we not formalize and extend this approach to include neuroscience? To explicitly incorporate inter-theoretic reduction into the economic, psychological, and neuroscientific endeavors? I think we can, if we are brave enough, and in the next chapter I begin to examine how.

6

Because, Not *As If*

Précis

In the preceding chapters I have made several arguments:

- I have suggested that a synthetic interdisciplinary approach to choice, if it could be accomplished, would prove valuable to its parent disciplines. I have made this argument on both historical and philosophical grounds.
- I have argued that such an interdisciplinary approach would be most powerful if it were an iterative attempt to generate reductive linkages between the different disciplines that seek to describe choice.
- I have provided some examples of what such a linked theory might begin to look like.

What I have not yet done is provide a clear paradigmatic statement of how one would go about structuring such a theory, nor have I responded to the well-developed theoretical corpus (present particularly in economics) that argues that interdisciplinary theories of this kind lie, by construction, outside the province or interest of practitioners in the parent disciplines. My goal in this chapter is to provide a high-level description of the explicit theoretical goals that should guide the neuro-economic (and I believe the economic, psychological, and neurobiological) study of choice.

We already know that the key organizational insights for inter-disciplinary synthesis tend to arise in the higher-level disciplines. Watson and Crick, to take an obvious example, were searching for the chemical manifestation of genes because biologists working at a higher-level of abstraction had already developed the concept of the gene and showed the predictive power of that construct. To take a more modern example, physicists studying the subatomic structure of matter know that it is atoms they are trying to explain. Their findings may stretch or alter our definitions of atoms, but as a general rule it is the structure of the higher-level abstractions that guides the more reduced-level inquiries. This is a key point: it means that insights from economic theory must provide the organizational structure for more reduced forms of neuroeconomic inquiry. This is a point I made in detail several years ago in my monograph *Decisions, Uncertainty, and the Brain* (Glimcher, 2003).

Recognizing that fact, however, poses a problem. Much of modern economic theory rests explicitly on the notion that mechanistic constraints are irrelevant to the study of choice and behavior. All young economists are trained to believe that the economic models they develop do not make any conceptually reducible predictions. This was a point codified into economics doctrine during the middle of the 20th century by Milton Friedman.

In this chapter I argue that while Friedman's approach may have been justified when it was presented, modern economic theory must begin to abandon the *as if* modeling tradition he fostered. For reasons that may be opaque to non-economists, in many economic circles the argument that economic theory should be constrained by the mechanisms of the human brain is nothing short of a heresy. The goal of the first part of this chapter is thus to defend my heretical view that economic theories must become explicitly sensitive to mechanism. The goal of the second part is to lay out the most basic structural details of a global theory of neuroeconomics, a structure that, after reading the first half of this chapter, will be obvious. It is a theory that proceeds *mechanistically* from axioms such as those used in GARP and expected utility.

Milton Friedman

What is the goal of an economic theory? In the 1950s Milton Friedman published one of the core documents of modern economics, a document in which he largely defined what an economic theory was and how one should go about testing it (Friedman, 1953). An economic theory was a "good" theory, he argued, inasmuch as it made accurate predictions about the behavior of human choosers and markets. It was a "bad" theory inasmuch as it made inaccurate predictions *or* the assumptions it relied upon could be falsified by empirical observation.

In making this argument, Friedman was responding to a growing class of criticisms of the neoclassical approach that were emerging in the middle of the century. When they had been developing the economic models of the 1940s and 1950s, scholars such as Friedman, Savage, and von Neumann were making highly stylized and quite mathematical predictions about human and corporate behavior. A typical parameterized form of expected utility theory, for example, might predict that human behavior *reflects* the product of outcome probability and a power function of outcome value. A subject is asked whether she wants to place a $5 bet on the New York Yankees that pays $6 or a $5 bet on the Boston Red Sox that pays $12. Expected utility theory describes her decision process as (1) taking the value of each win raised to a fractional power times the probability of that bet winning and (2) selecting the bet with the higher output from this calculation.

Critics of expected utility theory were beginning to argue that although human subjects did choose among bets like these, it seemed implausible that they actually knew the probabilities of the events on which they were betting, let alone that they could calculate the numerical value of $12 raised to the 0.6th power.

In support of the conclusion that models such as expected utility were unrealistic, these scholars produced evidence that, for example, most Red Sox fans cannot tell you the value of $12 raised to the 0.6th power. If they cannot verbally report the value of this mathematical operation, these critics wondered, how can we hope to characterize their behavior as dependent on this operation?

Friedman's response to this criticism is legendary and brilliant, although I will argue in a moment that it did not go far enough.

> Let us turn now to another example, this time a constructed one designed to be an analogue of many hypotheses in the social sciences. Consider the density of leaves around a tree. I suggest the hypothesis that the leaves are positioned as if each leaf deliberately sought to maximize the amount of sunlight it receives, given the position of its neighbors, as if it knew the physical laws determining

the amount of sunlight that would be received in various positions and could move rapidly or instantaneously from one position to any other desired or unoccupied position. Now some of the more obvious implications of this hypothesis are clearly consistent with experience: for example, leaves are in general denser on the south than on the north side of trees but, as the hypothesis implies, less so or not at all on the northern slope of a hill or when the south side of the trees is shaded in some other way. Is the hypothesis rendered unacceptable or invalid because, as far as we know, leaves do not "deliberate" or consciously "seek," have not been to school and learned the relevant laws of science or mathematics required to calculate the "optimum" position, and cannot move from position to position?...

The constructed hypothesis is presumably valid, that is, it yields "sufficiently" accurate predictions about the density of leaves, only for a particular class of circumstances...

A largely parallel example involving human behavior has been used elsewhere by Savage and me. Consider the problem of predicting the shots made by an expert billiard player. It seems not at all unreasonable that excellent predictions would be yielded by the hypothesis that the billiard player made his shots *as if* he knew the complicated mathematical formulas that would give the optimum directions of travel, could estimate accurately by eye the angles, etc... Our confidence in this hypothesis is not based on the belief that billiard players, even expert ones, can or do go through the process described; it derives rather from the belief that, unless in some way or other they were capable of reaching essentially the same result, they would not in fact be *expert* billiard players (Friedman, 1953, pp. 19–21).

For our purposes, the greatest strength of Friedman's argument was that he focused on the importance of bounded theory. If our goal is to predict only the shots of a billiard player at a billiard table, we can rely on a limited theory of his behavior: *He acts as if he computed the Newtonian physics of ball movement on the table surface.* The notion that one begins with a theory that explains only a portion of behavior and then builds outwards, generalizing and improving the theory so that it applies to more complicated situations, seems obviously attractive to scientists working in a new field. For a biologist, however, the greatest weakness of Friedman's argument was his conclusion that mechanism was irrelevant—that models made predictions only *as if* the equations they described were computed. What Friedman did, though tactically sophisticated for achieving his goal, was hopelessly frustrating from the point of view of a biologist.

> Under a wide range of circumstances individual forms behave as if they were seeking to rationally maximize their returns... Now of course businessmen do not actually solve the system of simultaneous equations in terms of which the mathematical economist finds it convenient to express this hypothesis...The billiard player, if asked how he decides where to hit the ball, may say that he "just figures it out" then also rubs a rabbit's foot just to make sure...the one statement is about as helpful as the other, and neither is a relevant test of the associated hypothesis (Friedman, 1953, pp. 21).

In essence, what Friedman propounds with these two points (that a theory is only designed to explain a limited portion of behavior and that its mechanistic implementation is irrelevant) is an argument I would call a "Soft theory" of economic behavior. Although our theory includes well-defined axioms about choice that imply a series of specifiable computations, we remain indifferent about whether or not these computations really occur. It is enough to say that our agent behaves *as if* these computations occur.

But why, a biologist might ask, give up this chess piece so easily? Surely we all believe that Friedman's billiard player is a physical system, a material device. Surely we believe that he gathers sensory data and uses these data to compute joint angles and muscle trajectories. If all of Friedman's billiard player's actions at the table reflect the computation of Newton's laws of motion, then surely every modern materialist has to believe that the brain of the billiard player does in fact compute, using its neurons and synapses, the very laws of motion Friedman uses in his theory (or at least some close approximation to those laws). If the Newtonian model really describes the player's behavior, it does so *because* it describes the mechanism that produces the behavior. Friedman is right that whether or not the player is verbally conscious of these computations is irrelevant to his theory, but it is *only* whether or not the player is *verbally conscious* of these computations that is irrelevant to the mechanistic validity of the theory.

The methodological limitations Friedman and his colleagues faced meant that they could test only the behavioral predictions and not the mechanistic claims of their models. Friedman argued that mechanistic claims were hence irrelevant; this conclusion gave rise to the *as if* school of economic modeling, born of necessity in the middle of the 20th century. But as neuroscience comes of age, it now provides us with the tools to test the mechanistic claims of models. We should be brave enough to accept the challenge of testably mechanistic models. We must trade *as if* models for their more rigorous *because* cousins.

An Example

Consider a billiard player being modeled by Friedman's method who faces the highly stylized pool table shown in Figure 6.1.

We observe that, faced with this table configuration, our player reacts by driving his cue ball towards the center of the right-hand corner pocket. This has the effect of driving the 8-ball into that pocket. As students of Friedman, we might propose that expert players behave in

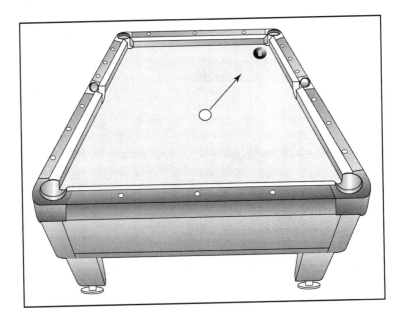

FIGURE 6.1

the limited world of this particular billiard table *as if* they simply drive the cue ball precisely towards the center of the right-hand corner pocket. Friedman is agnostic about what the brains of the players actually do; this is simply a limited model and the details about how the brains of real players achieve corner shots is, Friedman argues, irrelevant.

When we relax the conditions of our empirical observations and allow billiard balls to be placed at other locations, we discover that the theory we had been employing is no longer predictive of the behavior of expert players. Under these conditions we are driven to a richer theory in which subjects appear to maximize the number of balls that they drive into pockets by computing the Newtonian physics of ball motion. We come to that conclusion using the tried-and-true methods of social science, by observing behavior and modifying our theory accordingly.

Let us for a moment, however, imagine a harder form of Friedman's initial hypothesis. Let us imagine, just for a moment, that there was nothing "*as if* " at all about the theory of the billiard player. Let us imagine that Friedman's theory is a theory of both behavior *and* mechanism. Such a theory would predict that players in the first example drive cue balls towards corner pockets because their brains represent *only* the locations of right-hand corner pockets. A theory of this type can be tested in two ways. We can still examine behavior, of course, but we can also examine mechanism. In this simple example we can examine the theory either by making new behavioral observations or by demonstrating that neither the location of the right-hand corner pocket nor the straight-line trajectory of the pool cue towards that pocket is uniquely represented by the neural circuits that control behavior. A contemporary neurobiological inquiry of just this situation would identify in the player's brain the representations of many possible trajectories, each representation encoding the likelihood that this specific trajectory would result in a ball being driven into a pocket. What we would see is that the mechanistic analysis suggested a richer theory. The neural computations we would encounter are, in fact, more accurately described by the laws of Newton and a maximization algorithm specified by the rules of billiards than by the "shoot for the right-hand corner pocket" theory.

The most important point here is that there is no logical or empirical barrier to generating and testing *because* theories. One might argue that behavioral tests are less expensive and time-consuming than mechanistic tests, but one simply cannot argue that mechanistic tests are logically irrelevant to the goal of modeling behavior. We can make mechanistic tests irrelevant by assertion—"This is only an *as if* theory"—but that is a political rather than a scientific operation. As should become clear in the pages that follow, it is also an unproductive operation if one's goal is either to understand the world around us or to build accurate and predictive models of human behavior.

A Response to Friedman

If we, as scholars, were to be so bold as to discard Friedman's *as if* assumption and instead hypothesize that the computations businessmen, billiard players, and regular choosers *appear* to perform are actually *being performed* by their brains (where else they could be performed I myself simply cannot imagine), then we gain something important: we gain the ability to test our economic theories with both neurobiological and behavioral tools.

To this end, a neuroeconomist must propose, if he or she is serious, a "Hard theory" of economic behavior—a *because* theory. We must propose a theory without *as ifs*. We must propose an explicit theory of mechanism that can be tested simultaneously at the neural, psychological, and economic levels of analysis. That simply has to be the structure of any Hard theory of economic behavior that seeks to unite neurobiological, psychological, and economic explanations of behavior under a neuroeconomic framework.

Searching for the Hard Theory of Economics

How then, should we begin the search for a Hard theory of economic behavior that could serve as a foundation for neuroeconomic inquiry? What are the features that would be most desirable in such a theory? Our goal would be to begin with a theoretical construct at the core of modern economics—something that everyone would recognize as an economic object. It should also be as simple and parsimonious a theory as possible. It should follow Friedman's dictum of making accurate predictions about an important subset of behavior with as little complexity as possible.

We could then take such a theory and simply transform it into a *because* theory by testing, at a neurobiological and psychological level, whether the theory is implemented as proposed.

In this way we will likely falsify the initial theory, because all initial theories are easily falsified. But the study of mechanism may well yield new constraints on the theory, and as those constraints multiply they should yield both new behavioral predictions and a simultaneously richer and more constrained theory.

Let us begin then with the obvious core primitives of modern economics—expected utility theory and the theories of WARP and GARP from which it evolved. Let me stress again that we do not start with these axioms because we think any existing form of utility theory is correct, but because starting with utility theory allows us to begin with clear links between neurobiological, psychological, and economic levels of analysis, and because it allows us to cover well-trod ground as we begin.

Recall from Chapter 3 that if we say that we have a chooser who obeys in her choices the axioms of GARP, that turned out to be the same as saying that we have a chooser who behaves as if she had a monotonic utility function. Von Neumann and Morgenstern proved that if we have a chooser who obeys GARP plus the continuity and independence axioms, it is the same as saying that she has some monotonic utility function (as in GARP) and she computes the desirability of any lottery by multiplying the probability of the gains or losses presented in the lottery by the utility of those gains or losses.

If we are going to take expected utility as a Hard theory, then in essence we have to test the hypothesis that an expected utility compliant chooser behaves the way she does *because* she has a monotonic function that encodes the value of the lotteries among which she chooses and multiplies this internal valuation with her estimate of outcome probability. A *because* theory hypothesizes that phenomena observed at one level of abstraction arise because of mechanisms operating at lower levels of abstraction (Fig. 6.2).

For this reason, a *because* theory permits the direct examination and comparison of objects at different levels. It is a theory that, if well formulated, can be tested at any level. The Hard forms of expected utility theory or GARP would have to posit that subjects who obey the behavioral axioms of the theory do so because they neurally represent

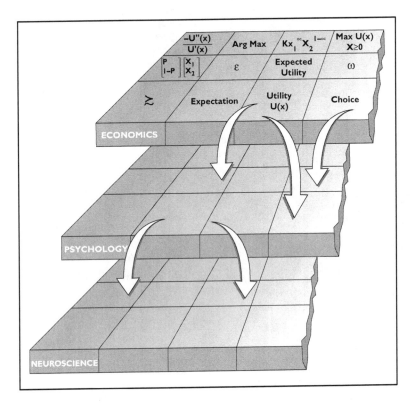

FIGURE 6.2

something having the properties of utility—a neural activation that encodes the desirability of an outcome in a continuous monotonic fashion. That is a clear and testable hypothesis.

Let me pause here to make a number of important terminological distinctions as we begin to specify a particular hard form of expected utility theory.[1] The first and most important set of facts to keep in mind is that utility, in the sense used by economic theories, is a fairly complex and quite specific object. Utility has the following properties:

1. Utility is ordinal, not cardinal. This is a very important point developed in detail in Chapter 3. Recall that Pareto pointed out that utility had

---

1. In the pages that follow, we will also encounter the hard form of GARP. When we talk about choice, GARP is often simpler than, and just as powerful as, expected utility. For the purposes of generality and exposition, I focus here on expected utility.

no "natural" units, and that even in expected utility theory the numbers we assign to objects as utilities are fairly arbitrary.

2. Utility implies welfare. If a chooser actually obeys the axioms of expected utility theory, then she is behaving as if she is maximizing a quantity called utility. But we can go a step further and even argue (as scholars from Pareto to Friedman have) that under these conditions this is the best possible course of action for her—this is the method that maximizes her welfare. This is true because in a traditional expected utility-compliant chooser, welfare derives from utility. They are the same thing in traditional expected utility theory.[2]

3. Utility is sometimes discussed even when subjects fail to obey the axioms of the theory. This is a subtle and important point. Consider a situation in which we observe a chooser who violates the axioms of expected utility theory: for example, she behaves intransitively. One possible explanation for this behavior is that she has made an error of some kind. If that is the case, she might still have a utility that she cannot use accurately to guide her behavior. The point here is that for some theorists utility can, under some limited conditions, have a life independent of choice.

With these properties of utility in mind, let us return to a simplified form of our inter-level diagram.

What are the properties of the unlabeled object linked to utility at the neural level in Figure 6.3? First and foremost, this is obviously some kind of neural firing rate, either the rate of an individual cell or a weighted function of the firing rates of a group of neurons. That is an important point because measurements of this object are necessarily going to be fully cardinal. The natural unit of measurement in the nervous system is action potentials per second. These measurements have a limited range (typically from 0 to 100 Hz and never exceeding 1,500 Hz) and fixed degrees of variance that are well understood and described in a later chapter. In this regard they are nothing like utility.

These observations thus tell us something about how serious *because* theories need to be structured. To generalize expected utility into a hard

---

2. This is a traditional viewpoint many behavioral economists are trying actively to relax.

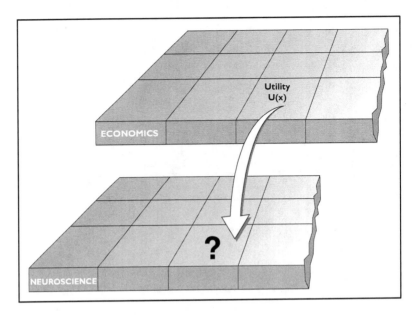

FIGURE 6.3

theoretical form, we have to posit the existence of a set of new (and measurable) empirical objects at the neurobiological level. Our theory then hypothesizes a link of a fully defined form between these two objects. For the *because* form of expected utility theory, I propose the following new object at the neurobiological level of abstraction:

> **Subjective Value**: Subjective values, at least for the purposes of this initial argument, are neurobiological objects having mean cardinal values ranging from 0 to 1,500. These firing rates also have finite variances that have been well described by neurobiologists and are known to be largely fixed properties of the mean rate. Mean subjective values are equal to the mean firing rates of populations of neurons (at least for this initial argument). For this reason, mean subjective values are linearly proportional to the BOLD signal (the signal of neural activity typically quantified by contemporary brain scanners) as measured in these same populations. Subjective values have a unique anchoring point called the baseline firing rate (again, a well-described neurobiological quantity). All subjective values are encoded cardinally in firing rates relative to this baseline.

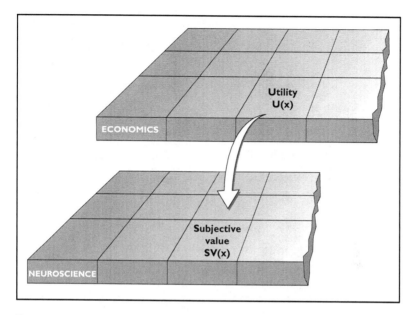

FIGURE 6.4

The next feature of the hard theory, which is critical, is that we specify the relationship between the economic object and the neural object in a way that captures the "because-ness" of the hard theory and that respects mathematical differences between the objects; therefore:

> **Subjective Value ↔ Utility**: Mean subjective values are linearly related to utilities. This describes the linking hypothesis relating the objects at the two levels of abstraction in a testable way.[3]

Conclusions

The neoclassical theorists of the mid-20th century argued that choosers who obey a few simple rules in their behavior acted as if they had an

---

3. This implies a linkage between expected subjective value and expected utility, which also rests on a neural representation of probability.

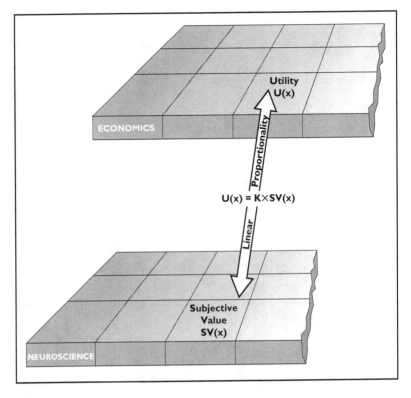

FIGURE 6.5

abstract representation of the values of the objects among which they were choosing and then selected that object having the highest value on this scale. Hard expected utility theory proposes that choosers who obey the axioms of expected utility theory do so because a group of neuronal firing rates in a valuation circuit encodes the cardinal subjective values (and/or expected subjective values) of each of the objects among which they are choosing. These values are linearly proportional to behavioral measurements of the utilities (and/or expected utilities) of these objects. That means that as long as behavior is expected utility compliant, these firing rates must obey all of the axioms of the original theory:[4] they must

---

4. Let me note that as soon as we examine real firing rates, we see variance in those firing rates. Here lies the first mismatch within Hard-EU. Subjective values have variance

obey independence and continuity and must be complete and transitive. Those are the necessary predictions of hard expected utility (Hard-EU). If we can identify the neural location at which these subjective values are encoded, we can begin to test Hard-EU at the neural level.

The testing of Hard-EU must therefore begin with an effort to identify the neural circuits for valuation. It must link activation in these circuits to choice behavior, and it must begin to examine the axioms of theory in these circuits. Let me presage the arguments that follow by revealing immediately that testing Hard-EU will reveal, as did the neoclassical testing of Soft-EU, that Hard-EU is demonstrably false. The tests of Hard-EU at the neural level, however, will suggest a new theory that captures many of the features of expected utility theory, of prospect theory, and of random utility theory in a hard mechanistic fashion. We begin the neuroeconomic process of theory development with Hard-EU not because expected utility theory is right, but because for a synthetic neuroeconomist, Hard-EU is the right place to start.

---

if they are neuronal firing rates and classical expected utilities do not. The implication of this is that any standard neuroeconomic theory will have to be anchored to a "because-version" of random utility models. This is a point to which we will return shortly.

Section 2

The Choice Mechanism

The first section of this book argued both that interdisciplinary syntheses between the natural and social sciences are possible, and that to have broad impact these syntheses will have to take a very specific form. I suggested that these syntheses will have to take the form of partial interdisciplinary reductions.

When biochemistry arose at the border of chemistry and biology, it began with biological definitions of the objects of study. Biologists had known since the time of Gregor Mendel (1866) that theoretical objects called genes served as the units of heredity. By the time Watson, Crick, Pauling, and others were engaged in searching for the hidden physical instantiation of these genes, quite complete mathematical models of their properties had already been developed, and these models guided much of the ensuing biochemical enterprise. Barbara McClintock's discovery of transposable genetic elements at the level of chromosomes in the 1940s (McClintock, 1950), for example, guided a host of linking hypotheses and interdisciplinary reductions after the identification of mobile genetic elements at the level of DNA in the 1960s (McClintock, 1983). When such interdisciplinary fusion occurs, theoretical insight from higher-level studies guides inquiry at lower levels of analysis. In turn, these lower-level analyses provide new constraints and lead to modifications of the higher-level theories that make them more powerful.

I have argued that just such a process has already begun between economics and psychology, that the first hints of a further partial reduction to neuroscience have already begun to appear in the literature, and that neurobiological studies of choice that ignore pre-existing higher-level theories succeed only in identifying patterns rather than in explaining important phenomena. In a similar way, I argued that economic scholars who ignore neurobiological constraints, scholars who ignore the physical limitations of the human brain, reject a host of powerful tools for the improvement and development of economic theory.

The previous section of the book ended by suggesting a very specific approach, rooted in the core theoretical tools of economics, for linking brain, mind, and choice. Economists have known for decades what macro-level phenomena are important for guiding human choice. They have developed theories of representation that describe hidden elements with well-described features that appear to guide choice under at least some conditions. They have also, as a matter of principle, argued that these hidden elements should not be a subject of inquiry, and some have even gone so far as to argue that were these elements to be identified, this identification would be of no interest to economics. I argued that this conceit must be abandoned if we are to seriously understand choice. We must take these powerful mathematical models at face value and begin to ask whether the hidden elements that they propose actually exist. On these grounds I concluded the previous section with an argument for what I called "because" models—hard interdisciplinary theories testable at multiple levels of analysis.

In the two sections that follow, I adopt this approach and begin a serious effort to develop an investigation of choice at several levels of analysis simultaneously. I begin with Hard-EU and identify pre-existing psychological and neurobiological data that link successfully, and unsuccessfully, to this theoretical corpus. Of greatest interest are incomplete or failed linkages. We can use these kinds of linkages to guide theory selection and development, a process described in detail in the pages that follow.

Section 2 of this book begins this process by first outlining general neurobiological observations relevant to choice. This is followed by an iterative examination of data and theory that leads to a surprisingly specific neuroeconomic theory of choice. The section concludes with a summary of the current state of the art, a hard theory of the human choice process as we understand it today. Section 3 expands that model into the domain of valuations, the hidden objects of economic theory that have recently been linked to well-studied frontal and basal ganglia circuits in the primate brain.

With these goals in mind, we turn next to the neurobiology of the human brain.

7

Neurobiological Kinds: Understanding the Abstractions of Neurobiological Thought

Précis

A serious effort to map Hard-EU onto the nervous system must start with a basic, and uncontroversial, outline of the well-understood input and output structures of the primate brain. Understanding the basics of how data are organized and processed in the primate neuraxis is essential if we want to use the many well-developed constraints imposed by contemporary neurobiology to build a serious interdisciplinary theory. We do not, for example, want to waste time and effort trying to map Hard-EU to the neural architecture that controls muscle force patterns simply because we did not take the time to absorb what is already known about these mechanisms. Neuroscience has already constrained the functions of many neural components in a way that makes them poor candidates for playing a significant role in economic choice, and any serious theory should incorporate that knowledge. A second class of neural constraint as we build this interdisciplinary approach is to acknowledge, and to employ, the global organizing principles of brain function that structure all neural computation.

We therefore begin with a brief tour of the sensory mechanisms of the human brain. The goal of this tour is to reveal several of the basic computational principles that recur throughout the mammalian brain. This is followed by a brief tour of the movement control (or *motor*) structures of the brain, which current evidence points to as a major component of the primate choice mechanism. The goal of this second step is to provide the anatomical foundations for understanding choice.

143

For practicing neuroscientists this section will be, necessarily, a review, and such readers might consider skipping this chapter. The first half of the chapter highlights key insights that underlie all of modern neurobiology. The second emphasizes the actual structural details of what one of the fathers of neurobiology, Charles Sherrington, called the "final common path" (Sherrington, 1947): the neural funnel through which choice must, of necessity, be expressed. For those completely unfamiliar with neuroscience, the sections that follow can serve as a starting point for further study of the brain or can simply be taken as an article of faith. Each section provides, at its end, a clear statement of the organizing principles that can be drawn from the insights presented in that section. For our purposes, these organizing principles are most important; the reader unfamiliar with neuroscience may take them, rather than the data preceding them, as the starting point for the discussions that follow.

Sensory Systems of the Human Brain

Nearly all of the sensory systems of the brain can be viewed as gathering data from the outside world in a three-step process: (1) transduction, (2) encoding and initial processing, and (3) cortical processing.

Transduction is the process that converts energy that arises in the outside world into the membrane voltages and action potentials that are the common currency of neuronal processing. When an electric bulb emits photons or an acoustic speaker sets up a pressure wave in the air, these are physical events in the outside world. In order for neurons of the brain to use those events to guide behavior, the energies those events produce must first be transformed into bioelectric signals that can be processed and analyzed by the circuitry of the nervous system.

In the retina (to briefly describe just one example), this transduction occurs in specialized cells called rods and cones. *Rod* cells transduce photons of many wavelengths into bioelectric potentials that underlie colorless night vision, while three types of more specialized transducers called *cones* transform photons in a wavelength-dependent manner that serves as the first step in daytime color vision. In the rod cells, this transduction occurs when a single photon of light collides with a molecule called 11-cis-retinal, which is embedded in a larger protein molecule called opsin. Opsin, like most important neural molecules, has been fully described at the level of its atomic structure (Nickle and Robinson, 2007). This is a molecule that, like many in the nervous system, has been sequenced, cloned, and identified in literally dozens of different species. The evolutionary relationship of this molecule to the opsins found in cone cells has been well described, as have the evolutionary relationships between the opsins found in literally dozens of species.

The energy of photons is physically transduced to a change in the *membrane voltage*[1] of a rod cell when a single photon is *absorbed* by 11-cis-retinal. This absorption is a quantum physical event that drives that molecule transiently into a higher energy state, which is reflected by a change in 3D shape. This unstable high-energy state (or shape) provokes a cascade of well-characterized biochemical events, each of which amplifies the number of molecules involved in the cascade. This cascade ends with the closing of *ion channels*[2] permeable to sodium ions in the rod cell membrane. Passive flow of these charged sodium ions through these ion channels drives the electric field existing across the cell membrane towards a higher voltage. Closure of these particular ion channels thus has the effect of shifting the membrane voltage towards a lower (a more negative) level—a bioelectrical event caused by the initial photon absorption. Single photon detection is thus accomplished at the level of a single rod cell, an engineering feat accomplished by evolution that places human vision at the physical limits of light sensitivity imposed by quantum physics.

I admit to belaboring this description of the first tiny step in the visual process, but I do so for a reason. For scholars unfamiliar with the nervous system, there is always a tendency to suspect that we know very little concrete information about the brain and almost nothing that could constrain an analysis of cognition. Colored maps of the cortical surface

---

1. An electrical potential produced by the active segregation of positively and negatively charged salt particles across the outer skin of a cell according to the well-described rules of electrochemistry.

2. Openable and closeable tubes that connect the interior and exterior of the cell. These atomic-scale tubes serve as a conduit through which specific salt particles can migrate, driven by the force of the extant electric fields and concentration gradients, from one side of the cell membrane to the other. It is this migration of charged particles that gives rise to changes in the membrane voltage.

presented by the lay press often reinforce this belief that no prior knowledge of neural structure need constrain neural models. Nothing could be further from the truth. The most basic first-year graduate textbook on neuroscience contains seven dense pages of text describing, down to the level of atoms, the outlines of this first step in the transduction process for photons that I have just described (Zigmond et al., 1999). Dozens and dozens of subsequent pages track the impact of this bioelectric signal as it cascades through the nervous system and gives rise to perceptual experiences at the level of human cognition. Just as no young economist would believe that one can practice economics without knowledge of Walrasian equilibria, one cannot practice neurobiology without knowledge of how the brain works. My goal in this chapter is, among other things, to provide a cursory understanding of a few critical elements in brain structure and function. My larger goal is to describe the logical kinds of neuroscience, and the transduction process is the first of these kinds we have encountered.

To continue, the transduced signal arising in the rods is next processed in the retina, where information content (in the formal information-theoretic sense) is known to be maximized with regard to the statistical properties of the external visual world (Atick and Redlich, 1990, 1992; Yan et al., 1996).

Signals from all locations in the retina (and hence in the visual world) are then topographically passed from the retina to a structure in the thalamus called the lateral geniculate nucleus (LGN) depicted in Figure 7.1. In the human, the LGN is composed of six layers. Each of these layers forms a topographic map of the retinal surface.

Points in the central retina project to the central point in each of these six maps (Fig. 7.2). Within each map, the organization of visual space is essentially logarithmic; magnification occurs such that the amount of space on the map dedicated to each square degree of the visual world drops as the logarithm of distance from the center of vision. It is this logarithmic magnification that underlies our greater visual acuity for central versus peripheral vision.

Across these six maps we also see tremendous structure, revealing a powerful kind of information sorting. Three of the six maps in the LGN receive information from the left eye and the other three receive precisely analogous information from the right eye. Within each of the three maps

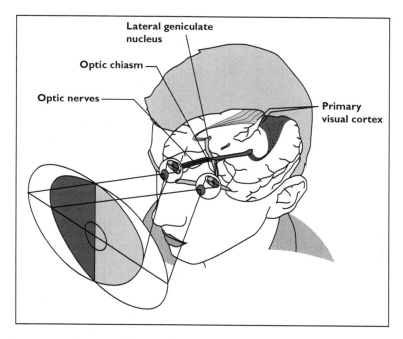

FIGURE 7.1   Anatomy of the visual system.

that encode information from a single eye, one of the maps is specialized for encoding information related to moving objects and the other two are specialized for stationary objects. (For a more detailed explanation of these processes at an undergraduate level, see Breedlove et al., 2007; at a graduate level, see Zigmond et al., 1999).

While there is much more detailed information about the anatomical and physiological specializations in each of these maps (as I write this chapter, the principal indexing service for scholarly biomedical articles lists over 8,000 scholarly papers that describe the LGN), two key points about the global organization of the mammalian brain are revealed here:

1. The topographic organization of information about the external world is a basic organizing principle of the brain.
2. Specialization of these topographic maps so that individual maps serve as modules that carry or organize information along discrete dimensions is a second critical feature of neural organization.

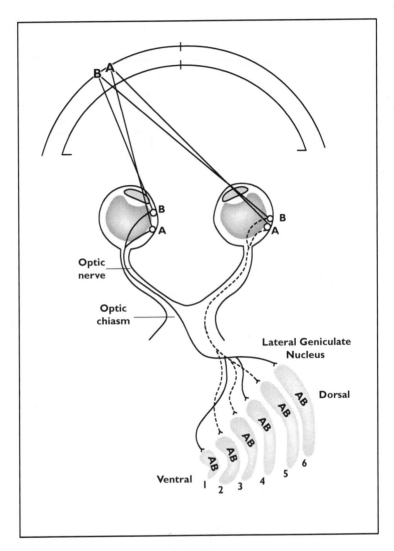

FIGURE 7.2   Retinal projections to the LGN.

These are the first two general principles of brain organization we have encountered, and keeping these principles in mind as we proceed will be critical for any deliberate effort to link neurobiology to the psychology and economics of choice.

Like the output neurons of the retina, which send bioelectric signals to the LGN via their axons,[3] the output neurons of the LGN send axons to a discrete area in the mammalian brain, in this case an area in the cortex known as visual area 1 (V1). Like the LGN, V1 forms a topographic map of the visual world through which nearly all visual information must pass. Since V1 is topographically organized, information from central regions of the retina projects (via the LGN)—again with a logarithmic magnification as a function of eccentricity—to central regions of area V1. In this way the neurons in V1 form yet another bioelectrical map of the visual world.

If we examine a tiny sub-region of this map, say an area 1 × 2 mm located at the central area of the map that encodes information arising in the central 0.1 degrees of the visual world, we reveal yet another degree of structure. This is a structure for organizing incoming information that arises for the first time in the cerebral cortex.

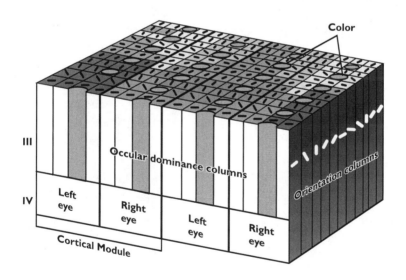

FIGURE 7.3   A segment of area V1.

_____

3. The long wire-like output processes through which neurons pass the biophysically computed integral of their input signals to their downstream targets.

We find in V1 that neurons cluster by the eye from which they receive information (and hence by the LGN sub-map from which their input arises). Neurons deep within each cluster receive input from only one eye, while neurons on the borders of these clusters encode information sourced from both eyes. (This is the first point in the visual processing stream at which information from the two eyes converges.) In a similar way, we find that a defined sub-region of this 1 × 2-mm area encodes information about color in a highly structured fashion. Also organized into this area are structural arrangements that segregate representations of light from representations of dark (or, to speak more technically, the phase of visual signals as measured in the Fourier plane), the orientation and spatial frequency of light and dark patterns, and even the speed and direction of visual stimulus motion.

The key principle here is that within this topographic map of visual space, a two-dimensional topographic map of the retinal world carried into cortex, are many additional dimensions of data arranged in a repeatable, highly structured, and well-understood manner. A pattern of action potentials at a single location on this map reveals not only the location of photons in the visual world but also the wavelength distribution of those photons and information about the spatial and temporal frequencies of the patterns of light and dark in the outside world. *Topographic maps with embedded high-dimensional encoding of secondary properties are another basic feature of neuronal organization* (Hubel and Wiesel, 1977).

Subsequent to area V1, action potentials[4] arising in V1 neurons pass along two roughly parallel, although interconnected, streams of processing in the visual system (Ungerleider and Mishkin, 1982). The first is a pathway of interconnected specialized topographic maps that passes dorsally (upwards) through the cortex away from V1. These dorsal areas are largely specialized for the analysis of the position of objects in the visual world. The second pathway of interconnected specialized maps descends ventrally and extracts information about the identity of the objects in the visual world. What we observe is increasing specialization as we move away from V1. The globally organized image of the world

---

4. The bioelectric pulses that travel down axons, thus allowing communication between neurons. Since nearly all inter-neuronal communication is mediated by action potentials, these signals serve as the common currency of neural communication.

encoded in V1 is first separated into what are known as "what" and "where" sub-pathways. Within each sub-path, further specialization can be observed. Within the dorsal stream, for example, one discrete sub-map encodes information only about the speed and direction of visual motion. This reinforces our second principle, *the existence of modular specialization across topographic maps.* Cortical areas often perform highly specialized functions, as revealed by their intrinsic topographic organization. For many maps this intrinsic organizational structure is not yet known, but for every area that has been well studied, such a structure (and the cell biological mechanisms for the generation of that structure) has been revealed.

I have described only the most basic (and important) features of the organization of the visual system (see Hubel, 1988, for a deeper lay introduction to these ideas). What has been revealed are a set of basic organizing principles for sensory encoding:

1. Topographic organization of information about the external world is a basic organizing principle of the brain.
2. Specialization of these topographic maps exists, such that individual maps serve as modules that carry or organize information along discrete dimensions.
3. Topographic maps with embedded high-dimensional encoding of secondary properties are another basic feature of neuronal organization.

A similar description can be provided for the organization and structure of information in the other sensory modalities. Each of these descriptions reveals unique properties of the neural encoding of that modality, but these three principles stand out clearly in our studies of all sensory systems (and, as we will see, all motor systems). The two most important points to take away from this discussion are the organizing principles described above and the simple fact that we know an awful lot about how information is—*and is not*—organized in the human brain.

Motor Systems of the Primate Brain

While the motor systems of the primate brain are built around these same organizing principles, some of the special problems faced by this set of mechanisms have very profound implications for any theory of decision making. The simple process of moving one's hand across the surface of a computer keyboard is an enormously complicated computational task. Allowing for the structure of the joints, the viscosity of the muscles, the pull of gravity, are all significant engineering problems that we overcome effortlessly. Once we decide what movement we want to make, billions of neurons must be mobilized to physically realize our movements. These billions of neurons, like the billions participating in the processing of sensory information, lie in highly organized and precisely interconnected movement control maps. These movement control maps thus form a "final common pathway" through which all the choices we make see their physical expression.

If the process of movement—the process of wielding a pencil, speaking a word, or pressing a key—were not computationally complex, then we could look to the neurons that control the musculature to understand how choice occurs. But we know that a huge portion of the primate brain exists for the realization of our choices. Choice itself must, of necessity, occur upstream of this final common path for action. This is a point first made by Sherrington (1947) when he invented modern neuroscience. As we develop theories that describe the neurobiology of choice, we must be mindful of the necessity of understanding the motor control circuitry. We therefore turn next to the movement control systems of the brain.

Studies of the motor system have revealed that the neural mechanisms for the control of action can be divided into two separate classes of mechanism: those that serve as the final common path for moving the body, and those that serve as the final common path for moving the eyes. It must be these circuits that our choices control. We begin our examination, perhaps somewhat counter-intuitively, with a brief tour of the eye movement system, because studies of the eye movement system have revealed many critical principles of neural organization. The greater mechanical simplicity of the eye movement system has allowed it to serve as a model for understanding the neural organization of the movement control circuit in general.

Eye Movements

While a number of classes of eye movements occur, and all have been well studied, we focus here on the rapid orienting shifts of gaze known as *saccades*. (For a complete review of eye movement control, see Leigh and Zee, 2006. For a review of the saccadic system, see Glimcher, 2003b, and Krauzlis, 2005.) Perhaps unsurprisingly, distinct neural circuits segregate eye movements into different functional classes, most of which are involuntary. Saccades, however, are largely voluntary eye movements and so are of particular interest to understanding how we express the choices we make.

When we look from one face to another or from one object to another, we do so by rapidly rotating our two eyes so that the centers of the retinas move from alignment with one object into alignment with the next. The actual high-speed rotations of the eyes induced by a dynamic contraction of the muscles are managed by a set of brainstem circuits that control both the position and the velocity of the eyes as they are in motion. These circuits decompose each movement into two orthogonal dimensions and then regulate the contractile forces produced by each of the six eye muscles to achieve these instantaneous velocities and positions. In turn, these brainstem circuits receive their primary input from an evolutionarily ancient midbrain structure called the *superior colliculus* (see Fig. 7.4).

Not unlike the LGN, the superior colliculus is arranged as a topographic map, but in this case that map (more formally, the intermediate layers of this seven-layer structure) encodes features of movements rather than features of the outside world (e.g., Robinson, 1972).

This means that activity at one location on the map might, for example, be associated with a 10 degree rightward shift in one's gaze. Activity at an adjacent location on the map would then be associated with a movement that shifted gaze 11 degrees to the right. Activity on the other side of the 10-degree position is similarly associated with a 9 degree gaze shift. As Figure 7.5 shows and as these examples communicate, patterns of activity in this motor structure topographically encode the repertoire of all possible shifts of the line of sight.

Interestingly, though, the activity that precedes a 10 degree rightward eye movement, for example, is not simply the activation of a single neuron at the 10 degree rightward location in the map. Instead, a broadly distributed spatial and temporal pattern of activity precedes this 10 degree rightward movement. As many as several seconds before the movement, one observes a gradual increase in the rate of action potential production over a broad portion of the map. This broad activation is highest at the

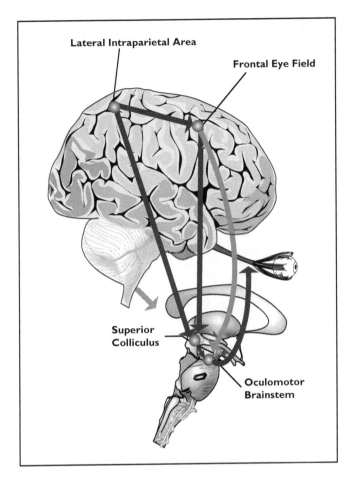

FIGURE 7.4   The eye movement system.

precise location in the map associated with a 10 degree rightward movement; as one moves away from this point, the rates of action potential fall off as a Gaussian function of the logarithm of movement amplitude (and as a linear function of physical distance in the map). Conceptually, one can think of this as a "hill" of activity on the map as shown in Figure 7.6. (It is a hill if one imagines the rate of action potential production as a vertical dimension.) This is, in fact, a broad hill that may span as much as one sixth of the map in the instant before each movement (Sparks, 1978).

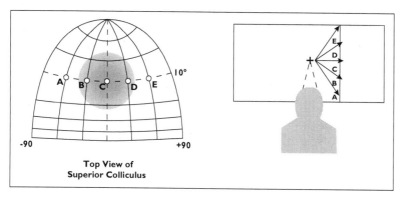

FIGURE 7.5   The superior colliculus.

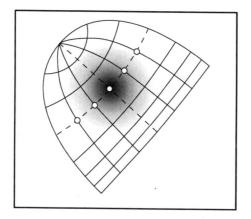

FIGURE 7.6   A 'hill of activity' in the superior colliculus.

One also observes that the temporal structure of this pattern of activity is very stereotyped and highly structured. Long before a movement occurs—this could be seconds or milliseconds, depending on the particular movement—the "hill" of activity centered on the topographic coordinates of the impending movement may be quite "low." Activity at the center of the hill may be characterized by action potential generation rates as low as 10 or 20 Hz. However, very shortly before a movement occurs—typically about 30 milliseconds before movement onset—activity throughout the hill increases suddenly from levels always beneath 100 Hz to levels as high as 1,200 Hz at the central location. This collicular *burst* reflects an interesting biophysical property of this tissue. In normal (or *tonic*) mode, the tissue has a maximal firing rate of about 100 Hz, and activity at this level is not sufficient to activate the brainstem circuits that actually move the eyes. However, once the strength of signals impinging on the colliculus from upstream exceeds a fixed biophysical threshold—once those signals drive the colliculus above about 100 Hz—then the tissue suddenly becomes much more active. A nonlinear (and essentially discontinuous) transition occurs that switches the tissue from its low-frequency tonic mode into a "bursting" state. In the bursting state, activity on the map becomes briefly self-perpetuating at this high level of activity. This higher level of activity in turn activates the brainstem eye movement execution circuits that generate, ballistically, the actual rotations of the eye called for by the collicular burst (Isa, Kobayashi, and Saito, 2003; Lee and Hall, 1995).

One can thus think of the collicular burst as the final deliberative event in saccade production. Once the burst occurs, a threshold has been crossed and the movement is produced. When we choose to make an eye movement, that choice becomes irrevocable once the collicular tissue transitions to its burst mode. So what, then, precedes this burst? Interestingly, it is often the case that when in tonic mode, before any burst is initiated, the colliculus maintains two or more distinct low-frequency hills of activation (Glimcher and Sparks, 1992). A number of researchers have observed that two or more sub-threshold movements may be entertained simultaneously in the collicular tissue when no movement is in active production by a burst (Basso and Wurtz, 1998). In fact, it has even been shown that the strength of activation in these two patterns—the heights of two hills of activity present in the colliculus at any time—can be quite different, with one "potential movement" showing much greater activation than the other (Dorris and Munoz, 1998).

As the tissue transitions to burst mode, however, the rising burst activates a strong *inhibition*[5] that spreads throughout the map and silences

---

5. This inhibition can be thought of as a negative image of the burst. The bursting neurons send, through their axons and through intermediate neurons contacted by their axons, a suppressive signal throughout the rest of the collicular map. This ensures that only one burst can occur at one location at a time.

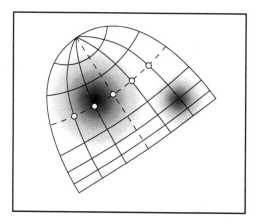

FIGURE 7.7   Two possible movements represented simultaneously.

all neurons outside the bursting region (Dorris et al., 2002; Ozen, Helms, and Hall, 2003). Thus, if two or more weak hills of activity arise in the colliculus at the same time, and one of those hills crosses the threshold for entering burst mode, this active hill effectively silences the other weakly active hills. In some sense, the interaction between the weakly active hills can be seen as competitive. Only one of those hills can conscript the actual eye movement circuitry at a time. In neurobiological circles, this kind of competitive interaction is often referred to as a "winner-take-all" mechanism (van Beuzekom and van Gisbergen, 2002). In purely mathematical terms, one can conceive of this interaction between the weakly active hills as a kind of "argmax" operation. Only the maximally active hill at any point in time controls what it is that our eyes actually do. When one active population receives sufficient input to drive it over the biophysical threshold for movement generation, all other candidate actions are temporarily silenced.

As a final note, the precise movement produced by the active population has been shown to be the vector average of the overall activity of the bursting population (Lee, Roeher, and Sparks, 1988). This tells us something about how the downstream circuits use the burst to structure the movements they actually produce. From the point of view of those downstream circuits, we can think of each neuron in the bursting colliculus as associated with a single movement based on its location in the topographic map. During the burst phase, each neuron effectively "votes" for its "best movement" and the strength of its vote is encoded by its firing rate. The movement actually produced by the brainstem circuitry can be shown (by experimentally manipulating the spatial structure of the burst) to simply be the weighted average of those votes— the movement at the center of the active population under normal physiological conditions. This process of vector averaging thus allows a broadly distributed pattern of activation to produce a highly precise movement.

To summarize, the critical features of movement generation revealed by this exposition are:

1. The process of generating a saccadic eye movement is driven by the activation of this single final common path.[6] Whatever deliberations we engage in about what movement we want to make, those deliberations must be complete before one passes through this final common point in the circuitry for motor control.

2. Within this topographically organized final common path, activity associated with a single movement is broadly distributed, but in a way that allows very precise control of the actual movement through vector averaging.

3. To actually produce a movement, activity at one location on the map must exceed a biophysical threshold. Once that occurs, a wave of inhibition suppresses all other possible movements until after the current movement is complete.

Understanding these features of the motor control circuitry is a prerequisite for the study of choice. The next critical point, then, is to understand what causes these patterns of activation in the collicular map. The colliculus is reciprocally interconnected with a small network of related areas that provide many (but not all) of the colliculus' inputs, so we next turn to these areas. Each of these areas also contains a topographic map of saccadic eye movements and each of these maps is connected, in

---

6. However, if the superior colliculus is removed surgically, saccades are abolished completely for only days or weeks (Schiller et al., 1987). In time, a second structure we will encounter shortly, the frontal eye fields, develops the ability to trigger the brainstem circuits directly through a weak but pre-existing pathway. Under non-pathological conditions there is, however, widespread agreement in the neurobiological community that the colliculus forms a single final common path for the generation of these movements.

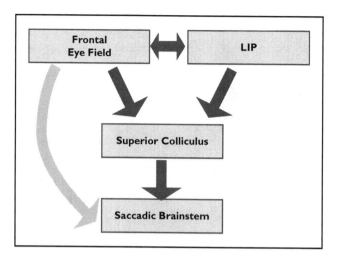

FIGURE 7.8   Saccade control areas.

a topographically organized fashion, with the collicular map. At least two cortical areas form this extra-collicular network: the frontal eye fields (the FEF) and the lateral intraparietal area (area LIP).[7]

Other areas also are closely interlinked with this three-area network, suggesting that these other areas also serve as components in the saccade control network. Connections among the FEF, area LIP, and the colliculus are very strong, suggesting that these are the primary control areas, but this primacy is a distinction of degree. The next most important member of the saccadic control network is almost certainly the supplementary eye field. In the discussion that follows, we focus on the FEF, area LIP, and the colliculus because this focus provides a clear pedagogical boundary. Other areas are important, and a more thorough treatment of the saccadic system generalizes the principles revealed here to those areas as well.

Returning to our focus on these three primary areas, it is important to note that activity in the FEF, area LIP, and the superior colliculus is

---

7. The precise features of the topographic organization in some of these areas remain subjects of active research. In the frontal eye fields, for example, movement dorso-ventrally in the map encodes saccade direction, but it is not entirely clear how saccade amplitude is encoded within the topography (Bruce and Goldberg, 1985).

almost always very tightly coordinated by reciprocal interconnections (Platt, Lau, and Glimcher, 2004). Indeed, in most models (e.g., Schall and Thompson, 1999) it is activity in the FEF map that provides the major input to the colliculus, and it is this activity that is presumed to drive the collicular map above threshold for burst production.

The area LIP of the parietal cortex, although also very closely interconnected with both of these areas, is widely believed to solve a slightly different but also critical problem in coordinate transformation that is a necessary part of the movement generation process (Andersen, 1987; Colby and Goldbeg, 1999). To understand the problem this parietal area solves, consider a subject who sees a visual stimulus 10 degrees to the right of his current point of fixation. He then decides to make a saccade that aligns his gaze with that stimulus. In principle it seems easy to understand how the neural circuits we have encountered might accomplish this sensory-to-motor process. The visual stimulus activates a point 10 degrees to the right of the center of the retina. This activity propagates to the 10-degree location in the LGN, then V1. and so on until it ultimately leads to activation at the 10-degree location in the FEF and area LIP maps. This in turn activates the collicular map and yields the appropriate eye movement.

Now consider a more complicated situation (which may appear a bit contrived for this example, but which communicates an important problem clearly). A firefly blinks on for one second 10 degrees to the right, just as the subject turns 10 degrees to the left to look at another person. What if he now wants to look at the firefly—a movement that we know humans can make accurately? The firefly activated a point 10 degrees to the right on the retina, but now to look at the firefly the subject must rotate his eyes 20 *degrees to the right*. How is that accomplished? The answer is that apparently rather bulky circuits in the posterior parietal cortex perform this transformation by storing the location of the firefly and updating that location to account for the intervening 10-degree movement of the eye. This is a particularly important process for the generation of accurate arm and hand movements (where the eyes are often in motion relative to the arms), and much of the anterior portion of the parietal cortex is dedicated to solving this class of "coordinate transformation" problems.

Movements of the eyes thus require the coordinated action of a final common network of areas that functions in a highly structured manner. The key elements in this network are the superior colliculus, the FEF, and area LIP. Each has been extensively studied, and their contributions to the control of eye movements have been carefully mapped. *Each can be viewed as a member of the final common path for saccadic control, although it is the biophysical properties of the burst circuit in the colliculus that act as the last element of this final common pathway. The burst is a threshold, or gate, that must be crossed for movement production to occur.*

Body Movements

Movements of the body (which include the movements of mouth, tongue, larynx, and lungs that generate speech) are controlled by a parallel network that obeys nearly all of the organizational features of the eye movement system, but faces some special challenges that heighten the importance of the coordinate transformation areas of the parietal cortex mentioned above.

Lying on the anterior bank of the central sulcus is a cortical area known as motor area 1 (area M1), which, in the case of skeletomuscular movements, serves as the final common pathway for that system. Like all of the areas we have encountered so far, M1 is topographically organized. Neurons in a specific region of M1 encode movements of the shoulder while adjacent groups of neurons on encode, for example, movements of the arm (Penfield and Rasmussen, 1950; Woolsey, 1952). While the precise details of the fine structural organization of M1 are under current investigation (e.g., Meier et al., 2008), it is beyond doubt that this is also a topographically organized area that sends projections into the spinal cord for the control of the musculature.

Much like the colliculus, the neurons in area M1 show activity long before movements are actually produced, and it can be observed that activity in M1 increases abruptly before movement onset (Tanji and Evarts, 1976). Like the colliculus, individual movements are encoded by populations of active neurons. Also like the colliculus, area M1 is embedded in a network of coordinated and interconnected cortical areas. The key players in this network are (1) the premotor cortex, a loose analogue of the FEF; (2) the parietal cortex (a suite of sub-regions in what anatomists call *Brodmann's areas 5 and 7*), which can be thought of as an analogue of the area LIP; and (3) the supplementary motor area, which is homologous to the supplementary eye fields of the eye movement system.

One important way in which the skeletomuscular system differs from the eye movement system is in the importance of the sensory motor transformations discussed above in the story of the firefly and the eye movement. To make it clear why this is an important (and computationally intensive) feature of this architecture, consider a subject lying on his back pushing a weight away from his chest with his arms. Here the subject produces rotations among the three joints of the arm along seven degrees of freedom that takes the center of the hand along a straight line projecting away from the body as shown in Figure 7.9.

To accomplish this movement, the subject's principal action is to contract the triceps muscle to push the weight against the force of gravity. Next consider the same subject making the same movement of the arm, but this time lying on his stomach, as in Figure 7.10.

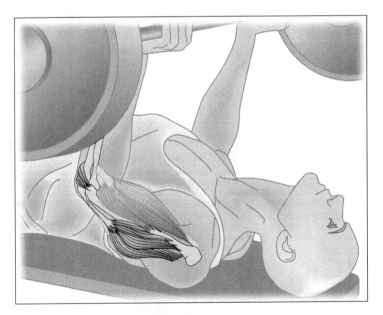

FIGURE 7.9   Extending arms against gravity. Triceps muscle shown in black.

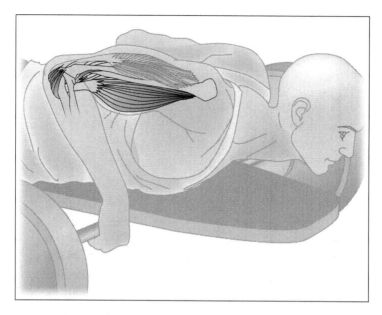

FIGURE 7.10   Extending arms with gravity. Biceps muscle shown in black.

Under these conditions the subject chooses to make the same movement, but because gravity now works with him instead of against him, he does so by relaxing the biceps muscle rather than contracting the triceps. In the most important sense, the weightlifter chose to extend his arm, so these are the same movements, but they require very different patterns of muscle force. We know that neurons in area M1 and in the premotor cortex treat these two movements very differently. Those areas encode the forces (and to some degree the first derivative of forces with regard to time) required for a movement (Evarts and Tanji, 1974). But when we choose to make a movement, as actors, it is with regard to the movement, not the force required to make that movement. Put another way, decisions about movements are made in what are called *kinematic*[8] terms, not in terms of muscle forces. Much of the complicated inverse mathematical modeling of the arm moving in a gravitational field that is required to derive the force required at any given moment as a movement

---

8. Or pure movement.

proceeds appears to occur in the anterior and middle parietal cortex as well as in MI and the premotor cortex. We know this because the neurons of areas 5 are the first place in the motor cascade that movements are represented in a force-independent way (Kalaska and Hyde, 1985; Kalaska et al., 1990). This places the neurons in these areas upstream of the computations about force that must logically follow any decision at a kinematic level about what movement to make. For this reason the MI network is slightly different from the eye movement network—for this system the parietal cortex plays an enormous and very complicated role in structuring the forces required for movement generation.

This is an important point for two reasons. First, it means that the bulk of the neural machinery in the anterior half of the parietal cortex has been well accounted for by current theory. In the absence of these circuits, movements are disordered, highly imprecise, and often not executed at all. Second, it clearly places these circuits inside the final common path (in the sense that the entire saccadic network is inside a final common path) for movement generation and thus at least partially downstream of any decisions we make about what movement to execute, a point to which we will return in a future chapter.

Conclusions

When we examine the structural features of the primate nervous system, we see a number of engineering constraints that shape how we have to think about the interactions of these circuits. We know, for example, that both sensory and motor systems arrange information topographically. We know that very large pieces of the nervous system have to be devoted to the initial processing of sensory signals and to the organization and production of movements. These circuits, which are evolutionarily quite ancient and can be thought of as constraints on models, must receive very specific kinds of inputs. We also know how these circuits change as multiple inputs compete to produce single outputs in the limited resource of the motor system. The challenge all of this information poses is whether we can use these neurobiological primitives, these "kinds" in the philosophical sense, to specify a primitive theory of choice that can be linked to expected utility theory in a way that yields a first version of Hard-EU.

8

Hard-EU and the Rudiments of a
Standard Model

Précis

The core goal of this chapter is to demonstrate how to directly link a pre-existing utility-based theory of choice to pre-existing neurobiological descriptions of the brain mechanisms that produce choice. Utility theory tells us that any subject who obeys even the limited constraints of GARP behaves exactly *as if* he had both a consistent internal representation of the subjective values of the options before him and a mechanism for selecting for execution the option having the highest of those values. Neurobiological studies conducted in the past 30 years have traced the pathways by which sensory information about multiple stimuli (or options) passes through the nervous system, and have demonstrated anatomically where these signals connect to the motor control circuits that produce actions. These are two sets of observations that remain largely unconnected.

This disconnection reflects two facts. First, until now utility-based theories have been silent about mechanism. It has been an article of faith among nearly all economists that if one says explicitly, "Any subject who obeys the axioms of GARP behaves exactly *as if* he had a consistent internal representation of the subjective values of the options before him," one does not mean that the subject actually has such a representation inside him. This is an article of faith, even though any decent economist could prove that such a neural representation would be the minimally complex tool for generating behavior that obeys GARP. Second, while neurobiological theories have been rich on mechanism, they have been extremely poor on theory. The standard "model" for describing the pathways that connect sensory processing circuits to motor control circuits remains the notion of the conditioned reflex and its direct intellectual descendants. These "stimulus-response couplings" remain the principal tools with which neurobiologists characterize their data and design new experiments. This is true despite the fact that we have known since the 1960s (e.g., Herrnstein, 1961; for an overview of this literature see Herrnstein, 1997) that these models cannot predict multi-option choice efficiently or accurately (Glimcher, 2003a).

Can these sets of observations be reconciled? Can Hard-GARP or Hard-EU actually be used to account for the existing neurobiological data in a way that both better explains what we already know and makes new predictions? Can a richer model of the nervous system anchored to utility theory make novel predictions about behavior? The first step towards answering those questions is to take what we already know about the neural structures that underlie choice behavior and try to look at those facts through the lens of utility theory. For neurobiologists, that means asking whether data traditionally viewed as compatible with stimulus–response style models could, at least in principle, be explained by the utility-style models we *know* to be more parsimonious at the behavioral level. For economists, it means asking whether the way in which data are stored and processed in the primate brain is compatible with the simplest possible algorithmic instantiation of something such as expected utility theory.

I believe that the single answer to these preceding questions is "yes." In this chapter I try to take a first step towards drawing that conclusion. I present, in chronological order, several of the key decision-related neurobiological results from the past three decades. All of these key early results come from single-neuron studies in awake-behaving monkeys. Almost all of these studies were constructed to trace stimulus–response relationships through the nervous system. What I hope to reveal is that they are all compatible with a simple algorithmic instantiation of expected utility theory (or in some cases GARP). This is a point I first made in a paper with my colleague Michael Platt (Platt and Glimcher, 1999), so this chapter ends with a discussion of the data presented in that paper. Subsequent chapters will offer significant refinements of these ideas.

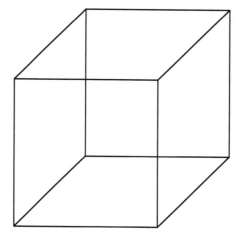

FIGURE 8.1   A Necker cube.

In those chapters I will show how additional data from neuroscience and psychology interact with theory from economics to specify a more intricate form of utility theory. For scholars from all disciplines, this chapter will probably raise more questions than it answers. What I ask is that you treat this chapter like a drawing of a Necker cube, relaxing your focus and allowing more than one interpretation of the image to coexist as you read. To allow that to happen, we begin with a statement of the key features of Hard-EU.

Hard–EU: A Simple Theory

Soft-EU is a list of axioms about behavior. The behavior of subjects is assumed to show a complete ordering of preferences among objects, transitivity, independence, and continuity. These are testable hypotheses, and saying a subject obeys these rules is equivalent to saying that he behaves *as if* he (1) possesses stable monotonic utility functions, (2) represents probability objectively, (3) takes the product of utility and probability, and (4) chooses between objects in a choice set by selecting the element in the set that has the highest expected utility.

By extension, Hard-EU is simply the theory that a subject obeys these rules *because* he (1) actually possesses stable monotonic utility functions that transform objective value to subjective value somewhere in the nervous system (a possibility discussed in Chapter 4), (2) represents probability implicitly or explicitly in the nervous system, (3) takes the product of utility and probability and represents this quantity in the nervous system, and (4) chooses between objects in a choice set by performing a neural operation that effectively selects the element in the current choice set that has the highest expected utility.[1]

As discussed in Chapter 6, we make one necessary addition to Hard-EU in order to respect the fact that the concept of utility embedded in Soft-EU (a behavioral measurement) is ordinal and "internal-utility," or "subjective value" (a neurobiological measurement) is fully cardinal with a unique zero (or baseline) point. To keep these concepts related but separate, we always refer to the neural form of utility as "subjective value."[2]

With that theory in hand, the very first question that arises is whether we can find *even preliminary* neural evidence for the existence of a representation of (1) subjective value, (2) probability, (3) the product of subjective value and probability (expected subjective value), and (4) a neuro-computational mechanism that selects the element from the choice set that has the highest "expected subjective value" and interacts with the movement control system to produce the physical movement that realizes that choice.

---

1. It is important for non-economists to remember here the difference between utility and expected utility. Utility is the subjective value of the objects of choice. *Expected* utility is the product of utility and probability, implied principally by the independence axiom.

2. Formally, what we want to do is to link a theoretical object constructed at the level of neurobiology called "subjective value" to a theoretical object constructed at the level of economics called "utility." The linking hypothesis that, in the sense used by Teller and Pugh (1983), joins these two objects is that subjective value is linearly proportional to utility. As a final formal note, the neurobiological theory also can be assumed to include an object called "action" that is constrained to be identical to (isomorphic to) the economic object called "choice." As hinted at by Gul and Pesendorfer (2008), the presence of at least one perfectly isomorphic object-pair in the two theories is required to guarantee that the interaction of neurobiology and economics can be bidirectional.

To begin to answer that question, we first have to ask where in the billions of neurons that make up the primate brain might such signals be found. At a purely causal level there seems one obvious starting point: in the circuits that are physically responsible for action—the motor circuits described in Chapter 7. These are the final common path, all action and choice must occur at, or upstream of, these elements.

If we were asking a human subject to choose between two options by pressing one of two keys on a computer keyboard (and those arm movement-produced decisions were observed to obey expected utility theory), then the last point in the sensory-motor chain at which we could plausibly begin to search for *expected subjective value* would be in such brain areas as M1, premotor cortex, supplementary motor area, and parietal areas 5 and 7. If we were searching for these neural signals with regard to an eye movement-expressed decision, we would naturally begin our search at the final point of convergence for the control of the movements that expressed those decisions: in the superior colliculus, the FEF, and the area LIP.

For purely technical reasons, in this chapter we will mostly ask this question in the voluntary eye movement control system. As mentioned in the preceding chapter, studies of that system have generally led studies of the arm movement system conceptually because of the reduced bio-mechanical complexity of the eye. Unlike the arm, which faces changing gravitational loads, the eye rotates around its center of mass and is a highly damped system that is thus insensitive to inertia. The result is that studies of the eye movement control network have largely served as a model for understanding how movements in general are produced.

It is also important to note that these movement control systems have been studied predominantly in the rhesus monkey. Our human genetic lineage diverged from these animals about 25 million years ago, which makes them fairly close evolutionary relatives. The only closer extant animals are the apes (animals such as chimpanzees and gorillas), and moral considerations preclude invasive experiments on such near relatives. For this reason, studies of both eye movement and arm movement control in the 1980s and 1990s were most sophisticated in single- and multi-neuron studies of this primate. It is to that pre-existing literature that we turn next.

Connecting Stimulus and Response

In 1976, Jun Tanji and Edward Evarts provided the first single-unit data on what could have been called a *decision*, albeit a very simple decision. In a now classic experiment, they recorded from neurons in area M1 related to movements of the arm while animals engaged in an almost trivial behavioral task (Tanji and Evarts, 1976). As the task began, the subject was informed by the illumination of a colored light that it would soon be offered a reward for either a pushing or a pulling arm movement, but not for both. Only later would it be told by another stimulus which movement was to be rewarded on this particular trial.

At the moment that a trial began, Tanji and Evarts found that activity in neurons associated with a pushing movement in the M1 topography became weakly active, as did neurons associated with pulling movements. After a brief delay, Tanji and Evarts signaled which movement would be rewarded on that trial with a "direction" cue and observed a marked change in firing rate: the neurons associated with the rewarded movement

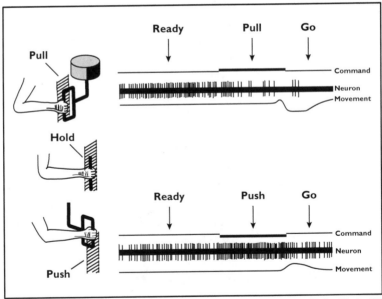

Adapted from Tanji and Evarts, 1976.

FIGURE 8.2   Tanji and Evarts, 1976 Expt on a "pulling neuron".

roughly doubled their firing rate and the neurons associated with the unrewarded movement reduced their firing rate to baseline. Finally, the experimenters signaled to the animal with a "go" cue that the previously identified movement, if made immediately, would yield a water reward for the thirsty monkey subject. At this point, the activity of the M1 neurons encoding the rewarded movement increased very rapidly and the movement was produced milliseconds later.

Let me add that there was little doubt (really no doubt) that these signals were causally related to the movements the animals were producing. There was a very tight temporal correlation between the high-frequency activation of these neurons and movement onset (Fromm and Evarts, 1982). These neurons were known to project into the spinal cord and to make direct connections with the motor neurons that directly activate the muscles (Cajal, 1909; Kuypers, 1960). Artificial activation of these neurons resulted in movements at short latency (Mackel et al., 1991), and the destruction of these neuronal populations eliminated finely controlled movements of the arms (Kuypers, 1960; Woolsey, 1952).

Although Evarts himself was quite hostile to stimulus–response style representations—see Glimcher (2003a) and Bernstein (1935) for Evarts' arguments—these experiments and the data they yielded are usually explained by neurobiologists using that set of conceptual tools. Here is how that traditional explanation goes. The directional stimulus is presented identifying a pushing movement as rewarded; this is followed by a pushing movement. We observe activity in the sensory neurons associated with the pushing stimulus, followed by activity in the neurons of the final common path for a pushing motion. Stimulus and response, a complete explanation. Alternatively, the directional stimulus is presented identifying a pulling movement as rewarded; this is followed by a pulling movement. We observe activity in the sensory neurons associated with the pulling stimulus followed by activity in the neurons of the final common path for the pulling motion. Stimulus and response again. The notion of "choice" invoked by economists seems irrelevant to these observations.

The weak activity observed before the "direction" cue is somewhat harder to explain within this framework, but not much harder. The weak activity observed early in the trial, activity Evarts called "preparatory," can be seen as a kind of "bias" to produce both of the potentially rewarded movements. This is a signal that arises from the onset of the trial-initiating stimulus. The weak preparatory activity can thus be seen as a kind of incomplete (or behaviorally unobservable) stimulus–response event that might, for example, serve to effectively reduce the reaction times during the upcoming stimulus–response event.

What I hope is clear from the preceding seven chapters, however, is that there is also another way to view this same sequence of observations. This is a view that emerges if we try to think like monkey economists just slightly outside the constraints of the traditional *as if* box. We begin from the monkey's point of view. The monkey is sitting in his chair deciding at each moment what it is that he wants to do. What he has learned is that when the light that signals the beginning of a trial is illuminated, there is a 50% chance that he will be able to obtain a fluid reward if he later pulls and a 50% chance that he will be able to obtain a fluid reward if he later pushes. When that initial sensory stimulus is presented, we observe that firing rates for both movement control circuits increment to a bit less than half of the threshold for movement production. When the directional stimulus, which identifies the rewarded movement, is presented, those probabilistic expectations about reward shift from 50%/50% to 100%/0% or 0%/100%. At that moment, we see activity in the circuit associated with the rewarded movement roughly double and activity in the circuit associated with the unrewarded movement drop to baseline. Shortly thereafter the "go" cue is delivered, firing rates radically increment at the remaining active site, and the movement is initiated.

Now, imagine that we knew that Tanji and Evarts' monkeys obeyed the axioms of expected utility in their behavior. This would mean that, for example, if given a choice between a movement that yields half a milliliter of water with a probability of 100% and a movement that yields half a milliliter of water with a probability of 50%, they consistently prefer the former. If given a choice between a movement that yields half a milliliter of water with a probability of 100% and a movement that yields half a milliliter of water with a probability of 0%, they consistently prefer the 100%-associated movement. Let us further imagine that in order to make such choices they kept track of the magnitudes and probabilities of all of the rewards that they had recently received. They would then know, at any moment, something about the expected utilities of their available actions. When we actually gave them the "go" cue they could use this information to select the movement having the highest expected utility at that moment.[3]

As a very first step towards examining that hypothesis in more detail, consider an experiment David Sparks and I performed in 1992 (Glimcher and Sparks, 1992). This experiment essentially repeated the original Tanji and Evarts experiments, but this time in the eye movement system. As in their experiments, our animals were told what movement would be reinforced and later told to execute their movement for a reward. The animals were thirsty and received a sip of fruit juice as a reward. The only significant difference between the two experiments was that we imposed a long delay between the time at which we indicated which movement would be rewarded and the time at which we cued the animals to execute that movement as quickly as possible. This allowed us, on occasion, to impose delays of up to 10 seconds between the time at which the monkey should know what movement to make and the time at which that movement should actually be made. We found that movements that would later be reinforced were associated with strong persistent activity in the superior colliculus during this entire 10-second period and that this activity was predictive of the actual movement that would later be made, even if that movement was an error. And like Tanji and Evarts, we found that the magnitude of this signal changed when we revealed to the monkey which movement would definitely be reinforced on that trial.

In 1997 Michelle Basso and Robert Wurtz extended this finding. In their experiment, a trial began with the presentation of one, two, four, or eight possible targets to a monkey. This was followed by a "direction" and "go" cue that indicated that a movement to one (and only one) of the targets would yield a reward. Basso and Wurtz found that the activity associated with each target on the collicular map during the initial presentation period was a function of the number of potential targets currently being displayed. As more targets were presented, the magnitude

---

3. Many economists will be troubled by the idea that expected utility-like signals might temporally precede the action. This is troubling to some economists because it suggests that valuation precedes choice and thus that these preceding valuation signals could occur even when a choice is not later expressed—an idea that Pareto rejected as untestable. Let me stress here that in the pages that follow, this will become very much a testable hypothesis.

of the preparatory activity associated with each target was systematically decreased. After the "direction" and "go" cues were presented, however, activity associated with the unreinforced movements rapidly waned and the activity associated with the reinforced movement grew rapidly into a burst.

In the language of stimulus–response associations, one could interpret these data as indicating that during the initial presentation period one, two, four, or eight stimulus–response circuits were weakly activated. We can think of this as some kind of early bias signal induced by the physical onset of the visual stimuli. This is followed by the "go" cue, which triggers strong enough activation in one of the stimulus–response circuits to evoke a behavior.

Put in the language of Hard-EU, however, we explain the same phenomena in a slightly different way. Basso and Wurtz observed that the firing rate of neurons in the colliculus during the initial presentation period was roughly proportional to the probability that a movement to that target would yield a reward. As Basso and Wurtz (1997) put it, "the activity of many saccade-related superior colliculus neurons changes substantially as the uncertainty of the target changes." After the "go" cue, the probability that the monkey will receive a reward for one target goes to 100% and the reward probabilities associated with the other targets go to 0%. At that moment the neurons associated with the rewarded movement increase their firing rate while the others become silent, and this is followed by the movement-producing burst of activity in the active neurons. One cannot help but notice that this quantitative pattern appears to track something like an instantaneous estimate of the "expected utility" of each movement, if we allow the notion of expected utility to precede in time the observation of choice.

Let me stress again, for economists who may be concerned that these signals might not be causally related to the actions produced by the animals, that activation of these neurons is followed, at a very short and repeatable latency, by saccadic movement onset (Sparks, 1978). Artificial activation of these neurons produces saccades (Robinson, 1972); destruction of these neurons eliminates saccades (Schiller et al., 1987). This is a structure that causes movement.

The next critical step, which occurred at about the same time that Sparks, Basso, Wurtz, and I were working on these issues in the colliculus, was the study of stimulus–response pathways in the parietal movement control area LIP conducted by Shadlen and Newsome (1996). Bill Newsome and his colleagues had, for some time, been studying a region in the dorsal stream of the visual pathway known to encode information about stimulus motion. Newsome and his colleagues had demonstrated the existence of a topographically organized map in the middle temporal area (area MT) that encoded the speed and direction of visual stimulus motion (Britten et al., 1993; Movshon and Newsome, 1992, 1996; Newsome et al., 1990; Newsome, Britten, and Movshon, 1989).

They and others found that one patch of neurons in this map became active whenever a visual stimulus included anything that moved at a location 10 degrees to the right of straight ahead. An adjacent patch of neurons responded to visual motion 11 degrees to the right of straight ahead, and so on. As in the visual cortex, neurons within a given patch showed a further organizational structure with sensitivities to specific directions of motion clustered in sub-patches. Newsome and others had hypothesized that activity in this map underlies our visual motion sense. Building on earlier work (Zeki, 1974), they hypothesized that under normal conditions activity here accounted for all of the motion-based perceptual judgments that we make, and that in the absence of these neurons we were incapable of motion-based perceptual judgments (although still capable of all non-motion-based visual judgments). To begin to test that claim, Newsome and colleagues (1989) refined a technique for matching neural and behavioral sensitivity functions

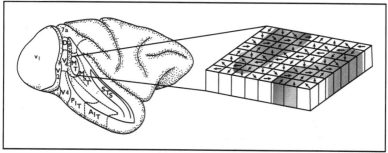

Adapted from Born and Bradley, 2005 and Maunsell and Newsome, 1987

FIGURE 8.3   Cortical area MT.

called the neurometric-psychometric matching technique (Parker and Newsome, 1998).

In their classic first experiments (Newsome et al., 1989), monkey subjects were trained to report the average direction of motion in an ambiguous and stochastic display. The monkeys viewed, for two seconds, a dark circular display filled with small flickering spots of light. On sequential frames of the video display, each spot was moved by the display computer in a random direction, and the overall impression one had was of watching a blizzard of tiny snowflakes. The critical manipulation of this display Newsome and his colleagues introduced was a systematic alteration of the directions in which the spots moved. Newsome's idea was to introduce a continuous independent variable that came to be called *coherence*. Under a 100% rightward coherence condition all of the dots moved coherently to the right. Under a 50% rightward coherence condition 50% of the dots moved to the right and the remaining 50% moved randomly. Under a 0% coherence condition all of the dots moved randomly. The coherence variable allowed them to systematically manipulate the perceptual strength of the visual motion in this field of moving snowflakes. They hoped to demonstrate that manipulating the degree of stimulus coherence influenced both the perceptual judgments of the subjects and the MT neurons *in an identical way*.

In a typical experiment, as illustrated in Figure 8.4, an MT neuron might be identified that responded to rightward motion with an increase in firing rate and to leftward motion with a decrease in firing rate. What Newsome and colleagues would do once such a neuron had been identified was to present, in random order, a sequence of displays containing all possible leftward and rightward coherences to the monkey. However, regardless of the degree of coherence, trials that presented leftward motion were those on which a leftward eye movement would yield a water reward for the monkey. Similarly, rightward motion identified a rightward movement as rewarded. After each display was presented, a rightward saccade target and a leftward saccade target were illuminated, and Newsome and colleagues waited to see at which target the monkey chose to look.

If one pauses to think about how an optimal decision-maker would choose in this task, it should be clear that the animals face a situation of limited information whenever the fraction of coherently moving dots is set to a small number. At the start of such a trial, the animal knows that

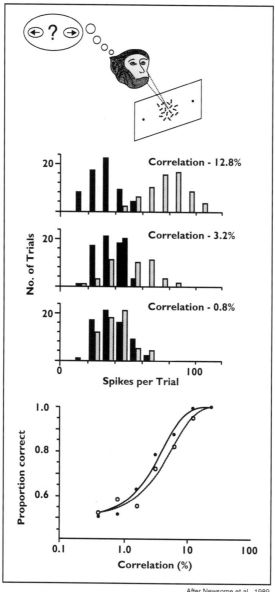

After Newsome et al., 1989.

FIGURE 8.4   Newsome's task.

there is a 50% chance a rightward movement will yield, for example a half-milliliter water reward, and similarly a 50% chance that a leftward movement will yield a half-milliliter reward; the expected values and expected utilities of the two movements are identical. As the monkey views successive frames on the video display, however, he gathers more and more information that allows him to refine his estimate of the reward probabilities.

In the Basso and Wurtz experiment mentioned above, the monkeys were told that the probability of a given target yielding a reward was either 100%, 50%, 25%, or 12.5% (depending on how many targets appeared). In Newsome's (1989) experiment, the probabilities always started at 50% and then changed continuously as the monkeys viewed the display. Under the 100% rightward condition the monkey could quickly gather adequate information to identify the rightward movement as rewarded with 100% probability, so the estimate of probability and expected utility would be expected to change quickly. Under the 3% rightward condition the estimate of the expected utility of the rightward target would be expected to grow much more slowly. The first critical point here is that the animals must continuously gather data over time to guide their choice, and this continuous stream of incoming data should allow the animals to update their estimates of the expected utilities of the two movements in a way that depends on the strength of the motion signal.[4] The second critical point is that both the display and the behavior were stochastic. Even in the 50/50 condition there is some net dot motion, just by chance, and the behavior of the monkeys under these conditions was observed to be stochastic. Based on behavioral observations such as these, Newsome and colleagues constructed choice curves that related the probability that the monkey would choose "right" to the percentage of rightward dot motion. What they showed in a subsequent neural analysis was that MT activity precisely predicted this behavior.

---

4. Motion information is presented in a way that makes successive samples from the display statistically independent. This is important because it means that each pair of frames presented to the monkeys provides equally valid data on the likely reward. Under these conditions it should be obvious that an optimal (Bayesian) monkey would simply compute the continuous temporal integral of the motion signal to derive the best possible estimate of instantaneous expected utility of each movement for this task.

Their data thus supported the hypothesis that the MT signal was sufficient to account for the observed motion judgment behavior.

What Shadlen and Newsome proposed was that an analysis of the neurons in area LIP (to which these MT neurons projected) might reveal the process by which the moment-by-moment motion signals documented in area MT were cumulated (or integrated) to guide choice. To that end, Shadlen and Newsome recorded the activity of LIP neurons while monkeys viewed the moving dot display, and they built a series of process-based models of the circuitry with which the animals made a decision about whether to look left or right at the end of each trial (Shadlen and Newsome, 1996).

What Shadlen and Newsome found, as shown in Figure 8.5, was that the firing rates of LIP neurons that encoded rightward movements grew gradually over the 2-second trial when rightward motion was presented. The greater the strength of the presented rightward motion signal, the faster the firing rates of the rightward associated neurons grew. Shadlen and Newsome interpreted this mechanistically as evidence that neurons in area LIP were effectively competing to trigger, in the superior colliculus, the stimulus–response pair they represented, as shown in Figure 8.6. The gradual rise in activity produced by a low-coherence rightward motion signal reflected, they argued, the growing probability that the rightward response would be triggered and could be represented as the aggregate integral of the visual motion signal presented to the monkey.

However, reading their work from the perspective of Hard-EU raises another interesting possibility. If the network of movement control areas that include the superior colliculus, the FEF, and area LIP represents something like expected utility (or, more precisely, *expected subjective value*) in the period before a behavior is produced, then Shadlen and Newsome's results take on new meaning. One is forced to consider the possibility that the instantaneous firing rates associated with the 10-degree rightward location in the LIP map might indeed encode the monkey's estimate of the instantaneous expected subjective value of the rightward movement. The steady growth of the LIP firing rate during a trial might well reflect the integral of MT firing rates as Shadlen and Newsome had proposed, but it would do so *because* the integral of those firing rates provides the best possible estimate of the expected utility of each eye movement the monkey could consider executing. The accumulation of

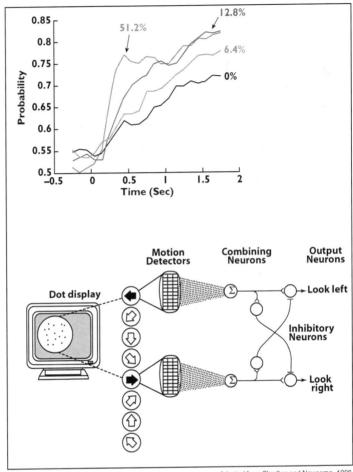

Adapted from Shadlen and Newsome, 1996.

FIGURE 8.5   Figure of LIP firing rates in the original Shadlen expt from Shadlen and Newsome, 1996 Shadlen, M.N. and Newsome, W.T. (1996).

information in area LIP firing rates would then reflect the fact that in this particular task, the most efficient way to compute the expected utility of each movement is to take the integral of the stimulus motion signal arising in area MT.

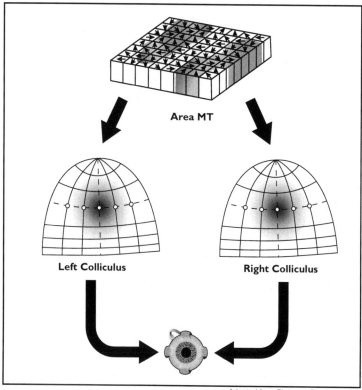

Area MT

Left Colliculus   Right Colliculus

Adapted from Platt and Glimcher, 1999

FIGURE 8.6   Newsome's proposed circuit.

To put that another way, imagine that the visual stimulus the monkeys were trained to observe was negatively correlated with the rewarded movement for the first half of the 2-second display and positively correlated with the rewarded movement for the second half. In other words, on trials in which a rightward movement would be rewarded, the visual dots would move first to the left and then later to the right. Under those conditions we might expect that LIP firing rates would be a negative integral of motion strength during the first second summed with a positive integral of motion strength during the last second. The firing rate in area LIP would serve as an efficient decision variable *because* it was linearly correlated with the expected utility of each movement, even though it was not globally related to the direction of stimulus motion.

To further explore these ideas, and to begin to test the hypothesis that neurons in area LIP might encode something like expected subjective value, Michael Platt and I developed an experiment (shown in Fig. 8.7) that allowed us to ask whether LIP firing rates were positively correlated with the probability of reward and/or the magnitude of reward in a simple lottery-like task familiar from traditional economics.[5]

We therefore first trained our monkeys to perform a "cued saccade task," in which animals maintained fixation of a central yellow target while two visual stimuli, one green and the other red, were presented on the screen. After a delay of unpredictable length, the fixation light would change to either red or green, unambiguously identifying one of the two stimuli as the endpoint of a reinforced saccadic eye movement. Shortly thereafter the central stimulus was extinguished and the animal was reinforced if it looked at the target that matched the final color of the central fixation light.

During the experiment, animals were presented with blocks of 100 sequential trials in which the probability that a movement towards the green target would be reinforced might be 80% and the probability that a movement to the red target would be reinforced was 20%. In essence, trials from this block presented (from the point of view of a green target-encoding neuron) an 80% chance of a reward. That block of 100 trials might then be followed by a second block in which these probabilities would be reversed. The monkeys could learn these probabilities as the block progressed, but, importantly, they did not have to do so in order to perform the task. However, if animals are predisposed to take advantage of opportunities to learn about the rewards in their environment[6] and these neurons actually encoded expected subjective value or something related to it, then activity in these neurons should track the probability of reward, as suggested by Shadlen and Newsome's experiments.

What we found when we analyzed the firing rates of these cells was surprisingly clear. When there was a high probability that a movement to

---

5. I use the term "lottery-like" because these particular lotteries resolved to degenerate cases at the end of the trial. Only in experiment 3 from that paper, which is described below, were non-degenerate lotteries presented.

6. In other words, if the expected subjective values of options are encoded before choices are actually made.

the red target would be rewarded, we found that LIP neurons encoding the red movement responded very strongly. When there was a low probability that a movement to the red target would yield a reward, the same LIP neurons responded weakly.

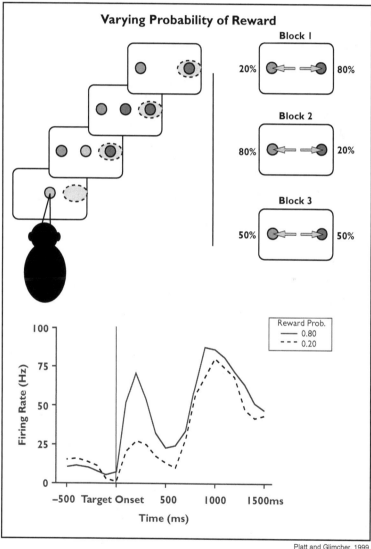

Platt and Glimcher, 1999.

FIGURE 8.7   Platt and Glimcher's 1999 experiment.

Figure 8.7 shows an example of how a typical neuron in area LIP responded during this experiment. Both the solid and dashed lines plot the average firing rate of the neuron on groups of trials in which the fixation stimulus turned red and the monkey looked at that target. Both the stimuli and the responses are identical in all cases. The trials plotted in the solid line were drawn from a block in which the central stimulus was 80% likely to turn red, while the dashed line plots data from a block of trials in which the central stimulus was only 20% likely to turn red.

To determine more precisely what information this neuron carried about the probability of reward, we presented the animal with seven different blocks of trials in which the probability that the fixation stimulus would turn red was systematically varied. As shown in Figure 8.8, firing rate and reward probability are strongly correlated even in this small dataset.

The other major variable that should influence the firing rates of these neurons if they really do encode expected subjective value would be the magnitude of the rewards offered to the monkeys in these "lotteries." This led us to wonder whether these same neurons in area LIP might also carry information about the value of each movement to the animal. To examine this possibility, we once again employed the cued saccade task. Animals were again presented with sequential blocks of 100 cued saccade trials, but for this experiment the likelihood that the fixation

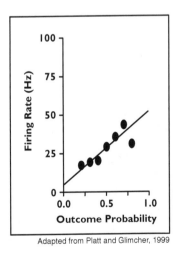

Adapted from Platt and Glimcher, 1999

FIGURE 8.8   Probability experiment data.

stimulus would turn red or green was always fixed at 50% each. Across 100 trial blocks we now varied the amount of reward that the animal would receive for looking at the red or green targets. In the first block the animal might receive 0.2 milliliters of fruit juice as a reward on trials in which he correctly looked at the green target and 0.4 milliliters of juice on correct red target trials. In a second block he might receive 0.4 milliliters on green trials and 0.2 milliliters on red trials.

Figure 8.9 plots the behavior of an LIP neuron under these conditions. Again, only trials that were identical in their sensory and motor properties were selected for use in this figure. The trials differ only in the value of the two movements. Note that the neuron fires more strongly during trials in which the animal could expect to receive a large reward (solid line) and more weakly during trials in which the animal could expect to receive a small reward (dashed line).

As in the previous experiment, we also examined how seven different movement values influenced the firing rates of these neurons early in the trials. Once again we saw that firing rate was well correlated with the variable we were manipulating. Finally, I should add that we were able to perform both of these experiments on a small group of individual neurons. All of these neurons, which were examined when both

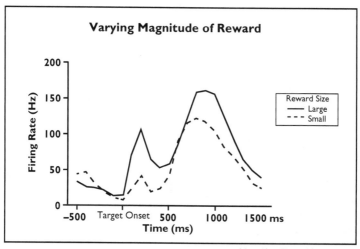

Adapted from Platt and Glimcher, 1999.

FIGURE 8.9   Reward magnitude experiment.

probability and magnitude of reward were varied, were influenced by both of these variables.

Taken together, these initial results pointed in a clear direction. They raised explicitly the possibility that expected subjective value may be represented in the firing rates of neuronal networks *known* to trigger actions, and that this hypothesized representation of expected subjective value arises before those actions are triggered. Indeed, taken with our understanding of the basic architecture of the primate nervous system, these data suggest a fairly structured mechanistic model of the very last stages of the decision-making machinery.

The limitation of these observations, however, is that the choices these trials examine are actually quite impoverished. At the end of each trial we resolved the reward probabilities, revealing which single movement would be rewarded with certainty on that trial. While there did seem to be evidence that an expected utility-like signal occurred in the nervous system, what was troubling was that the choice condition at the end of the trial was really quite unsophisticated. Anticipating this point, we also conducted a third experiment much like the first, which employed what we called a "free choice" task. In that experiment, red and green targets were illuminated in blocks where the expected value for each movement was systematically varied. In those trials, however, rather than identifying one of the targets as reinforced with certainty, we simply allowed the monkeys to choose between the two targets. Under the very specific behavioral parameters we employed in that experiment, we observed that the probability a monkey would look at a particular target was roughly equal to the relative expected value of the target. And we observed that the neurons continued, under these conditions, to linearly track the expected utilities of the two targets. This was an observation later borne out quantitatively in game theoretic experiments of this same general type (Dorris and Glimcher, 2004).

How, then, should we interpret these findings? One traditional approach would be to invoke stimulus–response explanations for all of these observations, except perhaps for those made under the "free choice" conditions just mentioned. Illumination of the red central stimulus triggers a rightward movement. Illumination of the green central stimulus triggers a leftward movement. Like Shadlen and Newsome, we could conclude that the properties of the visual stimuli trigger responses, and

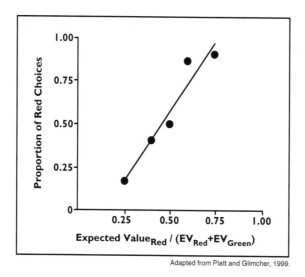

Adapted from Platt and Glimcher, 1999.

FIGURE 8.10   Experiment 3 figure from Platt and Glimcher, 1999.

that when we observe graded activity in these "trigger circuits" we can interpret this changing activity as growing or shrinking "trigger probabilities."

Hard-EU, however, would suggest an alternative interpretation. We know that with regard to voluntary eye movements, three interconnected topographically mapped brain structures serve as a final common path for triggering a movement. When activity in the superior colliculus crosses a threshold at any one location on that map, a movement is generated. We now also have compelling evidence that in the period before a movement is triggered by this mechanism, the activity of neurons in area LIP is correlated with both the probability and magnitude of reward in a topographic way (Dorris and Glimcher, 2004; Platt and Glimcher, 1999). What this suggests is really quite simple: the activity in the FEF, the LIP, and the superior colliculus serves as a topographic map of the instantaneous expected subjective value of each action in the animal's eye movement repertoire under all conditions. This would be true regardless of whether the monkey is in a simple one-target task, in Basso and Wurtz's (1997) eight-target task, in Shadlen and Newsome's (1996) motion task, or in Platt and Glimcher's (1999) "free choice" task.

Instantaneous firing rates under all of these conditions would encode expected subjective value.

Making a choice under these conditions would reduce to the process of identifying the single movement of highest expected subjected value encoded on these interconnected maps and executing that movement. When a movement is about to be produced, a transient increase in inhibitory connections within each map serves to force convergence to a single site of supra-threshold activation. Increases in inhibitory interconnections cause a winner-take-all calculation that is effectively an "argmax" mathematical operation, selecting and executing the movement of highest expected subjective value.

At the beginning of this chapter I said about Hard-EU, "With that theory in hand, the very first question that arises is whether we can find *even preliminary* neural evidence for the existence of a representation of (1) subjective value, (2) probability, (3) the product of subjective value and probability (expected subjective value), and (4) a neuro-computational mechanism that selects the element from the choice set that has the highest 'expected subjective value' and interacts with the movement control system to produce the physical movement that realizes that choice." I think it should be obvious that the answer to all of these questions is an unambiguous "yes." There is at least preliminary evidence for these four processes in at least one brain area.

Of course, it is not by chance that we have found these four properties; these are the core conceptual pieces around which Hard-EU would have to be organized. I recognize that this very brief presentation of the core of the Hard-EU model raises more questions than it answers, and I hope to address most of those questions in the pages that follow. This is a starting point from which the following chapters proceed to develop this model in more detail.

Before turning to a richer development of the theory, however, it may be valuable to respond to a few key questions that immediately arise from this presentation.

More Questions and Some Answers

How can Hard-EU be the right model if both choice and the neural architecture are stochastic as indicated by these data?

The simple answer is that these neural and behavioral data (and many that follow) make it clear that Hard-EU is not the right model. Instead, these data suggest (and I believe upcoming data prove) that hard economic models will have to be based on the random utility framework: Hard-RUM and Hard-REU will be the models of choice.

Why are these simple movements "choices" in any meaningful economic sense?

For any reasonable economist, really interesting choices are about things such as cars and refrigerators. Is there any reason to believe that the neural circuitry we use for choosing between goods and services is the same neural circuitry that evolved for choosing between actions? This is a great empirical question and one to which we shall return in a later chapter. Let me state here, however, that experiments such as these have clearly shown that these circuits encode expected subjective value-like signals even in more abstract decision-making tasks in monkeys (Gold and Shadlen, 2003, 2007; Horwitz, Batista, and Newsome, 2004) and in humans (e.g., Paulus and Frank, 2003; Rangel, 2008). In a later chapter I will describe similarities and differences between decisions about goods and decisions about actions. While the bulk of our available data say that these two classes of decisions conscript overlapping neural circuits, there is reason to suspect that these two classes of decisions may be partially distinct at a mechanistic level.

Do choice and the representation of subjective expected value occur exclusively in area LIP?

This is an excellent question to which the answer is "no." In the eye movement system we have growing evidence that signals such as the ones described here are present at least in the FEF, the superior colliculus, and area LIP. These heavily interconnected areas almost certainly work together with other areas both to represent expected subjective values and to produce choice. Subsequent chapters will present this evidence and will also generalize these findings beyond the eye movement system.

Where does expected subjective value come from; is it computed in these brain areas?

This is another key question to which we will turn shortly. A huge amount of data now indicates that expected subjective value is derived and stored in the frontal cortex and the basal ganglia. There are, however, significant differences between the expected subjective value representation in these areas and the expected subjective value representation in the decision circuits outlined above, differences described in the pages that follow. These are differences that can tell us much about behavior and how to construct predictive economic models.

We know that choice is often not predicted by expected utility theory. When expected utilities and observed choice diverge, does subjective value track choice or expected utility?

This is a critical question for many economists because expected utility has two important features: it can be used to predict choice, and it can be used (if subjects obey expected utility and one accepts the welfare assumption of that theory) to figure out how to maximize people's welfare. So this important question becomes: If subjective value tracks expected utility even when behavior does not, then can we maximize people's welfare by maximizing subjective value?

In answering this question I want to be very clear that Hard-EU and its descendents are first and foremost *positive theories*; they are meant to predict what people (and monkeys) do, not what people or governments should do. Identifying expected subjective value is the process of identifying a variable causally related to choice—that is the core goal of Hard-EU based theories. This causal relationship means that expected subjective value tracks choice regardless of whether or not choice is predicted by expected utility theory. Finding a condition (such as the Allais paradox) where expected subjective value and expected utility diverge is an opportunity to revise the theory so that the neural and behavioral objects remain as closely aligned as possible. Our goal is to produce a successor to Soft-EU that has greater predictive power. The degree to which this necessarily means that the new theory loses normative power will be a largely empirical, and to a lesser degree political, question.

Conclusions

The attraction of a utility-based analysis of choice in economics is parsimony. Under conditions in which a chooser can be described as maximizing something, a utility-based theory is the minimally complex systematic approach. That also means that it would describe the minimally complex system.

Over the past 300 million years, evolution has pushed vertebrates *towards* the efficient maximization of genetic fitness—there is no doubt about this simple fact. There is also no doubt that how much food we gather, how well we escape predators, and how effectively we obtain mates are features of our behavior that are tightly correlated with our genetic fitness. Put another way, evolution pushes all animals towards the maximization of a single function, and the evidence we have is that it pushes hard (Krebs and Davies, 1997). This means that nervous systems are pushed to effectively maximize fitness with efficient neural circuitry.

As the 20th-century behavioral ecologist John Maynard Smith put it in 1982:

> [T]he theory requires, that the values of different outcomes (for example, financial rewards, the risks of death and the pleasures of a clear conscience) be measured on a single scale. In human applications this measure is provided by 'utility'—a somewhat artificial and uncomfortable concept [an opinion Maynard Smith seems to share with Friedman at some level]: in biology Darwinian fitness provides a natural and genuinely one-dimensional scale. (Smith, 1982, p. vii-3)

If we were to take Maynard Smith's point to its natural conclusion at the boundary of evolution, biology, and economics, we would have to at least entertain the possibility that natural selection might have discovered the simplicity and power of a utility-based analysis somewhat before Samuelson and Friedman did. If that were the case, then the search for Hard-EU and its relatives in the nervous system might yield the foundations of a hard economic science. Indeed, our first exploration of the primate choice mechanism gives one hope (rather than frustration) in this regard. The question now is whether contemporary neuroeconomics can deliver a hard economic theory. In the pages that follow, I hope to convince you that the answer is "yes."

9

Stochasticity and the Separation of Utility from Choice

Précis

A key point, perhaps *the* key point, that Samuelson and his colleagues made when they invented the modern axiomatic method was that choices and utilities *are the same thing*. As technically defined objects they are inseparable.[1] Before Pareto, however, utility was thought of as a quantity hidden inside the head that we measured through behavior. Neoclassicists like Pareto railed against this approach *because utility itself was completely unobservable*. If economic theories were theories about something that could never be measured, they argued, then they were untestable theories, of no interest to a real scientist. After this point became clear to most economists, the only reason the concept of utility survived into the 20th and 21st centuries was because mathematicians such as Samuelson and von Neumann were able to demonstrate a perfect identity between the concepts of utility and observable choice through sets of testable axioms. These axioms were constructed to describe observable patterns of choice behavior and were connected to utility through the "argmax operation," the assertion that choosers always pick the best of their options. All of this reasoning made utility and its relation to choice explicit, but it meant that to talk about utility and observable

---

1. More precisely, when our key theorems of representation, axioms such as WARP, accurately describe behavior, then we know that the preferences of our subjects can be *equivalently* described with a utility function having certain well-defined properties.

choice as separate things was to engage in a logical fallacy: choice and utility were two sides of the same coin. We cannot speak, in this framework, of the utility of an object about which we have never asked our subjects to make real choices. If there was no choice then there could, *in principle*, be no such thing as utility.

This is a very important cultural and philosophical point that Hard-EU must address, because neurobiological notions of subjective value and action (unlike modern economic notions of utility and choice) are measurably distinct objects. Hard-EU, if it is to incorporate this mechanistic feature, must necessarily hypothesize that neurobiological notions of subjective value and action are linked by an observable mechanism. In Hard-EU, just as economic notions of utility and choice are linked by the argmax operation, neurobiological notions of subjective value and action are linked by a physical device. In this sense the neural mechanism and the argmax operation can be thought of as isomorphic in Hard-EU. If studies of the neurobiological mechanism, however, suggested that subjective value and choice were linked in ways that

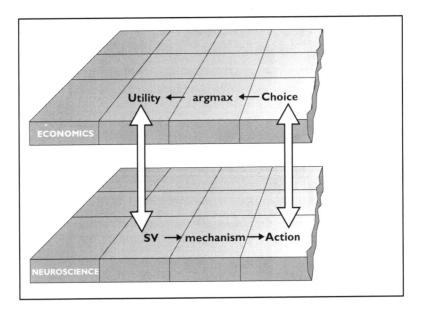

FIGURE 9.1

the argmax operation failed to capture, then this would reveal a critical first mismatch between the logical "kinds" of neuroscience and expected utility theory, a mismatch that would require modifications of Hard-EU. Even the simplest mismatch of this kind would present the first opportunity for a meaningful interdisciplinary interaction aimed at reconciling the neurobiological and economic elements of the theory.

A First Goal

We begin by reviewing what is known about the mechanism that links subjective value to action. The first and most important goal of this examination is to achieve a convincing mechanistic separation between expected subjective value and action. We must be sure that these two objects are mechanistically separable *and* causally related. Neurobiological evidence (by no means all of the evidence) that makes this point suggests that a single mechanism can account for this linkage both in traditional decision making and in reservation-price–based or reaction-time decision making. If we are convinced that we have identified expected subjective value and action, and that these objects map isomorphically to the economic-level theory, *then we can begin to treat utility and choice as separate objects within the framework of Hard-EU.* This profound fact means, among other things, that we can begin to discuss utility in the absence of choice through its linkage with subjective value.[2]

A Second Goal

The second goal of this chapter will be to identify mismatches between economic theory and neurobiological data within Hard-EU and to examine, as a test case, how neuroeconomics should deal with such mismatches. While clear evidence identifies at least a portion of the mechanism that links subjective value and action, the details of that linkage turn out *not* to be completely described by the argmax operation. As we will see, the neurobiological data clearly indicate that subjective

---

2. It may not be clear to non-economists how unattractive this assertion will be for some economists.

value and choice are linked stochastically, rather than deterministically as assumed in Soft-EU. The data furthermore allow us to characterize the details of this stochastic linkage with a precision unavailable in contemporary economics.

We can use this mismatch to see how neuroeconomic theories move through the process of inter-theoretic evolution. The revelation that the neural instantiation of the choice mechanism has highly structured stochastic features challenges us to reformulate the economic-level theory in novel ways so as to better align it with the underlying mechanisms of behavior. In this case we will accomplish that, in an admittedly uncontroversial first step, by replacing the axioms of Samuelson and von Neumann with the more modern axiom sets of random utility theory (Gul and Pesendorfer, 2006; McFadden, 2005). In a slightly more controversial move, we will also be forced by the neurobiological data to introduce an explicit notion of error into choice that is distinct from the notion embedded in random utility theory.

The neurobiological data thus drive us to select, from the existing economic corpus, a particular set of theoretical tools for further study at both the neural and behavioral levels. That is one of the central goals of neuroeconomics; here we see it happen for the first time.

Individuals who are already familiar with both economics and neuroscience may find few surprises here as we refine Hard-EU into a specific form of Hard-Random EU. The principal goal of this chapter is to explore a methodology for studying decision making and learning more about mechanism.

Linking Subjective Value to Action Through Mechanism

Is there a representation of subjective value in the neural circuits that is causally related to action? Yes: Activity in area LIP encodes subjective value in a way that predicts actions when they are later produced. The data from Shadlen and Newsome (1996) discussed in Chapter 8 show that up to half a second before a monkey acts, firing rates in this area are related to the subject's estimate of the likelihood that a given action will yield a reward. Later in the trial, milliseconds before the action occurs, a high-frequency burst of activity in this structure uniquely identifies the action that the monkey will produce an instant later. To take another example, the third experiment in Platt and Glimcher's (1999) paper tells us that when the probability an action will yield a reward is systematically manipulated, firing rates in area LIP track that probability early in the trial. Again, milliseconds before the movement occurs, this pattern of activity is transformed into a burst of activity that uniquely identifies the impending movement. Many experiments have identified this two-stage representation in area LIP (Sugrue et al., 2004), in the superior colliculus (Basso and Wurtz, 1998; Dorris and Munoz, 1995) and the FEF (Schall et al., 1995b).

The Neural Instantiation of the Argmax Operation

The obvious question that this raises is whether these kinds of neural circuits (circuits such as the LIP, collicular, and FEF network) actually mediate this transition from subjective value to action in the same way that the mathematical operation we call "argmax" relates utility and choice. Fortunately, the basic architecture of cortical map circuitry has been relatively well described, and a number of models have now been proposed that describe the general operation of these kinds of circuits. If, as the experiments described above suggest, interconnected maps such as those in LIP and the FEF topographically represent the expected subjective values of actions, then we already know quite a bit about the general computational features of these circuits and how they might perform the argmax operation that transforms a set of options into an action.

To begin to understand what we already know about these circuits, consider a single square millimeter, as in Figure 9.2, of one of these topographically organized maps. A single square millimeter reveals that the cortex is a highly organized six-layer structure with inputs from other brain areas entering in layer 4, predominantly inhibitory connections with adjacent areas of cortex being mediated throughout layers 2 and 3, and outputs from this square millimeter originating in layers 5 and 6.

To take a square millimeter, or *column*, of area V1 as an example, topographically organized inputs from the lateral geniculate nucleus of the thalamus enter the cortex and make synapses with the neurons in layer 4. Outputs to subsequent cortical areas such as MT come from the

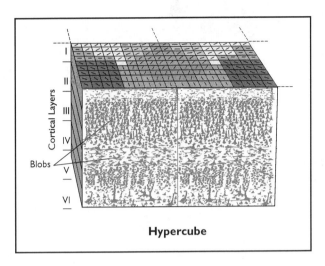

FIGURE 9.2   A cortical column.

large pyramidal cells of layers 5 and, to a lesser extent, 6. The upper layers of cortex serve to connect adjacent regions in a highly structured (Das and Gilbert, 1999; Ohki et al., 2005) and largely inhibitory manner that has now been well described at a cellular level of detail.

We know that the inhibitory connections, the intensity of which can be modulated, serve to "sharpen" the input signals. Put more formally, the inhibitory connections maximize the unique information at each point in the map by reducing the redundancy of cortical signals (Schwartz and Simoncelli, 2001). In the next chapter we will examine this computational process in greater detail, but for now the critical point is that changes in the overall level of inhibition increase or decrease overall activity in a very specific way. As inhibition is increased, the "hills" of activity we encountered in the preceding chapter therefore diminish in size—but in a competitive fashion. High levels of activity at one site in the map effectively work to suppress activity in adjacent sites. The result of increased overall inhibition is thus a process driven by regional competition in these maps. This is a general feature of cortex; one that theorists have argued can be used to implement what is called in neurobiological circles a "winner-take-all" computation (Hertz et al., 2001).

A similar structural feature can be observed in the seven-layered superior colliculus, where this computational process has been studied in even greater detail. In that structure, activity at one location in the topographic map serves to suppress activity elsewhere in the map—again a competitive feature that can effectively allow the map to shift from the representation of multiple input signals distributed across the map to the forced representation of the single strongest input. This shift from the representation of multiple inputs to the unitary representation of the single strongest input is the process referred to as "winner-take-all."

Standard neuro-computational models (Edelman and Keller, 1996; Van Gisbergen et al., 1987) indicate that the collicular network achieves this winner-take-all competitive interaction through two key network properties. First, adjacent neurons in the map tend to have locally positive interconnections that fall off as a roughly Gaussian function of distance. The result is that activity in one neuron tends to enhance the activity of adjacent neurons. Thus a strong input from the FEF or area LIP will result in a self-reinforcing peak of activity surrounding the point of input.

The second key property is remote inhibition. Although positively connected with adjacent neurons, neurons in the colliculus (more precisely, neurons in the central gray layers of the colliculus) are negatively connected with essentially all distant points in the collicular map. The strength of this inhibition rises to a plateau level as a roughly inverse Gaussian function of distance. The result is that a strong input from, for example, the 10-degree point in the FEF map will cause local activation at the 10-degree point in the collicular map *and will inhibit activity at all other locations in the collicular map.*

Three critical features thus determine the activity pattern at any single location on the collicular map: (1) the inputs it receives that excite that area, (2) the inputs other points on the collicular map receive that inhibit that area, and (3) the current overall strength of the inhibitory and excitatory networks of connections throughout the collicular map. Because of these structural features, standard models propose that a movement can be triggered from pre-existing activity either by increasing the strength of a single input until activity at that location rises high enough both to suppress all competing activity and to cross the threshold for burst initiation, or occurs when the overall strength of the inhibitory connections increases until a single winner-take-all site of activation

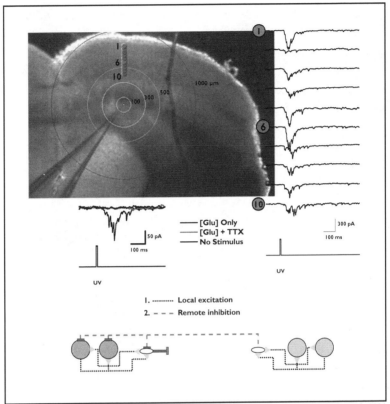

Adapted from Helm et al., 2004

FIGURE 9.3   Pattern of excitation and inhibition in the colliculus.

remains and triggers the burst mode.[3] (As we will see in a moment, these two mechanisms can, in principle, account for both simple choice of the kind discussed so far and very rapid "reaction-time choices" of a kind heavily studied in neurobiology.)

All of these data point in a single direction. One is almost forced to hypothesize that the winner-take-all mechanism studied by neurobiologists in the superior colliculus, LIP, and other areas is isomorphic to the argmax operation proposed in economic-level theories of choice.

_____

3. This begs the question of what mechanism dynamically adjusts the strength of the inhibitory and excitatory networks. We simply do not know the answer to this question yet.

At least as a starting point we can entertain the serious possibility that three key objects in an economic-level theory—expected utility, the argmax operation, and choice—all map directly to three logical "kinds" at a neurobiological-level theory: pre-action activity in areas such as LIP or the superior colliculus, the winner-take-all mechanism, and the bursts of activity that directly generate actions.

If these objects are really isomorphic, that has profound implications for what we can study in *because-style* theories of decision making. Consider a situation in which we offer a subject two options between which she must choose, but we withdraw those options (or alter them) before she can express her choice. *As if-style* economic theories tell us we can, in principle, know nothing about utility under these conditions. In contrast, a theory such as Hard-EU lets us make perfectly reasonable statements about utility, even under these conditions. If, after the initial offer, we observe an expected subjective value signal in area LIP, the logical isomorphism between expected utility and that signal lets us make perfectly reasonable statements about expected utility *even under those conditions.*

For many economists this will be a troubling idea. Economics spent the past century moving away from the idea that "utility is something in the head" because when that notion was first proposed it was fiction. With serious *because-style* theories in hand, that is no longer the case.

Understanding Alternative Models in Neuroscience

While the explanatory story presented in the preceding section reflects one of the central strands in the neuroscientific study of choice, it makes only passing reference to a second body of work that has played a huge role in the neurobiological study of decision making over the past decade and that also turns out to be important for the development of Hard-EU. That second body of research has focused on the study of fast and highly practiced perceptual decision making. We turn next to the powerful implications of that second area of research.

To understand this second body of work, consider a monkey trained to perform the Newsome moving dot discrimination task mentioned in the preceding chapter. In those experiments, monkey subjects chose to produce one of two actions based on the average direction of motion they observed in a field of small flickering spots of light. I argued that we could view this visual signal as a stimulus from which the monkeys computed the expected utility of the two possible movements, and then made their selection based upon that computation.

More recently, Michael Shadlen and his colleagues (e.g., Gold and Shadlen, 2007; Roitman and Shadlen, 2002) have explored a new version of this task in which the monkey is free to make his movement at any time instead of being required to wait for the end of the 2-second display to express his choice. Under these conditions, Shadlen and his colleagues have made several interesting observations about both the behavior of the monkeys and the activity of neuronal cell groups. First, when the motion stimulus is unambiguous, monkeys make their choices quite quickly, never waiting for the full 2 seconds of the display. Second, as the motion signal becomes more ambiguous, the monkeys take longer to make their choices. Third, and most important, under all of these conditions the firing rates of LIP neurons grow towards a specific "threshold level." Once that threshold level of neural activity is crossed, an action is produced irrespective of the ambiguity of the display. Finally, when the motion signal is ambiguous, growth towards that threshold is generally slow, but when the motion signal is unambiguous, growth towards that threshold is generally fast.[4]

Based upon these data, Shadlen and others argue that the process of making a decision can be modeled as the process of mathematically integrating the motion signal (or any evidentiary signal) until a threshold is crossed, at which time an action is triggered. They have captured this idea in a carefully parameterized computation called the *drift diffusion model* (Palmer et al., 2005) that is based on a psychological theory of memory developed in the 1970s by Roger Ratcliff (1978, 1980).

While there is no doubt that we can describe the activity of LIP neurons as integrating the motion signal presented to the monkey as Shadlen has proposed, it is also true that we can view these neurons as computing the precise probability that each of the two actions will yield a reward in a way compatible with Hard-EU. Computing the integral of

---

4. Closely related results have also been obtained in the FEF by Jeffrey Schall and his colleagues (Schall and Thompson, 1999).

the motion signal and computing the expected subjective values of the two responses are, in this task, exactly the same thing; these two statements are empirically equivalent. But what is especially striking about these data is the existence of the fixed threshold for movement generation. Unlike the slow decisions we have encountered so far, where an argmax operation relates subjective values to actions, here a fixed biophysical threshold appears to directly connect some fixed level of expected subjective value to the generation of an action. Why does that make sense?

At the neurobiological level the answer to that question comes, at least in part, from the work of Wei Ji Ma, Alex Pouget, and their colleagues (Beck et al., 2008; Ma et al., 2006). Ma and colleagues were able to show that for a monkey trying to guess which movement would yield a reward, the activity of the neurons in area LIP provided a near-perfect Bayesian estimate of reward likelihood (and thus expected subjective value) at each moment in time. To understand this, consider a monkey who knows in advance (from extensive training) the distribution of trial conditions he will encounter. What, one might ask, should a perfectly efficient monkey do if he wants to maximize the reward he obtains for a given hour of work? The Ma analysis indicates that such a monkey should, in principle, set a *criterion level of expected subjective value*, a threshold, and should make a choice as soon as that criterion is met. In more economic terms, the monkey should set a reservation price[5] for making a movement, and whenever that reservation price is crossed, an action should be triggered immediately.

That suggests an entirely different mechanism for making Hard-EU-like choices under these kinds of conditions. It suggests a mechanism based not on the argmax operation, but rather on a reservation price of the kind described by Herbert Simon (1957), realized neurobiologically as a threshold level of activation. The key idea revealed by the Shadlen experiments is that under these kinds of reaction time conditions we see

---

5. One can think of a "reservation price" as the minimal value at which choosing an option is profitable. What sets the reservation price in expected utility-like theories are such factors as the cost of action and the cost, to the chooser, of time lost waiting for more information. Economists will be familiar with these ideas from the work of Herbert Simon on *satisficing* (Simon, 1957).

a different mechanism at both the neural and the economic levels of analysis. Neurally we see this biophysical threshold; economically we see evidence for a fixed reservation price.

Like the winner-take-all mechanisms discussed above, very complete models of the biophysical process that underlies these kinds of reaction-time decisions have also been developed for areas including the cortex and the superior colliculus (Wang, 2002). Comparing these models to the winner-take-all models proposed for these same structures turns out to be quite instructive. In these neurobiological models, the overall inhibitory and excitatory tone, the level of intrinsic activation present in the network before the trial begins, effectively presets a threshold firing rate for movement initiation. For a given level of excitation and inhibition in the network, there is a fixed threshold for action production. Recall that in the decisions we have encountered so far, the choice network initially holds a fixed set of subjective values. Increases in the activity of inhibitory neurons, for example, is argued to cause increasing competition between these "hills" of activity until only one super-threshold hill remains with activity above a fixed biophysical threshold for action. Theories such as Wang's and Shadlen's suggest that under reaction-time conditions, the level of excitation and inhibition can be effectively preset (presumably based on prior experience) so that whenever a specific minimum level of expected subjective value (a reservation price) is crossed, the biophysical mechanism for action is automatically triggered. This implies that changes in the level of excitation and inhibition in these networks can effectively shift the computation of these networks from performing a winner-take-all operation to selecting for threshold-crossing at any prespecified level of input. In economic terms this would be isomorphic to a shift between the argmax operation and a reservation-price-based mechanism. This is a point first made by Wang and colleagues (Wang, 2002, 2008).

It should be stressed that these models of the cortical and collicular network I have described here, though quite standard features of neuro-biological discourse today, are also undergoing continual refinement and testing. We know, for example, a good deal about the patterns of excitation and inhibition that precede and follow a saccadic eye movement (Glimcher, 2003b; Krauzlis, 2005). We know quite a bit about the microcircuitry of the cortex and the colliculus and how these mechanistic interactions operate. There are many fine details, however, that are subjects of significant debate. Which cell types are the sources of long-range inhibition (Tepper et al., 2004)? How is the strength of inhibition adjusted? There is even some debate about whether long-range inhibition or short-range excitation should be considered the dominant threshold-setting feature of these networks (Hall and Moschovakis, 2003). But the basic structure of these networks, the existence of thresholds that must be crossed for movements to occur (Hall and Moschovakis, 2003), the computation of vector averages with an active region of a topographic map to specify action properties (Lee, Roher, and Sparks, 1988), and the use of inhibitory connections to enforce a winner-take-all decision seem now to be well-established features of these components of the neural architecture. As a result, we can draw the tentative conclusion that these networks instantiate two "choice primitives": an argmax-like operation of the kind encountered in von Neumann and Morgenstern (1944) and

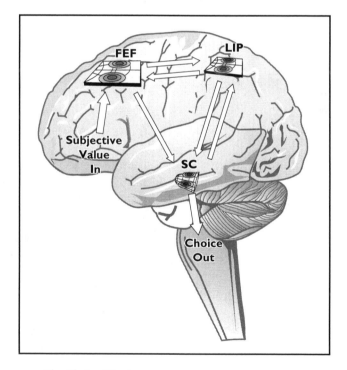

FIGURE 9.4   The Choice Circuit.

a preset reservation price of the kind explored within an extended neoclassical framework by Herbert Simon (1978).

Summary

There are three key features of Hard-EU that we have encountered so far that have important implications for both neuroscience and economics. The first of these key points is that we can think of the standard choice process of economics *Expected Utility* → *argmax* → *Choice* as mapping isomorphically to *Expected Subjective Value* → *Winner-Take-All* → *Action*. Second, Shadlen's and Wang's studies suggest that we can take this a step further and map *Expected Utility* → *Reservation Price* → *Choice* to *Expected Subjective Value* → *Threshold* → *Action*. We can accomplish this secondary mapping in the same neural system responsible for the winner-take-all mechanism, with a single network property controlling both mode transition (argmax or reservation) and the level of the reservation price. Finally, and perhaps most importantly for economics, these data suggest that we can begin to separate utility and choice within the context of Hard-EU.

Stochasticity, Local Correlation, and a Critical Failure of Hard-EU

Neuroscience

We began Hard-EU with the modeled assumption that we choose by activating a circuit that either forces a winner-take-all operation among actions in a choice set, or sets a value threshold for reaction-time responses. What we know about the saccadic network indicates that either function can be implemented as one of two modes of operation that occur in the same circuit, the current mode being set by the activity level maintained in the inhibitory and excitatory components of the circuit. The question that follows, then, is how we should think about the detailed relationship between expected subjective value signals and actions in these networks. Are those relationships fully deterministic, as I have implied so far? To begin to answer that question, we need to examine the properties of cortical neurons in more detail.

Neurobiologists often refer to the firing rate of a neuron as a determinate quantity: "The neuron was firing at 100 Hz." In fact, this badly misstates the actual behavior of neurons. To a first approximation, neurons behave much like statistical Poisson processes (Dean, 1983; Werner and Mountcastle, 1963). Neurons do have a mean spike rate that can be measured over long periods of stable conditions. Measuring these same spike rates over short intervals, however, reveals a tremendous degree of structured moment-to-moment variability that statements such as "The neuron was firing at 100 Hz" fail to capture. For a true Poisson process (Moore et al., 1966; Rodieck et al., 1962; Shadlen and Newsome, 1998; Softy and Koch, 1993), we can characterize this variability in *firing rate* (the number of spikes observed per second) most accurately by describing the inter-spike intervals (the time between successive action potentials) that we actually measure during any given period of observation.

A "Poisson process" is a process that generates events (in this case spikes) with the same fixed probability at each instant of time, a fact captured in Figure 9.5. To keep things simple when exploring this concept, think of time as passing by in fixed intervals of 1 millisecond. Under these conditions we can think of a Poisson process as a mechanism that generates spikes with a fixed probability, say a probability of 0.05, in each millisecond of passing time.[6] If one were to plot the inter-spike intervals of a true Poisson process, one would observe that the intervals between successive events showed an exponential distribution, and the speed with which this distribution dropped effectively to zero would be a function of that probability (Fig. 9.6).

As with any distribution, one can characterize this distribution both by its mean and by its variance (or the square root of variance, also known as the "standard deviation"). For a true Poisson process, an interesting fact is that mean and variance always have the same value. As the average inter-spike interval of a Poisson process neuron shrinks, so does its variance, and at exactly the same rate. Interestingly, the same

---

6. Readers familiar with Poisson processes will notice that I present a discrete-time version of these events. In fact, neurons are not best described in this way, but the discrete-time analogue captures the essential features of the process without significant loss of generality.

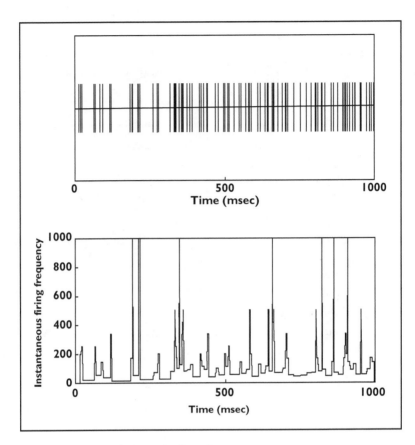

FIGURE 9.5   An actual neuronal spike train.

cannot be said when we analyze the number of action potentials per unit time (see Johnson [1996] for a review). The variability in the number of action potentials per unit time shows a one-to-one relationship between mean and standard deviation. To put all of this more compactly, we can take the ratio of standard deviation to mean, a measure called the "coefficient of variance" (CV). For a Poisson process this number is 1.

The first scholars to carefully examine the actual relationship between variance and mean in cortical neurons were David Tolhurst, Tony Movshon, and Andrew Dean (1983). What they found was that cortical neurons did approximate Poisson processes. As mean firing rates increased, so did variance, but variance grew slightly faster than the mean,

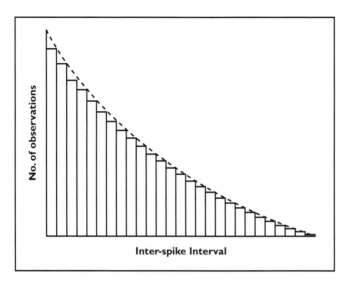

FIGURE 9.6   Idealized inter-spike interval histogram.

yielding an empirically measured CV of 1.1 or 1.15 over the intervals and rates they studied. Their work and subsequent studies revealed that this high CV reflects a Poisson process constrained by incompletely independent sequential events. Neurons cannot fire two spikes at the same time, nor can they fire two spikes one immediately after another, because once a neuron has fired a spike it enters a silent period of mechanical recovery called the *refractory period* that may last as long as 2 or 3 milliseconds for some types of neurons. Neurons also, however, tend to produce spikes in short bursts when the refractory period begins to constrain firing rates. The result is that the true inter-spike interval histogram is truncated and slightly deformed, as shown in Figure 9.7. For all of these reasons, cortical neurons are reasonably approximated by Poisson processes but in fact have variances slightly higher than Poisson.

Let me rush to add that this is a feature of cortical neurons, but not a feature of neurons in general. The dopamine neurons that play such a large role in learning and that we will encounter in a subsequent chapter, for example, have a CV of only about 0.6 (Bayer, Lau, and Glimcher, 2007), a much lower degree of variance than a cortical neuron evidences. In fact, some neurons in the spinal cord have CVs as low as 0.3, a degree

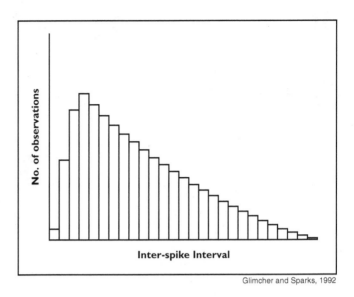

FIGURE 9.7   Real inter-spike interval histogram.

of variance so low that they really are best described as *clock-like* in the regularity of their inter-spike intervals. This is a tremendously important point because it means that neurons are not of necessity high-variance devices. Cortical neurons appear to have evolved to have this feature. Clearly, other classes of neurons have evolved not to have this feature. That is a constraint for modeling to which we shall return, but one that must constantly be borne in mind. In recent years it has become fashionable in some neurobiological circles to see this high variance as a limitation that cortical neurons cannot overcome, a "bad" stochasticity that the brain struggles to defeat when it performs computations. There is no reason, however, that one has to think of this high variance as a necessarily bad thing. Cortical neurons have evolved this variance structure; the question is, what does it buy and what does it cost?

To begin to answer that question about cortex, we next have to think about these individual Poisson-like elements embedded in the large-scale topographic maps we encountered in Chapter 7. Each square millimeter of a topographic map contains about 100,000 of these Poisson-like elements. How are they coupled? Consider a square millimeter of area LIP projecting to a square millimeter of the superior colliculus.

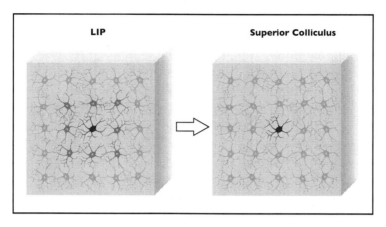

FIGURE 9.8   A square millimeter of LIP projecting to the superior colliculus.

We know that the distribution of synapses from each neuron in LIP to the neurons in the superior colliculus is roughly Gaussian. As Figure 9.8 shows, one neuron makes its strongest contact with a single matching neuron, but it makes some contact with as many as 1,000 neurons in the collicular map. Said from the point of view of the colliculus, a single collicular neuron "sees" the activity of 1,000 roughly adjacent LIP neurons in a topographically weighted fashion; the farther the broadcasting neuron is from the "strongest contact" neuron, the less influence it has on the collicular neuron's firing rate, see Figure 9.9.

Now, consider a situation in which every one of the 1,000 input neurons to our single superior collicular neuron behaved as *independent* Poisson processes, but fired at the same mean rate (encoded the same expected subjective value). By this independence I mean that the fact that one of these neurons is firing at a given microsecond tells us nothing about whether any of the other neurons are firing at that moment. Although all of these neurons fire at the same average rate, they are independent in the sense that their actual spike trains are not correlated spike for spike. If we were to plot the time of spike occurrence in neuron 1 against the time of spike occurrence in neuron 2, we would see no systematic relationship.

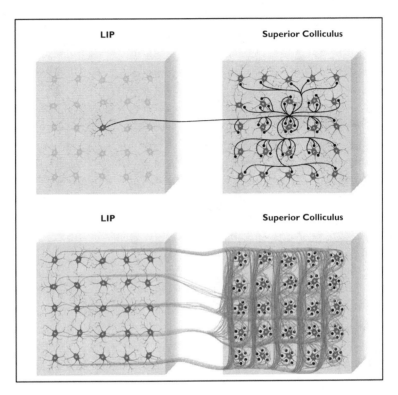

FIGURE 9.9   Connection strengths.

The important point here is that this independence of the spike trains of these neurons would have a profound effect on any downstream neuron listening to all of them: the Poisson variability would be averaged out by the voltage integration occurring in the dendrites of the postsynaptic neuron. If we were to look at the membrane voltage of the postsynaptic neuron—or the spike rate of that neuron, which is known to be a fully determinate function of membrane voltage (Mainen and Sejnowski, 1995)—then we would see the mean firing rate of the broadcasting neuronal *cluster* in LIP in the instantaneous firing rate of the collicular neuron even though each of the individual broadcast neurons was fluctuating randomly in its inter-spike intervals. The fact that each of the independently fluctuating input neurons had nothing but mean rate in common with its neighbors would allow the target neuron to extract the average firing rate perfectly from this noisy signal.

In contrast, however, if these adjacent neurons in area LIP were coupled in their firing rates, if the spike times in the adjacent neurons were correlated, then the membrane voltage we observed in the collicular neuron would fluctuate as a function of the variance of the Poisson process operating in LIP. If the inputs to our target neuron were correlated in both mean and in their variable spike times, then there would be no way for the target neuron to instantly extract the mean rate from its inputs alone. To take an extreme example, consider a situation in which adjacent neurons in LIP were perfectly coupled so that they fired at exactly the same time. If that were the case, the firing rates of target collicular neurons would show exactly the highly variable firing rate structure of the antecedent Poisson process implemented identically in each of the broadcasting neurons.

To put that with greater precision: given that neurons in area LIP have Poisson-like variance, the degree of correlation between the spike trains of adjacent LIP neurons would effectively control the variance of their target neurons. If adjacent neurons were perfectly correlated, their targets would see a very stochastic input signal from which the mean rate of a cluster of LIP neurons could be extracted only over very

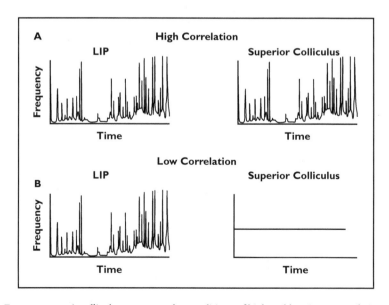

FIGURE 9.10   A collicular neuron under conditions of high and low input correlation.

long time-courses. If adjacent neurons were completely uncorrelated, then the opposite would be true: superior collicular neurons would extract the mean rate of the input LIP population instantaneously and deterministically at every moment in time.

So how correlated are the variances of cortical neurons? The initial answer to that question came from the work of Ehud Zohary (Zohary et al., 1994) when he was in Newsome's lab studying the activity of MT neurons while monkeys made perceptual decisions about moving dot displays. He knew in advance that neurons far apart from one another in a cortical map are typically uncorrelated. Recording from pairs of physically adjacent neurons located within area MT, however, Zohary found a spike train correlation of about 0.12. A correlation of 0.0 would have indicated complete independence of the adjacent neurons and a correlation of 1.0 would have indicated perfect correlation. Using Zohary's measurement as an upper bound on inter-neuronal correlation we can, for simplicity, assume that neurons within a single cortical sub-patch have a maximal correlation of 0.12 and that correlations must decline with distance.

A second observation made by Kristine Krug and Andrew Parker in 2004 (Krug et al., 2004), however, suggests that the story of inter-neuronal correlation may be a good deal more complicated than this initial observation might suggest. Krug and Parker trained a group of rhesus monkeys to perform two motion-based perceptual decision-making tasks that had slightly different reward structures. The first task they taught their monkeys was the standard Newsome moving dot task. The second was a task in which the animals viewed dots moving in front of them that lay on the surface of an invisible rotating cylinder, depicted in Figure 9.11.

When one views displays of this kind, it is often hard to tell whether one is viewing a cylinder rotating clockwise or counterclockwise. The monkey's job was to determine whether he was viewing a clockwise or counterclockwise rotation; if he chose correctly, he received a reward. What is important for our purpose, however, is what this revealed about the inter-neuronal correlation. Krug and Parker were able to record from the exact same MT neurons during both tasks and they found that pairs of adjacent MT neurons had different correlation coefficients depending on which task the animal was performing. When the animals were

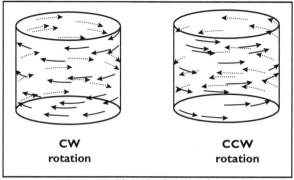

CW
rotation

CCW
rotation

Adapted from Dodd, Krug, Cuminary & Parker 2001.

FIGURE 9.11

performing the Newsome task, pairs of adjacent neurons showed a correlation of about 0.12, as Zohary and Newsome had shown. When the monkeys switched to the rotating cylinder task, that correlation jumped to 0.43. *These data indicate that the inter-neuronal correlation is adjustable as a function of what task the subject faces.*

Now let us put these neuronal studies of variance and correlation together with some behavioral studies of stochasticity and behavior. Consider a human subject choosing between two objects of highly different expected utilities, such as a first lottery with a 50% chance of winning $5 and a second lottery with a 25% chance of winning $5. We observe highly deterministic behavior under these conditions: basically all subjects always choose the 50% chance of winning $5. But what happens when we increment the value of the 25% lottery? As the amount one stands to win from that lottery is incremented, individual subjects eventually switch their preference. Exactly when they make that switch depends on their idiosyncratic degree of risk aversion. What is most interesting about this behavior for these purposes, though, is that actual human subjects, when presented with this kind of choice repeatedly, are never completely deterministic. As the value of the 25% lottery increases, they begin to show probabilistic behavior—selecting the 25% lottery sometimes, but not always.

As shown in the central line of each panel in Figure 9.12 for three typical human subjects facing choices of this type, human subjects show

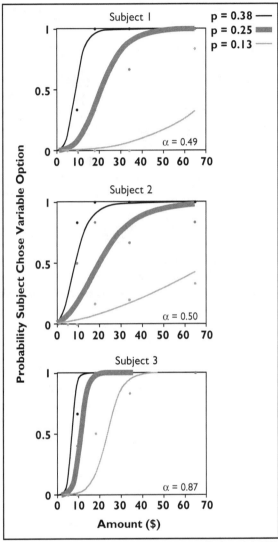

FIGURE 9.12

a *stochastic transfer function*. They gradually shift their preferences from the 50% lottery to the 25% lottery as the value of the lottery increases.

This is a class of behavior that has been well described, and economists typically analyze this kind of behavior in one of two ways. The first technique employed is called a *random utility model*; this class of models has its origin in the work of economist Daniel McFadden, who won the Nobel Prize in economics for their description (McFadden, 2000). The second method is to characterize this gradually transitioning function as a series of errors induced by the choice mechanism. An excellent description of this approach can be found in the Nobel Prize-winning game theoretic work of Reinhart Selten (1975), who called this behavior *the trembling hand.*

McFadden's random utility approach explains this kind of behavior by arguing that when a chooser asks himself what an option is worth, he does not get a single fixed answer when he consults his internal valuation, but instead a variable answer that reflects an actual variability in his preferences. Mathematically, this means that his expected utilities for the 25% lottery (more precisely, his utilities for the monetary prize) are drawn from a distribution of possible expected utilities that have a mean with (typically) Gaussian variance. In this regard, McFadden's approach is essentially the approach of classical psychophysics, discussed in Chapter 4, from which he drew his inspiration. One interesting feature of McFadden's approach, though, is what it says about the meaning of this stochasticity. Stochasticity in choice under random utility theory reflects stochasticity in true subjective value. If I am offered a choice between a 25% chance of $35 and a 50% chance of $5, and I pick the $5 one-quarter of the time, this is because the $5 lottery actually was better for me on that quarter of trials. That conclusion has profound implications for policy, because it means that we do not want to second-guess our choosers even when they behave probabilistically.

Selten's approach to this same problem, although mathematically similar, has very different implications. Selten hypothesizes that subjects have single-valued utilities but that when we ask them to choose, the choice mechanism itself behaves stochastically and this leads choosers to make what we can explicitly consider errors. Put more precisely, Selten hypothesizes that when we compare two utilities, we do so noisily. If the two objects being compared are close in their utilities, our hand trembles as we choose. The closer these two utilities are, the more this trembling is likely to induce errors.

How can we map these behavioral theories, these economic kinds, to the neural architecture? Consider the saccadic choice maps described in the winner-take-all section above. In that section I described the maps as encoding (in their firing rates) the expected subjective values of each option in a choice set. Now let us make that a bit more complicated by acknowledging that the firing rates on those maps—the physical instantiations of expected subjective value—are stochastic. Individual neurons in area LIP and the FEF can be described as Poisson-like objects. That means that for neurons in the superior colliculus receiving inputs from LIP and the FEF, expected subjective values fluctuate stochastically. The degree to which the collicular neurons observe this fluctuation depends critically on the intrinsic variance of these inputs and the inter-neuronal correlations between these input neurons. If the winner-take-all operation is conducted at the biophysical threshold of the collicular units, then this means that the choices we make reflect the well-documented biophysical stochasticity of this system. If that degree of stochasticity is adjustable within limits, then the degree of stochasticity in choice is adjustable by this mechanism.

Let us then look over all of these biologically defined elements and see what constraints they place on behavior. The saccadic choice network

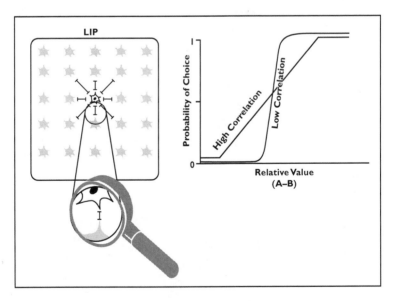

FIGURE 9.13

receives as inputs expected subjective value signals from other parts of the brain. (These signals are the subject of several upcoming chapters.) By definition these incoming signals are stochastic neuronal signals. As we will see, some of these signals arise from stable synapses in the basal ganglia, an area with a low CV. Others arise from stable synapses in the frontal cortex that have a higher CV, likely fixed at 1.15. If, as I will argue later, these are the physical instantiation of stored preferences, then variance in these signals can truly be interpreted in the terms of random utility theory.

These incoming signals then enter the saccadic choice network. Individual neurons in the saccadic choice network receive these signals and encode them in their mean firing rates. Downstream neurons, like those in the superior colliculus, see these mean firing rates (these random utility-like signals) contaminated by the Poisson noise of the individual FEF and LIP neurons that is in turn moderated by the degree of inter-neuronal correlation.

When the inter-neuronal correlation is low, choice robustly reflects the incoming utilities. These are circumstances in which the slope of the stochastic choice function shown in Figure 9.14 is as high as possible and choice is as deterministic as possible. Under these conditions the slope of the choice function is limited by the stochasticity of the random utility signal originating in the frontal cortex and the basal ganglia. When the

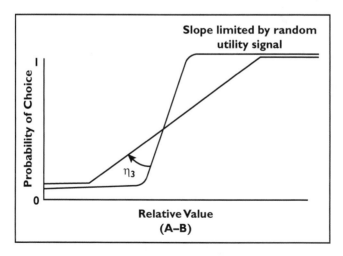

FIGURE 9.14   Flow diagram showing this sequence of events.

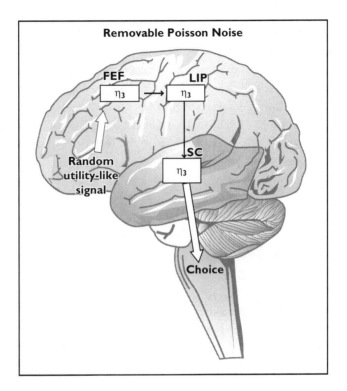

FIGURE 9.15

inter-neuronal correlation is high, then the opposite is true: collicular neurons receive a highly stochastic signal and the slope of the choice function is very shallow. Under these conditions the decisions the device makes do not reflect underlying randomly utilities very accurately; a large fraction of the slope of the stochastic choice functions can be seen as errors—things people ought not to have done if they were trying to maximize subjective value.

Conclusions and Implications

Let me stop here to underline what these findings require of us theoretically. This next step is the critical feature of the neuroeconomic exercise that makes it powerful for economics, psychology, and neuroscience.

We began this section at a philosophical level with two sets of theories. At the economic level we began with Soft-EU and a suite of neuro-biological observations about the mechanistic structure of the circuits that actually make simple choices. In this context Hard-EU was essentially a proposal for mapping these two sets of philosophical objects to one another.

The winner-take-all and reaction-time studies of the saccadic network (and the related networks for moving other parts of our bodies) provided very encouraging information about Hard-EU. Hard-EU requires that the brain represent expected subjective value and that it be able to implement something like a mathematical argmax operation or a reservation-price–based decision. Physiological studies of the brain areas described here provide very strong support for the existence of mech-anisms that perform exactly these operations. From these data we can begin to conclude that Soft-EU-like behavior arises *because* of expected utility-like properties in the human nervous system. There does appear, at least at first blush, to be an expected utility-like object (expected subjective value) in these areas, and the neural circuitry for performing an argmax-like operation does appear to exist. We also found, however, that this same circuitry can be used to set an expected utility threshold for action. Once the expected subjective value of any action in the choice set crosses some threshold, the action is produced when the circuit is set to this reaction time mode. This physiological observation immediately suggests a specific reservation-price–based extension to the core elements of Soft-EU; importantly, the selection of this extension to traditional argmax forms of expected utility comes (at least in part) from the con-straints of neurobiological theory. Here is a place where new behavioral theory is suggested, if admittedly not quite completely described, by neurobiological observations.

The studies of stochasticity are equally enlightening, but in a very different way. Studies of the nervous system tell us that all signals (and expected subjective value is a neural signal by definition) are stochastic. This is immediately a point of dissonance with Soft-EU, a fundamentally determinate theory. It says fairly unambiguously that Hard-EU is the wrong theory. If we want to develop a theory of human choice behav-ior that crosses the boundaries of economics and neuroscience, then Hard-EU fails. Instead we have to modify the objects we employ at the economic level of our theory to make them stochastic. *The observation of stochasticity in the neuronal architecture thus falsifies Hard-EU.*

This comes as no great surprise, which is why I am starting here with this uncontroversial example. Our behavioral data also tell us that expected utility is wrong in this regard. If we want to unite neural and behavioral data into a single framework, we have to shift the economic objects to a stochastic form. Fortunately that form already exists in random expected utility (REU) theory (Gul and Pesendorfer, 2006). To preserve the mapping between the neural and economic levels of the theory, we thus must abandon Hard-EU in favor of Hard-REU. That has to become the next stage in our evolving theory.

On a slightly more controversial note, this specific form of Hard-REU also explicitly includes an adjustable error term that regulates a portion of the stochasticity observed in behavior. This adjustable stochasticity, which arises in the neural architecture, maps to a variable error rate in the economic-level model. Here I intentionally use the word "error" in the economic sense: decisions subjects make that cannot be construed as maximizing expected utility (or expected subjective value). This is, of course, a statement that has policy implications for real economists.[7]

An equally interesting question that this raises is: How is the degree of stochasticity adjusted? What is particularly interesting about this conjoint neuroeconomic theory is that one can ask this question about the adjustable degree of stochasticity at either the neural level or the economic level. How, neurobiologically, is the inter-neuronal correlation adjusted by other brain circuits? How, economically, is the slope of the stochastic choice function adjusted as choice conditions change? These are asking the same question. Although we do not yet know the answer to this question, the answers derived in either the economic or the neuroscientific domain constrain the theory in the other domain.

The neuroscientific data thus tell us unambiguously that Hard-REU is a better theory than Hard-EU. Should we care? If, as economists, we decide to keep using Soft-EU, is that really a bad choice? It depends on

---

7. We already have behavioral evidence for the existence of adjustable error rates of exactly this kind. Daw and colleagues (2007), for example, have demonstrated that some kinds of suboptimal sampling behavior observed during bandit tasks can best be described as errors of this kind.

what we are using our theory to accomplish. If we have a pressing policy question and Soft-EU is adequate, and simple, then we should use it. If we are trying to understand, as scientists, how choice works, then the answer is no, we should not use it. It is a theory that we know is incompatible with the physical mechanism by which choice is produced. It is not simply, as some economists have argued, that Soft-EU is the right theory and measurements of human behavior are imprecise. Hard-REU is simply a better, if admittedly more complicated, theory. If the goal of a theory is, as Milton Friedman put it, "the development of a 'theory' or 'hypothesis' that yields valid and meaningful (i.e., not truistic) predictions about phenomena not yet observed," then the preceding chapter has provided the first gentle evidence that Hard-REU can be such a theory. Hard-REU makes predictions about the structure of our preferences (they are stochastic) and our choices (they include an adjustable degree of error). It provides both behavioral and neurobiological tools for measuring these preferences and errors. It makes novel behavioral predictions about the structure of reaction-time decision making that arise from studies of the underlying mechanism for these decisions. There is no getting around the fact that this theory is more complicated than traditional Soft-EU, but it is also far more constrained by many different kinds of data than is Soft-EU.

10

The Implications of Neuronal Stochasticity and Cortical Representation for Behavioral Models of Choice

Précis

The data reviewed in the preceding chapter suggest that the fronto-parietal choice circuits, at least for the eye movement system, represent the expected subjective values of actions long before a choice is made. Neural data suggest that these networks produce choices either by performing an argmax-like operation or by triggering an action whenever a reservation price is met. Our understanding of choice at both the neural and economic levels of analysis seems consistent.

However, while Hard-REU does seem to reconcile the logical kinds of economics with the logical kinds of neuroscience, we already know that Hard-REU incompletely predicts behavior. That has to be true because the traditional economic models from which it descends incompletely predict behavior. This is an important point. The central premise of the neuroeconomic endeavor is that the iterative process of reductively linking neuroscience, psychology, and economics through theoretical modifications to each discipline will maximize predictive power. Is that true? In this chapter we examine further neurobiological, psychological, and economic constraints on the choice mechanism to test that premise.

First, we will examine in greater detail the relationship between expected subjective value and expected utility, focusing on the inter-relationship between neuronal and behavioral stochasticity as revealed by existing psychological models. We know from economics that efficient organisms are often stochastic but that the degree of stochasticity evidenced by behavior can vary. We also know from neuroscience that the variability of signals extracted from populations of neurons can be adjusted. These two sets of observations can be linked if we accept a small set of interdisciplinary constraints in both neuroscience and economics.

Second, we will examine the precise nature of cortical representation in the nervous system. Theories of cortical representation anchored to normative models of efficient coding identify constraints all neural representations must acknowledge. As we will see, these constraints predict a specific class of choice behaviors that violate traditional Soft-REU, behaviors that have already been observed but not yet linked to the structure of the choice mechanism. This will suggest that a version of Hard-REU that incorporates these constraints has significantly greater predictive power at both the neural and behavioral levels than a model more closely aligned with traditional Soft-REU. These are the final issues we need to engage before summarizing what is known about the mechanism of choice and turning to the mechanisms for valuation.

Expected Subjective Value and Stochastic Choice

In 2004, Dorris and Glimcher explored the firing rates of LIP neurons while monkeys engaged in a repeated-plays mixed strategy economic game, the classic inspection game (Dorris and Glimcher, 2004; Kreps, 1990) developed during the Cold War. In that game, monkey subjects chose between two actions. The first of those actions, *working*, yielded a fixed payoff of a half-milliliter of juice. The second action, *shirking*, yielded either a payoff of 1 milliliter of juice or a payoff of 0 milliliters of juice. The relative probabilities of these two outcomes were, in turn, controlled by the monkey's game theoretic opponent. In preliminary studies with human subjects, a computer opponent had been developed for the monkeys that played the inspection game so as to rationally maximize its own winnings and closely mimic the behavior of a real human player.

Each round of the game for the monkeys began with the illumination of a centrally located yellow fixation target. Once subjects were looking at this target two eccentric targets were illuminated, the red "shirk" target that was positioned so that the neuron under study was active when the monkey picked that target, and a green "work" target that appeared opposite to the red target. Halfway through each round (or trial), the fixation point blinked; when it reappeared colored yellow, the subject had half a second to express a choice.

The payoffs available to the computer opponent on each round (in virtual dollars) were adjusted across blocks while the payoffs available to the monkey were always held constant. Nash (1951) defined the class of optimal solutions to this kind of problem as equilibrium strategies. The Nash equilibrium strategy for the game that the monkeys were playing, in this case, changed from block to block while the equilibrium strategy for the computer was, by construction, held constant. In this way, the block-by-block structure of the game theoretic payoff matrix effectively controlled the probability that the monkey would receive the 1-milliliter reward if it chose the red "shirk" target. The equilibrium probabilities observed ranged from about 20% to about 80%. Under such conditions, what are known in economics as mixed strategy equilibria, the desirability of the actions in equilibrium must be equivalent. *During the inspection game the expected utilities of working and shirking must be equal at equilibrium.*[1]

If LIP encodes expected subjective value, and this physiological form of expected utility is the substrate from which choice is produced, then we can make a novel prediction: at behavioral equilibrium (when the strategies of the players have stabilized during an extended block of trials),

1. This is a rather subtle point that deserves some exposition for non-economists. Nash (1950, 1951) pointed out that in single-round games, the best a subject could do was to select the option that maximized his return (more formally: there is no alternative strategy that yields a higher return) given that the opponent also seeks to maximize his return in the same way. For many games this resolves quite simply. In the well-known prisoner's dilemma, according to this logic the "best" one can do is to "defect." For some games, however, and the inspection game is one of these, one does better (obtains a higher expected utility) by playing a probabilistic (or mixed) strategy. In fact, under mixed strategy conditions it can be shown that the two options being "mixed" must have exactly equal expected utilities. It is probably obvious that this must be the case; if one option had a higher expected utility, then that option would be played exclusively. For a repeated game of the type used here, this is demonstrated formally using a refinement of the Nash approach called a *sub-game perfect equilibrium* that was developed by Selten (1965, 1994). For more on game theory, the reader is referred to Fudenberg and Tirole's classic text *Game Theory* (1991).

the expected subjective values of working and shirking should be roughly equivalent. This should be true even if the actual magnitudes of the rewards earned for working and shirking are very different. It should be true regardless of the probability that the monkey will shirk.[2] As long as the two behaviors are in equilibrium, they should give rise to roughly the same expected subjective value, as long as expected subjective value (the neural object) predicts expected utility (the economic object).

Dorris and Glimcher examined LIP neurons while subjects played the inspection game. Figure 10.1 plots the average activity of a single LIP neuron during four blocks of inspection game trials in the bottom left panel. Across blocks, the prescribed equilibrium strategy (as determined by a simplified Nash equilibrium calculation and shown in the inset) ranged from choosing the "shirk" target 10% of the time (pale gray) to 70% of the time (black). Although the proportion of choices directed towards the "shirk" target differed across these blocks, the relative desirability of the choices should, according to Nash, have remained constant. They found that across these four equilibrium conditions, the firing rate of this neuron, which was strongly modulated by reward magnitude outside of a game in the first two blocks of trials (Fig. 10.1), remained fairly constant.

These observations are significant for us because they conform to, and extend, the hypothesis developed in the preceding chapter in a number of ways. First, like Nash's (1950, 1951) and Selten's (1975) hypotheses about expected utilities in games with mixed strategy equilibria, the activity in these neurons seems to be roughly equal for all conditions, conditions in which the expected utilities *should* be constant and equal. Two other more important features, however, stand out that should help to flesh out the basic theory of choice described in the preceding chapter. First, although not shown on these average firing rate plots, the firing rates are not completely constant; instead, they fluctuate slightly from trial to trial. Second, they fluctuate around a mean value of about 50 Hz at behavioral equilibrium. What is interesting about that number is that it is almost exactly half of the maximal firing rate of a typical cortical neuron. This observation that firing rates at Nash equilibrium are roughly

---

2. And it should also be true in a repeated-plays environment like this one.

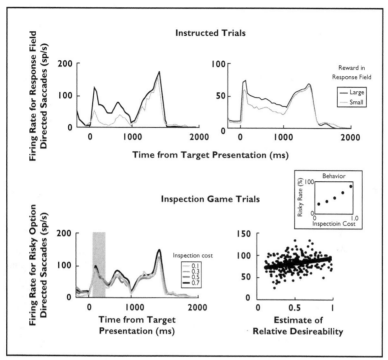

Adapted from Dorris & Glimcher, 2004

FIGURE 10.1   The activity of an LIP neuron in Dorris & Glimcher's inspection game.

half the maximal firing rates of cortical neurons was a widespread feature of the data; nearly all neurons studied had this property.

Neuronal and Behavioral Stochasticity

Of these two findings, the first is easiest to understand within the framework of the theory presented so far. Recall that this is a repeated-play game. The monkeys must learn the value of shirking from experience, and this value changes from block to block as the behavior of the opponent is adjusted. One possibility is that these fluctuations in firing rate reflect trial-by-trial changes in the learned estimates of the expected subjective values of the target, and that it is these trial-by-trial changes in expected subjective value that drive the mixed strategy behavior we observe.

To begin to test that hypothesis, Dorris and Glimcher used a standard model from reinforcement learning psychology (see also Lau and Glimcher [2005] and Sugrue et al. [2004] for more on this standard psychological model) to estimate, at a trial-by-trial level, the monkey's expected subjective values for working and shirking. They then asked whether that model could account for the trial-by-trial fluctuations in firing rate that they observed. Interestingly, they found that the answer was both "yes" and "no." The model could capture a statistically significant fraction of the variance, but not all of the variance. A very large amount of variance remained that could not be captured by the model (which probably was not terribly surprising, but which still has important implications that are discussed below).

At Nash equilibrium, our economic models tell us that subjects must behave unpredictably. When playing rock–paper–scissors it is not enough to simply play each action with probability one third on average by playing rock, then paper, and then scissors, in sequence: one must be completely unpredictable from trial to trial to play efficiently.[3] That the model we used to compute expected subjective value (our psychological model) did not entirely capture all of the trial-by-trial fluctuations in firing rate is thus essentially *required* by the theory presented in the preceding chapter. It is this residual stochasticity unexplainable by any model, these trembles of the trembling hand, that makes behavior at mixed strategy equilibrium unpredictable.

Let me be very clear here about what I am saying. The *mean* expected subjective values input into the fronto-parietal network by antecedent valuation systems are hypothesized to fluctuate from trial to trial. These particular fluctuations (which I am referring to as fluctuations in the mean firing rate) are driven by the recent history of rewards the subject has encountered—a product of the actual choices of the player and his opponent. But these particular fluctuations should not be thought of as random fluctuations in utility (although those almost certainly also occur in these signals), nor are they errors. These particular fluctuations are learning-driven changes in the subject's best estimate of the subjective values of working and shirking that drive behavior towards equilibrium

---

3. Players have to be random in their behavior to keep their opponents guessing.

in repeated play encounters. If that were the whole story, however, these monkeys would be very poor game players. To another species of monkey who knew (or learned through evolution) how their valuation systems derived estimates of the subjective values of working or shirking, their behavior in any game would be easily predicted *and defeated*. To defeat prediction when these learning and valuation mechanisms operate in a strategic game, these monkeys must make their behavior truly random, at least to a degree.[4] That is a behavioral requirement for efficient play in games. In a similar way, we know that the cortical neurons in the fronto-parietal choice networks are highly stochastic and that they have a variable degree of inter-neuronal correlation. The logical consequence of these observations is that the degree of stochasticity evidenced by behavior is controllable. When an animal plays a game and requires a high degree of stochasticity, then the inter-neuronal correlation should be high in these areas. These are situations in which, as Selten might have put it, the monkey's hand *should* tremble. The critical point here is that the cortical stochasticity observed by neuroscientists and the behavioral stochasticity observed during game play can be linked.

Neuroscientists have tended to argue (see Chapter 9) that the stochasticity of single cortical neurons poses an unsolved puzzle. Why are single neurons so variable? Isn't stochasticity in a computational system an undesirable feature? The standard model provides a simple response to this question: we know that behavior must, under some conditions, be stochastic. We have already encountered two examples of this: when sampling during learning and when behaving unpredictably in compe-tition. The stochasticity of individual cortical neurons, and the variable inter-neuronal correlation, provides a mechanism for generating this requisite stochasticity in behavior.

The high degree of stochasticity evidenced by these neurons does not place an upper limit on the accuracy of neuronal calculation (as some have argued), but instead places an upper limit on the stochasticity

---

4. The critical idea here is that there are two kinds of true stochasticity that one might expect to encounter in a system of this type: a fixed stochasticity associated with random utilities, and a variable stochasticity associated with the trembling hand. I am arguing here that we have neurobiological evidence for two such systems: stochasticity in the valuation circuits of the brain (which we encounter explicitly in the next section), and adjustable stochasticity in the fronto-parietal choice circuits.

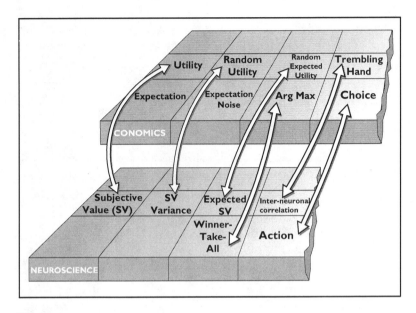

FIGURE 10.2

of behavior. As I have argued elsewhere (Glimcher, 2005) and in Chapter 9, stochasticity is easy to average out by reducing the inter-neuronal correlation in a network of neurons.

Stochasticity is hard to add in, however, at that same level, the level of networks of neurons. The stochasticity of individual neurons has its origin in fluctuations of the membrane potential driven by the true thermodynamic stochasticity in presynaptic release mechanisms and postsynaptic receptors (Stevens, 2003). Stochasticity at the level of these tiny objects, which operate at the scale of thermal noise, is easy to add in. The scale of neuronal stochasticity is thus almost certainly a thermo-dynamic mechanism that places an upper limit on stochastic computation of any kind, and on the essential stochasticity of behavior.

Figure 10.1 (bottom right panel) captures this to some degree for the monkeys and neurons in the Dorris and Glimcher experiment (2004). This figure plots the relationship between firing rate and Dorris' estimate of expected subjective value for the "shirk" target. The solid line is the highly significant best linear fit. The fact that the observed firing rates do not all fall on that line means that there is residual variance not accounted for by the model of expected subjective value we employed. Some of that huge amount of residual variance comes from the inadequacy of Dorris and Glimcher's model, but some also comes from the stochasticity of the neurons, the substrate for the irreducible stochasticity of the animal's behavior—an irreducible stochasticity in behavior that has been documented again and again in human and animal subjects (Neuringer, 2002).

Relative Subjective Value

The observation that firing rates at Nash equilibrium seem well centered in the dynamic range of the neurons is, however, a finding not as easily reconciled with the model presented in Chapter 9. How is it that this was observed? Was it just luck that the particular juice rewards offered in that experiment were worth exactly 50 Hz, or was some mechanism actively centering the firing rates of these neurons within their dynamic range? One obvious possibility is that neurons in area LIP do not encode the absolute cardinal subjective value of each action, but instead encode the *relative subjective values* of these actions. It is possible that the neuronal firing rates are, in fact, actively centered in their dynamic range when the animals were behaviorally at Nash equilibrium.[5]

We thus hypothesized that LIP neurons encode the relative expected subjective values of movements under current consideration, rather than some more absolute notion of subjective value. Dorris and Glimcher tested this hypothesis by examining LIP neurons while monkeys completed a block of trials in which the magnitudes of both working and shirking rewards were doubled and comparing this to a standard block. If LIP activity is sensitive to absolute expected subjective value,

---

5. For an economist, this distinction between absolute and relative subjective value may seem odd, and for good reason. Utility is an ordinal object. Even expected utility is largely ordinal, and such phrases as "relative expected utility" cannot really be said to have any very clear meaning. To understand why the idea of relative subjective value captures something important, we have to recall first that subjective value is a fully cardinal object and must ultimately account mechanistically for transitive choice behavior. Second, and more importantly, subjective values have Poisson-like variance. An economist should keep these two facts in mind as this section progresses. The combination of these two features has important implications for behavior.

the neurons should fire more for blocks in which all the rewards are doubled in value. If, however, LIP activity is sensitive to relative expected subjective value, the firing rate should be the same for both blocks of trials. Dorris and Glimcher observed no significant change in the firing rate of LIP neurons when absolute reward magnitude for both actions in the choice set was doubled.

So what does this mean? One possibility that has been raised by several neuroscientific groups is that this means that *only* relative expected subjective value is encoded in the brain. Schultz and colleagues (e.g., Tobler, Fiorillo, and Schultz, 2005), for example, have argued that the core learning system in the brain (the dopamine system examined in Section 3 of this book) works in such a way that we learn and encode the values of actions only relative to the other actions we could have chosen at that same time. Behavioral studies by economists, however,

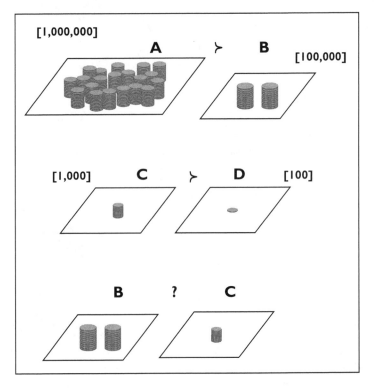

FIGURE 10.3

allow us to immediately dismiss this possibility: any system that stored only relative expected subjective value (the values of actions relative to the other actions in the same choice set) would routinely violate the axiom of transitivity, which humans and animals mostly obey. This is a critical point that is often overlooked. Economic theory heavily constrains neuroscience here.

To make it clear why this is so, consider a subject trained to choose between objects A and B, where A is $1,000,000 worth of goods and B is $100,000 worth of goods (Fig. 10.3). A system that represented only the *relative* expected subjective value (SV) of A and B would represent SV(A) > SV(B). Next, consider training the same subject to choose between C and D, where C is $1,000 worth of goods and D is $100 worth of goods. Such a system would represent SV(C) > SV(D). What happens when we ask a chooser to select between B and C? For a chooser who represents only *relative* expected subjective value, the choice should be C: she should pick $1,000 worth of goods over $100,000 worth of goods because it has a higher learned relative expected subjective value. In order for our chooser to be able to pick B over C, or in more complete theoretical terms, in order for our chooser to construct transitive preferences across choice sets (and to obey the continuity axiom), then it is required that somewhere in the brain she represent the absolute (or as we will see in a later chapter the more nearly absolute) subjective values of her choices.[6] The argument that subjects learn the values of their actions through the activity of dopamine neurons, and that they learn these only as relative values, is incompatible with the observation that humans are largely transitive in their choices.

So what does this mean? The Dorris and Glimcher data suggest that neurons in the choice circuit represent some form of relative expected subjective value, but the fact that humans and monkeys are largely transitive and largely obey continuity suggests that something more like an absolute subjective value must guide choices. How do we reconcile these observations? First and foremost this means that if the neurons in

---

6. By "absolute" here I do not mean to invoke any notion of uniqueness; I merely mean to capture the notion of continuity. An absolute representation of subjective value in the sense I use it here is simply a representation that is not significantly influenced by the composition of the current choice set.

the choice circuit do represent relative subjective value, then somewhere else in the brain a more absolute form of subjective value must be encoded—a representation of the subjective values of actions relative to more than just the options in the current choice set. Second, they suggest immediately that what these neurons in the fronto-parietal choice network encode is the relative expected subjective value of actions only with regard to the current choice set. To economists, this may seem a trivial point with little behavioral implication, but that is not the case: the variance structure of cortical neurons means that if these cells encode relative expected subjective values, errors will arise in a way highly dependent on choice set size. With this in mind, we turn next to variance, cortical normalization, and relative expected subjective values.

Cortical Normalization

Studies of cortical topographic maps have proceeded with greatest speed in the study of the primary visual cortex (area V1) and its immediate targets in the dorsal and ventral streams of the visual system. Early studies of V1 suggested that single neurons in this area could be viewed as template-like *feature detectors*. A particular neuron might, for example, respond to a vertically oriented dark bar on a light field. One way to think of that kind of sensitivity is to imagine that the neuron is essentially searching for a vertical line at the location in space it examines. Adjacent neurons perform a similar search for alternative orientations at that same location in space. For the first decade or so in which these neurons were studied, that was the dominant view: neurons in each patch of V1 were essentially a set of templates, a kind of primitive visual alphabet, that analyzed each point in the visual world (Fig. 10.4).

While a powerful and interesting idea, this kind of approach immediately leads one to ask: How are these templates picked? How does the brain, or our genetic code, from the infinite number of possible templates, select the relatively small finite number that are the neurons of V1? Once that question became clearly stated, a small group of scholars began to look for a more normative way to think about V1. If the neurons of V1 were evolved to encode the stimuli in the visual world, then what would be the optimal technique for performing that encoding?

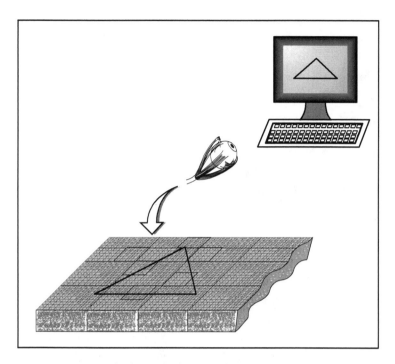

FIGURE 10.4   A cortical column "looking" at a line drawing.

One answer to that question comes from the work of the 18th-century mathematician Jean Baptiste Joseph Fourier. Fourier demonstrated mathematically that any complex waveform, such as the sound pressure wave produced by a musical instrument, could be mathematically described as a sum of sine waves. Sine waves, he proved, can serve as a perfectly efficient alphabet for representing any possible sound. In the mid-1900s the Hungarian mathematician Dennis Gabor (1946, 1971) extended those ideas by describing in precise detail the optimal structure of just such an alphabet for use in the encoding of both sounds and more complex two-dimensional signals such as images.

In the 1970s and 1980s, a small group of neurobiologists (Daugman, 1985; Jones and Palmer, 1987; Jones et al., 1987; Movshon et al., 1978a, 1978b; Webster and DeValois, 1985) reasoned that what was true for Gabor's Fourier alphabet in theoretical terms ought to also be true for image encoding by area V1. There ought to be a normative way to encode the two-dimensional patterns of light and dark that make up visual images, which could structure how we think about V1. Accordingly, they succeeded in demonstrating that the template-like neurons of V1 in fact employ a template alphabet very similar to the normative alphabet predicted by Gabor's work on two-dimensional patterns.

Further study, however, revealed over the next decade that things were a bit more complicated than this early Gabor-based theory had hypothesized. The most significant deviation from the theory was that cells in adjacent patches of cortex were not as independent in their activity as the purely linear Gabor approach had hypothesized. It was found that if a single vertically oriented line was placed in front of a subject, the Gabor detector specialized for that object (and looking straight ahead) became highly active. So far, so good. But if many vertical lines were then placed elsewhere in the visual field, the activity of the initial cell was found to be unexpectedly suppressed. In other words, when a single stimulus was presented in the visual field, the template for that stimulus became active. Under these conditions the high level of activity in that cell indicated unambiguously that a dark vertical line was located straight ahead. However, if there were other dark vertical lines nearby, the firing rate of the cell was reduced in a way that was not predicted by the Gabor model. What a large number of empirical studies began to indicate was that neurons in V1 encoded something about the *relative* properties, not just the absolute properties, of the image.

David Heeger (1992b, 1993) formalized this insight when he proposed that the neurons in V1 encoded a *normalized* response to their template image. Heeger's idea was that the firing rate in V1 could be described as the response to the template image divided by the sum of the activity of all nearby neurons sensitive to the same template image. Thus, Heeger proposed that the firing rate of a neuron could be described as

$$\text{Firing Rate} = \frac{A_i}{\sigma^2 + \sum_j A_j}$$

where A_i is the closeness of the match between stimulus and template for the studied cell, and all the other A_js are the closeness of the match between template and stimulus for nearby cells (Fig. 10.5). In this way, the neuron's firing rate encodes not only whether it "sees" its template image, but also how unique that image is in the current visual world. Finally, Heeger added to his equation the term σ, the *semi-saturation* constant. If Heeger had simply divided the activity of each neuron by the

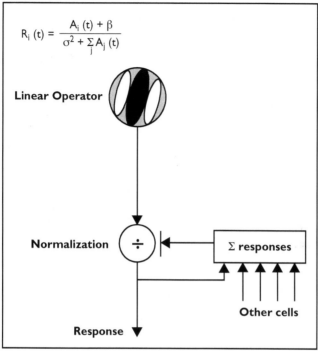

$$R_i(t) = \frac{A_i(t) + \beta}{\sigma^2 + \sum_j A_j(t)}$$

Linear Operator

Normalization ÷ ← **Σ responses**

Other cells

Response ▼

Adapted from Heeger, 1993

FIGURE 10.5   Heeger Normalization.

average activity of the adjacent neurons, then under some conditions the equation would call for unphysiologically linear increases in firing rates. Heeger knew, however, that V1 neurons have a peak firing rate of about 100 Hz and converge roughly exponentially towards that maximum rate, so he added the semi-saturation constant to ensure that the firing rate went smoothly from 0 to a maximum of 100 Hz.[7]

Subsequent studies of V1 have revealed that Heeger's equation does in fact do a remarkably good job of predicting firing rates. Physiological measurements of σ have been made by a number of groups (Carandini and Heeger, 1994; Carandini et al., 1997; Heeger, 1992b, 1993; Simoncelli and Heeger, 1998) and there has come to be widespread agreement that Heeger normalization provides a compact description of the difference

---

7. Heeger also captured the idea that neurons cannot have negative firing rates. He did this by half-squaring the output of the normalization equation and using matched pairs of neurons to encode positive and negative values.

between the idealized alphabet of Gabor and the firing rates that are actually observed (Carandini et al., 1997; Heeger et al., 1996).

If one thinks about it, it should be clear that Heeger's mechanism is also tremendously efficient at reducing the cost, in the number of spikes (which cost us energy), of encoding visual data while not reducing the information being encoded in the overall visual system. Consider yourself viewing a bounded field of vertically oriented lines. What is the information that you want to extract? The edges of the field are the only places where anything really changes in the image. What Heeger normalization does is maximize firing rates at the edges of a field such as this and strongly reduce the firing rates in the center of the field where nothing is changing. Formally, Heeger normalization increases the *joint information* (a technical term from *information theory*)[8] across the encoding elements—the V1 neurons.

Subsequent studies have revealed that Heeger normalization is a general feature of cortex. Heeger normalization has been observed in area V1 (Carandini and Heeger, 1994; Carandini et al., 1997; Heeger 1992b, 1993), in area MT (Britten and Heuer, 1999; Simoncelli and Heeger, 1998), in the temporal lobe (Zoccolan, Cox, and DiCarlo, 2005), and in portions of the parietal lobe (Louie and Glimcher, 2010). Basically, anywhere it has been looked for, this form of relative encoding has been observed.

More recently, neurobiologists and mathematicians Eero Simoncelli and Odelia Schwartz have generalized Heeger's insight to the study of efficient encoding systems of any kind. They recognized that an *optimally efficient encoding scheme*[9] would have to be sensitive not to an "alphabet" of *all* possible images, but only to an alphabet for the kinds of images that

---

8. Using information theory, it is possible to quantify the amount of information carried by any system. Of course, if two neurons carry exactly the same information, then the amount of joint information carried by the two-neuron system is exactly the same as the information carried by each single neuron. To maximize joint information, the second neuron must carry signals that are completely uncorrelated with those in the first, and thus signals that provide new information. For a biological system, this same idea can also be seen in reverse: if we have a fixed amount of information that we wish to encode, and we assume a system that maximizes joint information, we can ask, what is the minimum number of neurons required to carry that information?

9. A system that maximized joint information.

occur in the real world. Consider a visual world where vertically oriented dark lines are ubiquitous. For an animal living in a world of this kind, it would simply be wasteful to fire action potentials to represent the presence of vertical lines. It would be more efficient (in the information theoretic sense, which assumes that spikes cost animals something to produce) for that animal to represent the absence of those lines. Working from this kind of insight, Simoncelli and his colleagues were able to show that a slightly more complicated form of Heeger normalization could be developed that mathematically optimized the information content of V1 neurons, *taking into account the real visual world in which the animal operates.*

Simoncelli and Schwartz demonstrated that to formally maximize information in the V1 array, one needs to represent a weighted form of Heeger normalization:

$$R_i = \frac{L_i^2}{\sum_j \omega_{ji} L_j^2 + \sigma^2}$$

where R_i is the response of neural element i. L_i in the numerator is the response of "detector" i (which is the primary input to L_i) to a stimulus (in our case the un-normalized value of a particular option i). This is divided by the sum, over all other detectors j (options in the choice set in our case) weighted by a term, ω, for each individual detector's influence on element i (which captures the degree of correlation between each j and the common i), times the response of the jth element squared plus the semi-saturation constant. This is a process known simply as the Schwartz-Simoncelli (2001) equation. Simoncelli and his colleagues also went on to show, at an empirical level, how to compute these weights for any given visual world. This will turn out to be a very important point for studies of the systems that store valuations in upcoming chapters.[10]

To summarize, the Heeger normalization story tells us that firing rates in every piece of cortex studied so far represent relative, not absolute,

---

10. The insight here will be obvious to many economists. The Schwartz-Simoncelli equation defines a truly unique scale for subjective value encoding given the set of all possible choice objects and the frequency with which those choice objects are encountered. My suspicion is that this simple equation may provide the central tool for fully cardinalizing utility (via subjective value) in a way that, many believe, largely escaped Allais.

stimulus properties. The Simoncelli story tells us that the precise details of the normalization process can be tuned so as to incorporate the statistical structure of any set of stimuli being encoded by that area. If one needs to encode properties of a choice set with maximal efficiency, the Schwartz-Simoncelli equation tells us how to do that. If one needs to encode the properties of all of the options we have ever encountered, the Schwartz-Simoncelli equation also tells us how to do that. One final note, however, is that both of these approaches tell us only about the *mean* firing rates of cortical neurons. The full *theory of cortex* of course includes the fact that each of these neurons incorporates Poisson-like variance and that nearby neurons are correlated in their firing rates to an adjustable degree. So what does all of this mean for choice?

Choice and the Theory of Cortex

Dorris and Glimcher demonstrated that the representation of expected subjective value *in area LIP* appears to be in relative terms (relative to the current choice set), at least to some degree. When they doubled the values of both options in the animal's choice set, firing rates remained roughly constant, even though we know that when one increases the value of one option, firing rates associated with that option increase.

The pre-existing theory of cortex developed initially in V1 can provide some insight into how this might arise, especially if we add one more feature often proposed in the *theory of cortex* literature. The standard neuroeconomic theory described so far suggests that neurons in area LIP encode the expected subjective value of actions. If, like all other cortical areas studied so far, area LIP employs a normalization of the type Heeger described, then activity in area LIP would be described by something like

$$\text{Relative Expected Subjective Value}_i = \frac{ESV_i}{\sigma^2 + \sum_R ESV_R}$$

where ESV_i is the subjective value of the action encoded by the neuron under study (as supplied to LIP from a more absolute encoding system elsewhere), ESV_R indexes the set of all subjective values in the current choice set (which includes ESV_i), and σ is the semi-saturation constant.

When equations like this one have been studied empirically in the visual system, however, it has been generally agreed that one last term is required to capture the fact that neurons have a non-zero baseline firing rate. Under conditions in which no inputs are provided to a typical cortical neuron, that neuron tends to continue firing at a baseline rate of about 8 Hz. Recall that neurons are physical objects that cannot have negative firing rates. Having a baseline rate above zero thus allows these neurons to encode decreases from the status quo, a kind of "negative value," under some circumstances. To incorporate the non-zero baseline feature into the standard Heeger model, most researchers (Heeger included) have added a baseline firing rate term, β, to the numerator of the Heeger equation (e.g., Reynolds and Heeger, 2009):

$$\text{Relative Expected Subjective Value}_i = \frac{ESV_i + \beta}{\sigma^2 + \sum_R ESV_R}$$

The full theory of LIP would thus be that individual neurons in the topographic map receive inputs that encode a more absolute form of expected subjective value and that the LIP map, and/or its immediate cortical antecedents, normalize that input so as to represent relative expected subjective value as shown in the equation above. Such a normalization would have a number of interesting features with both neuronal and behavioral implications.

At a mechanistic level, one advantage of such a system is that it would always center the firing rates of the choice circuit neurons within the middle of their dynamic range. To make that clear, consider a monkey asked to choose between 1 milliliter of juice and 1,000 milliliters of juice (Fig. 10.6).

Given that these neurons have a dynamic range of about 100 Hz, a baseline of about 10 Hz, and Poisson variance, what would the function that maps milliliters of juice to firing rate look like? If the LIP neurons encoded the absolute amount of juice being offered to the monkey, then the mean firing rate for 1 milliliter might be about 11 Hz and the mean firing rate for 1,000 milliliters might be 50 Hz. The job of the choice circuit would then simply be to identify 50 Hz as greater than 11 Hz using the winner-take-all mechanism described in the preceding chapter. But what happens if, on the next trial, we ask the monkey to

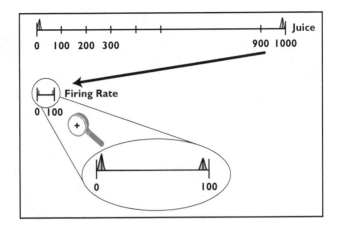

FIGURE 10.6   Mapping of two number lines, one to the other, with variance.

choose between 1.0 milliliter and 1.2 milliliters of juice? We know, as a well-validated empirical fact, that monkeys can make this judgment accurately (e.g., Platt and Glimcher, 1999). If LIP encoded absolute expected subjective value, then we would be asking the LIP architecture to choose between something like 11 Hz and 11.4 Hz. Given that firing rates have Poisson variance, the architecture we have described would make a huge number of errors when faced with this choice, and we simply do not observe errors of this kind.

If, however, the neurons in area LIP represent relative expected subjective value, then this problem does not arise. Under these conditions the normalization process effectively forces the two options apart in units of firing rate. For the first choice set, the two mean firing rates would be separated by something like 90 Hz and, importantly, this would also be true for the second choice set. In the first choice set, the mean firing rate for 1 milliliter might be about 15 Hz and the mean firing rate for 1,000 milliliters might be 90 Hz. The critical point here is that the normalization mechanism ensures that roughly this same gap in firing rates also distinguishes the 1.0-milliliter and 1.2-milliliter choices. The normalization mechanism has the effect, in these two alternative choices, of distributing the firing rates of the neurons in LIP in a way that roughly maximizes the discriminability of the two options in the choice set given the existing cortical variance. That seems a very powerful and useful feature of the architecture that may have significant implications for how we make errors when faced with choices between two objects of varying value.

Even more interesting, however, is how such a mechanism would perform as the number of elements in the choice set grows. Consider a situation in which a subject is asked to choose between two options, A and B. Given that the firing rates of individual neurons are highly variable, we can think of the firing rate we observe at any moment as a draw from a random distribution centered on the mean firing rate with a variance equal to that mean.

Figure 10.7 shows a single such distribution. The average value we will observe on a single trial is, of course, the mean value. But how the value we actually observe changes from trial to trial is specified by the distribution. Now consider a real choice problem. A monkey is asked to choose between 3 milliliters of juice and 5 milliliters of juice. These two options give rise to two such distributions, one centered on roughly 30 Hz and another centered on 90 Hz. These distributions are non-overlapping, so the animal should not make any errors. Now let us add an irrelevant alternative, say an option to consume 2 milliliters of juice. In a system representing absolute expected subjective value, the addition of this third irrelevant option would have little effect, but in a system representing relative expected subjective value its effect will be quite significant because the irrelevant third option is added to the denominators of all other options to determine the firing rate. What that means is that

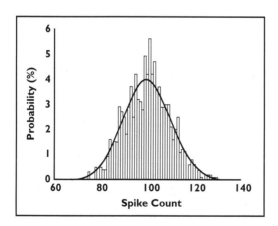

FIGURE 10.7

the firing rate decreases for both the 5-milliliter option and the 3-milliliter option, simply because the 2-milliliter option has been introduced. Importantly, this decrease in mean rate *is not* accompanied by an equally large decrease in variability. Recall that real neurons have CVs greater than 1. The result of this is that as the means fall due to normalization, the *effective neuronal variability* grows. Errors by the chooser thus increase in frequency as the size of the choice set grows, and the quantitative properties of these errors should, at least in principle, be computable from neuronal measurements of the Heeger normalization equation.

To summarize, the relative encoding system employed by cortex has a number of features of interest, if we conclude that choice occurs in this kind of tissue. The normalization mechanism suggests that behavioral errors on small choice sets should be rare—rarer than might be predicted by standard random utility models, rarer than might be predicted from a simple estimation of value experiment, and much rarer than might be expected from multi-option studies of valuation. But the converse is also true: this architecture would perform very poorly as choice set size grows. Error rates would increase with choice set size, and beyond a certain point, choice would appear largely random.

There does seem to be some evidence that choice set size can have an impact on error rates, and this has recently become an active area of research in behavioral economics.[11] In perhaps the most famous study of

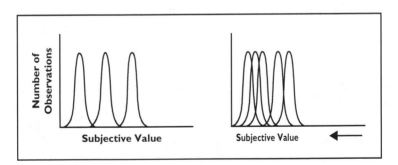

Figure 10.8

---

11. This area of research is controversial. No irrefutable study has demonstrated that having more options in a choice set increases error rates more than might be predicted by simple additive models of choice among objects having random expected utilities. However, many studies conducted over the past three decades hint at this possibility.

this class, Sheena Iyengar and her collaborator Mark Lepper (Iyengar and Lepper, 2000) examined the effects of choice set size in supermarket shoppers. In that study, Iyengar set up a table in a supermarket and displayed either 6 or 24 flavors (the number varied from day to day in a random manner) of an up-market brand of jellies, jams, and marmalades. They offered people visiting the supermarket the opportunity to taste as many of the flavors as they liked, and then gave the participants a coupon that offered a $1 discount on any flavor of the jellies, jams, and marmalades made by that company.

Iyengar found that subjects who had come on days when they displayed only 6 flavors had about a 30% chance of buying a jar. In contrast, subjects who had visited their sampling table on days when 24 options were presented had only a 3% chance of buying a jar! Adding options decreased the chance that the subjects would make a purchase.

Perhaps more directly relevant is the observation by these same scientists that the likelihood subjects will report satisfaction when asked to choose among chocolate truffles depends on the number of types of chocolate truffles from which they must choose. In that study, subjects were asked to select a single chocolate from among either 6 or 30 options. Subjects who chose from among 6 options were more satisfied with the chocolate they chose and were more likely to buy a $5 box of chocolates at the end of the experiment.

These data, and data like them about hypothetical choices studied explicitly with random utility models (DeShazo and Fermo, 2002), suggest that as the size of the choice set grows, the number of errors increases and the likelihood that a given option will rise above threshold for purchase drops. It seems hard to believe that this is unrelated to the structure of the choice mechanism that has been observed empirically by neurobiologists. Even more interesting is the possibility that neuronal measurements could be used to provide quantitative models of this process.

Empirical Measurements of Relative Expected Subjective Value

To begin to examine these issues empirically, Louie and Glimcher (2010) examined the effect of choice set size on mean firing rate in LIP in an effort to test the hypothesis that Heeger normalization described LIP firing rates. To do that, monkeys were presented with one, two, or three targets while fixating on a central point. The three targets, A, B, and C, each had a unique value: A yielded 0.5 milliliters of juice, B yielded 1.0 milliliter of juice, and C yielded 2.0 milliliters of juice. Louie and Glimcher measured the response of a neuron encoding the expected subjective value of target B as a function of what other targets were present. They found that the Heeger equation did an excellent job of characterizing the firing rates of these LIP neurons.

When the B target was the only target present, they observed a high firing rate that was diminished when a second, larger-value target appeared and diminished further when a third, lower-value target was also presented.

In more quantitative detail, what they were able to do was to measure the responses of LIP neurons under seven different relative value conditions. They found that firing rates under all of these conditions were well described by the Heeger equation, and they were able to derive estimates of σ and β from their neuronal measurements.

One interesting feature of the estimates of σ and β that they derived is that they suggest the choice mechanism should show low error rates

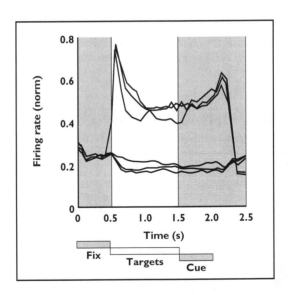

FIGURE 10.9   Single Neuron from Louie and Glimcher.

when choice set sizes are smaller than around six elements. Their data suggest, however, that once choice set size grows to above eight elements under conditions such as these, error rates should start to become quite significant. That is of particular interest because work by people such as Iyengar suggests that human choice mechanisms become particularly error-prone when choice set size begins to exceed eight, an observation that may be a coincidence, but that does suggest that quantitative studies of neuronal mechanism may be of value in predictive modeling.

Together, these data call for another revision of the standard model we have been developing. Chapter 9 made it clear that the standard model would employ a random expected subjective value signal, with an adjustable error term, to predict behavior. Inter-theoretic linkages thus require that the behavioral form of the standard model is a hybrid form of random expected utility theory, Hard-REU.

These data suggest a further constraint that is more startling. The precise variance structure and normalization mechanism in standard models of cortex make novel predictions about choice behavior. These data suggest that as choice set size increases, error rates increase. Formally, one must note that this model thus predicts stochastic violations of the independence axiom and, in very large choice sets, essentially predicts that the independence axiom is ignored by choosers.

This is a tremendously important point, a turning point in this presentation, and one that differentiates the standard model presented here (and the neuroeconomic approach in general) from traditional neoclassical economics and traditional behavioral economics. Traditional neoclassical economic models suggest that set size is irrelevant. Objects such as the traditional independence axiom (or perhaps more accurately the separability axiom) capture this idea. For some time, behavioral economists have observed that choice set size does seem to have a profound effect on behavior. Most efforts to describe these effects have relied on heuristic models of choice that have neither explicit axiomatic foundations nor quantitative mechanistic features.[12]

---

12. Although Emir Kamenica (2008) has developed a neoclassical model in which the existence of large choice sets signals to choosers that there may be problems in the marketplace that are best addressed by refraining from choosing.

The standard model of cortical function, when applied to topographic choice structures, provides a different way of thinking about these same issues. It is a fully described mechanism, which can be modeled down to the level of molecules, that makes a clear prediction about behavior. It says that the degree to which choices obey a stable preference ordering depends on set size, σ, and β—*all of which are observable variables* for a neuroeconomist.

Of course, in any real sense, the Heeger normalization model and the "standard" formulation of that model for choice presented here are only first-pass approximations. For example, we do not yet have a testable set of axioms describing how neuronal variance and set size influence behavior. Of course, we could have such a model; there is no intellectual barrier to the generation of such models, only a social one.

11

Putting the Choice Mechanism Together: A Summary

Précis

Over the past two decades, a tremendous amount of data has been gathered both about how the mammalian brain performs computations and about the final common path for movement control. The combination of these neurobiological data, what we know about the behavioral properties of mammalian decision making and what we know about the logic of choice, imposes serious constraints on any algorithmic model of this process. In this chapter we review the major features of any model that respects these constraints, and in subsequent chapters we turn to the valuation circuits of the brain that provide the inputs upon which the final common path for choice operates.

It is important to note that much of the specific neurobiological data that shapes our understanding of the structure of the final common path comes from studies of monkeys making eye movements. The general computational principles that the model I present here employs are central features of any mammalian brain, but many of the specific computational details of the choice-making architecture are extrapolations from studies of the saccadic system. That, of course, raises many questions about the generalizability of the model. Can the model be extended to predictions about arm movements? Does the model apply to humans making choices? Can the model be extended to more abstract choices between "goods" rather than simply choices between concrete actions? There are compelling reasons to believe that the answer to each of these questions is "yes," and this chapter includes answers to those questions.

Before answering those questions we conclude our examination of the choice architecture by reviewing the key features of the model.

Summary of the Choice Mechanism

Two parallel networks govern the generation of skeletomuscular (hand/ arm) and eye movements. In the case of eye movements, the key elements in this network are the area LIP, the FEF, and the superior colliculus. These areas are heavily and reciprocally interconnected. In the case of arm and hand movements, the key elements in the control network are the anterior parietal cortex (areas 5 and 7 including the parietal reach region), the premotor cortex, the supplementary motor area, and area MI.

While there is important specialization within each of the sub-areas, the outputs of these networks (principally through the colliculus and MI) unarguably lead to the generation of movements. These networks are the final common paths through which all actions flow and through which all choice must be expressed.

Activity in these topographic maps defines the broad structural features of the final stage of any model of choice and action. Before movements occur, more than one movement is often represented

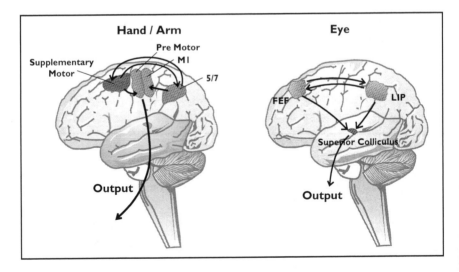

FIGURE II.I   The two motor control systems.

simultaneously in each of these areas. This is true in the monkey eye movement areas (e.g., Glimcher and Sparks, 1992), in the monkey skeletomuscular control areas (e.g., Tanji and Evarts, 1976), and even in the human brain (Curtis and Connolly, 2008). Just before a movement is produced, one pattern of activity dominates all of the component maps within the arm or eye movement circuitry, and that pattern of activity predicts the mechanistic features of the upcoming movement. This is a fact that first became apparent as long ago as the late 1970s (Tanji and Evarts, 1976).

Biophysical studies of these areas, and particularly of the superior colliculus, tell us quite a bit about how this transition from multiple movements to single movements occurs. The different locations within each of these topographic maps are connected to one another in two different ways. Short-range connections within the maps are excitatory, while long-range connections are inhibitory. The result is that single foci of activity within the map recruit the activity of their immediate neighbors while inhibiting the activation of other areas in the map. This architecture, which has been observed throughout the primate neuraxis, effectively causes foci of activity in each map to compete for control of overall map activation.

Movements arise in the colliculus when activity at one focus exceeds the fixed biophysical threshold of the burst neurons, triggering movement generation. That threshold can be crossed either because the input signals to one focus drive that region of the map above a critical firing rate, or because sudden changes in network *tone*, the static state of the short-range excitatory and long-range inhibitory connections, force an acute intra-focal competition for control of the burst neurons. Similar processes appear to occur in the interaction between M1 and the spinal cord.

The inputs to these networks, inputs that ultimately set the firing rates in the colliculus and M1, thus govern what movement will be produced. If we look at activity in these maps long before a movement is generated and see two movements represented, it is now clear that the movement associated with the higher firing rate is the movement more likely to be produced (e.g., Shadlen and Newsome, 1996). The larger the difference in firing rates between these two foci, the more lopsided is the likelihood that the more active focus, rather than the less active focus, will yield a movement. The strength of activity at a single focus and the likelihood that the movement encoded by that focus will be produced are positively correlated. This is a robust and uncontroversial finding.

If we increase the magnitude of reward associated with one movement, we increase both the probability that the movement will be made and the activity associated with that movement focus in the maps of the final common path (e.g., Platt and Glimcher, 1999). If we increase the probability that a particular movement will yield a reward, both the firing rate associated with that movement and the movement likelihood increase together. If we indicate with an ambiguous and temporally continuous signal, such as a field of moving dots, the probability that a particular movement will be rewarded, then both the firing rates of the neurons associated with that movement and the likelihood of that movement being produced grow continuously together in time (e.g., Gold and Shadlen, 2001). None of this is controversial.

Perhaps the most striking features of these observations are the similarities they show to the kinds of "as if" models developed by economists in the first half of the 20th century. Samuelson, Friedman, von Neumann, and those who followed them argued that human choice behaves *as if* a quantity called expected utility were associated with each action available to a chooser. The actions we choose to take, they hypothesized, are those among our options that have the highest expected utility. Indeed, they demonstrated mathematically that, at least under some conditions, it is exactly as if the options in a choice set each had an expected utility associated with them and then the action having the highest expected utility somehow gained control of a chooser—it was realized in choice. Again, none of that is really controversial.

Surely, for anyone who believes that our actions are the product of events occurring in the physical world, these two sets of observations, the neuroscientific and the behavioral, must be related. Human choice must behave the way it does *because* of these patterns of activity in the movement control networks.

The Choice Mechanism in Action

In an effort to demonstrate the operation of the choice mechanism, Louie and Glimcher (2010) performed a simultaneous behavioral and

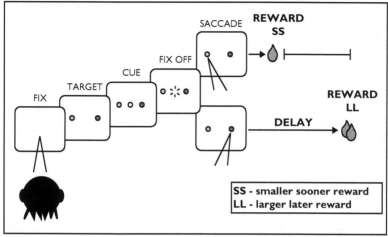

Adapted from Louie and Glimcher, 2010

FIGURE 11.2   The Louie and Glimcher Task.

neurobiological experiment on monkeys making economic choices between two options. In their experiment, the monkeys were asked to choose between a small immediately available fruit juice reward and a larger reward available after a variable delay.

On a typical day, a monkey might be asked to choose between 0.13 milliliters of immediately available juice and 0.2 milliliters of juice available after a delay of 0 seconds, 2 seconds, 4 seconds, 8 seconds, or 12 seconds. A typical monkey might be willing to wait 2, 4, or 8 seconds for this larger reward, but not 12 seconds.

From many measurements of this type made on each of two monkeys, Louie and Glimcher were able to describe the *discounted utilities*[1] for fruit juice rewards for each of their two animals. They were able to show that the animals behaved exactly as if the value of juice to the animals declined as a fixed function of delay. Interestingly, they found that each of the two

---

1. "Discounted utilities" are utilities that have been corrected, in terms of subjective value, for the fact that any reward is worth less if you have to wait for it. Patient people are those for whom utilities decline slowly with delay. Impulsive people are those for whom utilities decline rapidly with delay. These functions have also been related, by Lee and colleagues, to activity in the dorsolateral prefrontal cortices of monkeys (Kim, Wang, and Lee, 2008).

monkeys was different. One was more patient: he behaved as if the discounted utilities of the juice declined slowly with delay. The other was more impatient: he behaved as if the discounted utilities of the juice declined rapidly with delay.

At the same time that these monkeys were making these behavioral choices, Louie and Glimcher also measured the activity of LIP neurons. On each trial they started measuring LIP activity when a choice was first put to the animals and continued their measurement until the monkeys actually expressed their choices with an eye movement. They found that the activity in LIP *immediately after a pair of options was presented* to the animals was a very specific function of delay. When 0.2 milliliters of juice was offered at a delay of 0 seconds, the neurons were highly active, but the firing rates of the neurons were lower if that same reward was offered with a delay of 2 seconds and even less active if the same reward was offered at a delay of 4 seconds. Firing rate in LIP declined as a measurable function of delay, and those functions were different for the two animals. For the patient monkey, these firing rates declined slowly with delay; for the impatient monkey, the firing rates declined rapidly.

Perhaps most strikingly, when the neuronal firing rate as a function of delay for each monkey was compared to the behavioral discounted utility function for that monkey, the two functions were found to be truly identical. The monkeys were behaving exactly "as if" the firing rates in area LIP measured immediately after option presentation were guiding their later choices.

Louie and Glimcher next followed the activity in area LIP during the course of each trial. What they found was that the activity in the LIP network evolved as the time of behavioral choice, the time at which the animal expressed his action, approached. The less active focus declined slightly in strength shortly before the action was produced and the more active focus increased rapidly and strongly in strength until it reached a high peak of activity a few tens of milliseconds before the movement was produced. It appeared as if the monkeys were behaving the way they were *because* the initial firing rates in area LIP were driving a winner-take-all operation that produced their choices.

At its core the experiment was a validation of the hard-neoclassical approach first presented in Chapter 6. There was very little "as if" about these findings. Behavior seemed to occur *because* of these firing rates.

But these findings (like many before them) also challenged the detailed axioms of traditional Hard-EU in two ways. First, the firing rates of the neurons were highly stochastic, and this stochasticity was reflected to some degree in the behavior. Second, the functions that related *both* firing rate and choice to delay were hyperbolic—a class of function that violates most neoclassical axioms for understanding inter-temporal choice (e.g., Fishburn and Rubinstein, 1982). So the Louie and Glimcher experiments did two things. They seemed to validate the general kinds of theories embodied by Hard-EU while violating many of the specific axioms of which Hard-EU is built. Of course, those are the two core features of the neuroeconomic approach. The data make it clear that a hard-economic theory is possible, but they also make it clear that our current economic theory, Hard-EU, is inadequate.

Hard-EU, Hard-REU, and Relative Expected Subjective Value

What experiments such as the Louie and Glimcher study tell us is that the basic structure of the choice mechanism is broadly similar to the one imagined by the neoclassical program, but some modifications to that theory are required.

Topographically organized neurons in the choice circuit represent, in their *mean* firing rates, the *relative expected subjective value* of the action they encode. This signal is supplied from the valuation areas of the brain and is therefore stochastic. The degree of stochasticity in this input signal reflects the properties of the valuation circuits, which are described in coming chapters. The input subjective values are thus reasonably well described as random expected utilities; input subjective values are linearly correlated with random expected utilities when (but *only* when) random expected utilities stochastically predict choice.

Once these stochastic subjective values are in the fronto-parietal choice network, they are normalized.[2] Mean normalized activity at any topographic point in the network can be described by the equation

---

2. Exactly where this normalization occurs first is not yet known.

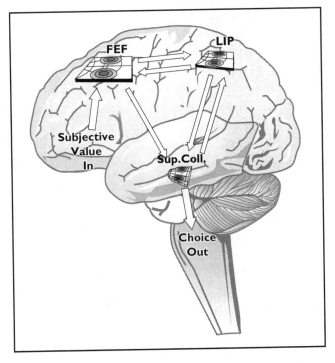

FIGURE 11.3   The Saccadic Choice Architecture.

$$\text{Relative Expected Subjective Value}_i = \frac{ESV_i + \beta}{\sigma^2 + \sum_R ESV_R}$$

where ESV_i is the instantaneous expected subjective value of the action encoded at that location in the map, ESV_R are the instantaneous expected subjective values of all of the actions encoded on the map, β is the baseline firing rate of the neuron, and σ is the semi-saturation constant.

For each individual cortical neuron, this describes the instantaneous mean rate of that neuron.[3] The instantaneous firing rate, however, reflects two different sources of variance: the first is variance in the valuation signal and the second is variance intrinsic to the choice network. We know that these neurons in the choice network are Poisson-like devices

---

3. "Instantaneous mean" refers to the fact that the input subjective values do in fact fluctuate stochastically; they are essentially random utilities.

with coefficients of variation of about 1.15. To simplify things for this presentation, we can approximate them as having Poisson variance. This means that *inter-spike intervals* (the reciprocal of instantaneous firing rate) can be thought of as showing an exponential distribution around this mean with a variance equal to that mean and a standard deviation equal to the square root of that mean.

It should be noted that at the level of the superior colliculus, which receives input from both the FEF and area LIP, the stochasticity of this relative expected subjective value signal attributable to the choice circuit can be reduced. The stochasticity of the relative expected subjective value signal coming from areas such as LIP can be reduced back towards the stochasticity of the input valuation signal by de-correlation of the cortical neurons. When adjacent neurons are highly correlated, the collicular threshold receives a relative expected subjective value signal that has Poisson variance. When adjacent cortical neurons are completely uncorrelated, the only residual variance is that of the random-expected-utility–like signal that served as the input to the choice network. At a behavioral level, this means that the slope of the "logit" or "softmax" function that relates the relative values of two options to choice probability can be actively adjusted by the inter-neuronal correlation within some limited dynamic range.

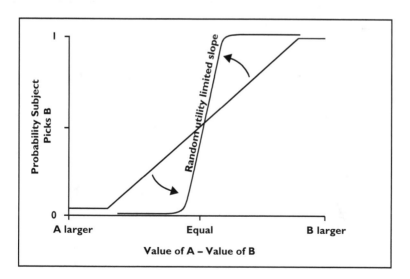

FIGURE 11.4   Limits to the adjustable stochasticity of behavior.

Choice occurs, in this circuit, when activity at one point in the topographic map exceeds a biophysically defined firing rate threshold, above which a choice is triggered. This does not mean that choice necessarily occurs when input expected subjective value has a particular magnitude. This is because the inhibitory and excitatory tone of the collicular network is adjustable. At the level of the collicular thresholding neurons (a class of cells called the *burst neurons*), the noisy relative expected subjective value signal at one focus of activity is subjected to inhibition by all other active foci. It is also subject to self-excitation. The result of these two degrees of freedom is that the threshold for movement generation by the burst neurons can effectively be adjusted, a point first made clearly by Xiao-Jing Wang and his colleagues (Liu and Wang, 2008; Lo and Wang, 2006). The system can thus operate in two modes. In the first mode, a sudden change in inhibitory and excitatory tone can be used to force the selection of a single action for execution at a given time as a winner-take-all operation. This is a mode that corresponds to traditional utility-based choice models that employ an argmax-like operation. In this mode, a sudden change in inhibitory and excitatory tone effectively forces the selection of a single action for execution at a given time as a winner-take-all operation. The rate at which this change in tone occurs, effectively the time window of integration for the convergence process, may also serve to adjust the stochasticity of the observed choice function. This is the mode in which the circuit operates in, for example, the Louie and Glimcher experiments described above. In the second mode, a minimum instantaneous expected subjective value "trigger level" can be set. Whenever the input signal exceeds that level, a movement is immediately generated. This mode corresponds to reservation-price–based models of Simon (1955, 1978), and this is the mode in which the circuit operates in, for example, the Roitman and Shadlen (2002) studies of reaction-time decision making. These are the basic features of the choice circuit as we understand it today.

Beyond Eye Movements and Monkeys

It is clear that we know a lot about monkey saccadic decision making. How much do we know about the mechanisms humans use to choose spouses (typically a threshold-crossing decision) or cars (perhaps more frequently a winner-take-all decision)? The model of choice presented up to this point defines an option in a choice set as an eye movement for a monkey, and for any serious economist that has to be troubling, for three reasons. First, we humans make very few economically relevant choices with our eyes under natural conditions. Second, we are not monkeys. Third, the objects of choice in the standard neuroeconomic model are actions, and it is not immediately clear that choices between actions and choices between spouses or cars are really the same thing. Before turning to the valuation circuits of the brain (which have been heavily studied in humans), we review these limitations of the standard neuroeconomic model.

We Do Not Make Choices with Our Eyes

There is no doubt that we make behavioral choices, on a moment-by-moment basis, about where to look. We do not stare at strangers on the subway; we glance at them only briefly. We stare deliberately at potential mates. Can we really build a mechanistic theory of choice on this limited saccadic foundation? My answer to this question, unsurprisingly, is "yes." Over the past two decades, it has become more and more apparent that when we identify a computational principle in one brain area, it is almost always at play in others. When we observe a general computational principle at work in three brain areas, it has almost always turned out to be of broad significance. It is for this reason that what we have learned about the saccadic decision-making system can almost certainly be broadly applied to the study of choice.

The paradigmatic example of a general computational principle revealed under very specific conditions that can be broadly applied is probably the principle of the topographic neural map. Topographic maps were first discovered in the motor cortex over 100 years ago. Since that time, hundreds of topographic maps have been discovered in the brains of mammals. We now understand what topographic maps look like in both sensory and motor systems. We understand how these maps are structured in fine detail, and we understand the cellular biology that guides their development. We know that those topographic maps occur in nearly all brain areas, definitely in both arm and eye movement control systems. It thus seems absolutely no stretch to argue that the decision-making architecture of humans involves the topographic representation of options.

A second example of a broadly applicable computational principle that guides the standard model is the process of cortical normalization. This is a general computational principle that has been observed again and again in cortical systems of many kinds. Within the domain of the final common path and studies of choice, it has been observed in the saccadic system, which is why it has been incorporated into the standard model. We do not know for sure that movements of the arm employ cortical normalization, but the fact that cortical normalization is a core feature of the general theory of cortex and has been observed in saccadic choice means that it merits inclusion in the standard model. A third example of a computational principle incorporated into the standard model is the variance structure of cortical neurons. All cortical neurons ever studied have the same variance structure. A fourth example is the winner-take-all computation. All of these are computational principles that we know are at work throughout the mammalian brain, and it is for this reason, not simply because each of these has been observed in the saccadic decision-making system, that these features merit inclusion in the standard model.

Perhaps surprisingly, even the notion that firing rates are correlated with decision variables is something that seems to be a broadly documented phenomenon. In retrospect, Tanji and Evarts (1976; Evarts and Tanji, 1974, 1976) were probably the first to observe this in their studies of the hand movement region in the M1 map. Since that time, signals that encode choice likelihood have been observed in arm and shoulder portions of the skeletomuscular system (Cisek and Kalaska, 2002) and throughout the saccadic system. The notion that something like expected utility is encoded in the firing rates of neurons in the final common path also seems a necessary feature of any model of the choice process.

What is unique about studies of the saccadic system, though, is that we simply have more data both about the interactions between the parts of the system and the final thresholding process for this system than for any other system. This set of findings is fairly unique to the saccadic system, but it is an assumption of mine that, like the other computational process described above, these patterns of computation that have been observed in the saccadic system will turn out to be general properties of the decision-making architecture. (Of course this is certainly a conjecture that requires additional testing.) So, while it is true that we do not usually make important choices with our eyes, and that I have used the saccadic control system as a model for drawing general conclusions about choice architectures, the basic principles employed by the model do not stray too far from well-trodden ground. My own guess is that the standard model does a good job of describing both arm and eye movement-related decision making, but of course that is meant to be a hypothesis.

We Are Not Monkeys

The standard model of the choice architecture rests heavily on studies of monkeys making choices. That reflects a technical limitation: we simply do not have the ability to observe high-speed dynamic neural systems in humans with any precision. Our neurobiological studies of human decision-makers are typically made with functional magnetic resonance imaging scanners, which have extremely limited spatial and temporal resolution. While in a monkey we can observe the activity of single neurons performing computations in real time and at the resolution of single action potentials, we have no way to do this routinely in humans. Brain scanners tell us about the average activity of hundreds of thousands of neurons at a time scale of seconds. That makes scanners ill-suited to the study of dynamic networks during choice.

Given that limitation, how can we assure ourselves that the phenomena we observe in monkeys can serve as a model for the phenomena we hope to predict in humans?[4] I think we can do this in several ways. First, we must demonstrate that the behaviors we study in monkeys are good models of human choice. Second, we must convince ourselves that the general computational principles we observe in monkey brains are broadly distributed throughout the mammalian clade

---

4. I want to acknowledge that for many neurobiologists the goal of understanding how monkeys make decisions is reason enough to study decision making in these species. For economists and for many psychologists, however, that is not the case. For these members of the neuroeconomic fraternity (and I include myself in that group), we study monkeys because of what they can tell us about ourselves.

and not a unique feature of one or two species. Third, wherever possible we need to check the predictions of these models and verify the existence of our general computational principles in humans—at least as far as that checking and testing is possible.

Progress has been made in each of these areas, which suggests that the basic outlines of the choice model presented here should apply to humans. At the level of behavior, there is growing evidence that we share with monkeys not only our rational but also our irrational features as choosers. Dorris and Glimcher (2004) showed, for example, that human and monkey game players could not be distinguished statistically. Laurie Santos and her colleagues, in much more comprehensive work, have demonstrated a host of "human" behavioral decision-making anomalies in monkeys. They have demonstrated loss aversion (Chen et al., 2006), endowment effects (Lakshminarayan et al., 2008), and price sensitivity (Chen et al., 2006), among other phenomena, in these near relatives. All of these data suggest that under many conditions, monkeys offer an excellent behavioral model for humans.

At the level of general computational principles, we also have good reason to be optimistic. Topographic maps have been demonstrated in species ranging from rats to apes. Cortical normalization has been documented in species ranging from cats to monkeys (e.g., Carandini, Heeger, and Movshon, 1997; Heeger, 1992b). Poisson-like variance has also been shown in the cat (Tolhurst et al., 1981) and monkey (Britten et al., 1993; McAdams and Maunsell, 1999). More recently, subjective value-like signals have even been observed in the rat (Kepecs et al., 2008). We have every reason to believe that the modeling tools and constraints described in the standard model reflect core features of the mammalian nervous system.

Finally, we do have some evidence that the things we have learned from monkeys are also true in humans. Humans have, for example, all of the same anatomical structures described in the standard model. They have FEF, an LIP-like area in the parietal cortex, and superior colliculi. The connectivities of these areas in humans largely match those of the monkey. Humans have an M1, a supplementary motor area, a premotor cortex, and areas 5 and 7 in the parietal cortex (see, for example, Bailey and von Bonin, 1951; Brodmann, 1909; Kaas, 1987; von Bonin and Bailey, 1947). As in the monkeys, these areas show a topographic organization, and we know that these areas serve as the final common paths for movement control in humans. Damage to each of these areas in humans, for example, produces well-described deficits in behavior that are identical to the deficits produced by the surgical removal of these areas in monkeys.

Of course, humans and monkeys are different. In the following chapters we will see evidence of this in the valuation circuits of the human and monkey brain. Language is unique to humans and clearly plays a role in human decision making, but the general computational principles and neural circuits that guide our decisions about what movements to make seem to be highly conserved. The circuits of choice, to the limited level of detail available to us today, seem to be very similar in these two closely related species.

Are Actions Choices?

This is probably the most important question that remains unanswered about the standard model. What we know about choice arises principally from the study of actions and our pre-existing knowledge of the final common path for the control of actions. How do these actions map to choices about spouses and cars? This is a critical question and one about which we have only limited information at this time. It is also a point to which we shall return repeatedly in our examination of the valuation systems of the human brain. To make it clear why this is such a major issue, consider the following.

A human chooser is given a choice between two retirement investment plans on a computer keyboard. If he presses the number 1, he invests his portfolio in a stock fund; if he presses the number 2, he invests in a bond fund. Can studies of the circuits that control hand movement really tell us about how he values stocks over bonds? Or does some anatomically unidentified process run to completion in some other part of his brain, and then trigger one of the movement control circuits in a way that simply does not involve the encoding of relative expected subjective values in motor control circuits under these conditions? Are choices about investment portfolios and choices about delayed juice rewards so different that they employ completely separate neural architectures? This is a question that forces us to consider two very different (and both possible) descriptions of the circuitry for human choice.

One possibility, the one I have advocated so far, requires that valuation circuits in the frontal cortex and/or the basal ganglia compute and represent the values of any two options in an action-independent way. These action-independent valuations are then connected with the fronto-parietal choice circuits and choice occurs, from the point of view of an electrode, simultaneously in all of these interconnected circuits. Of course, that description begs an important question: Where in this network of areas does that convergence process begin? One very reasonable possibility is that it begins in different topographic maps for different kinds of decisions. For very rapid orienting eye movements, that convergence might begin in the superior colliculus and flow outward to influence activation in the FEF and area LIP. For more abstract decisions, it might even begin in more anterior regions of the frontal cortex. We simply do not know, perhaps in part because the time course of the intra-areal convergence is so fast.

The alternative possibility, and it is very much a possibility, is that decisions between abstract alternatives are completed in another, unidentified brain area that replicates many of the general computational features of the choice circuit I have described here. In this model, we have two choice circuits inside our brains, one for decisions about actions and one for more abstract, action-free decision making. This hypothesis proposes that under some conditions, the ones we have mostly studied, decision making occurs in the action-specific circuits of the final common path I have described. Under other conditions, however, this hypothesis proposes that the action-free decision-making circuit operates and then passes its single choice to the final common path for implementation.

Both models have advantages. The advantage of the first is simplicity. Heavily redundant interconnections between valuation and action circuits allow simultaneous convergence to choice in a single multi-area network. There is no need, in this model, for evolution to have nurtured two parallel and redundant mechanisms for choice. Nor is there a need, in this model, for a controller that selects a decision-making mechanism from among the two available systems depending on the features of the task at hand. The advantage of the second hypothesis, the two-system model, is that it honors our subjective experience. We often do feel like we have chosen things such as investment allocations long before we have to produce actions that select or implement those allocations, and the standard model seems to ignore this psychological fact.

At the moment we have insufficient data to discriminate between these hypotheses in humans. We do, however, have some information about how the monkey brain deals with a simplified kind of action-free choice; those data do seem to support the standard model. Horwitz and his colleagues (Horwitz and Newsome, 2001a, 2001b, 2004) as well as Gold and Shadlen (2003) have both gathered data that bear on this point. In Horwitz's experiments, monkeys were trained to choose between two options identified by color rather than by action. Monkeys were asked to keep track of a "green" option and a "red" option that had different values and were selected with different actions on every trial. In one block of trials, to take a simple example, the "red" option might offer a large reward at a low probability and the "green" option might offer a small reward at a high probability. On each trial the "red" and "green" options would appear at random locations in front of the monkey on a

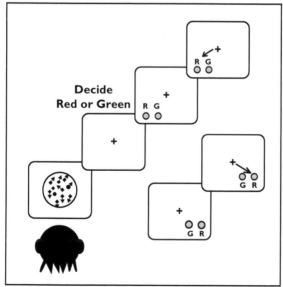

Adapted from Horwitz et al., 2004

FIGURE 11.5   The Horwitz Experiment.

computer screen and the monkey would indicate which he preferred with a saccade.

Horwitz and his colleagues found that the activity of neurons in the superior colliculus still showed basically the same pattern of activation under these conditions as had been seen in more traditional action-based choice tasks. As soon as the targets appeared, the firing rates of collicular neurons aligned with the target locations on that trial encoded what appears to be the expected subjective values of both of those targets. As the trial progressed, the firing rates changed gradually until only a single movement was represented in the network. At that point, a movement predicted by the location of the burst of activation in the collicular map was produced.

This finding tells us that while the learning and valuation circuits can store more abstract valuation information, such as the value of a colored target wherever it appears, these more abstract valuations can be mapped to the final common path as decisions are being made. This mapping process is apparently extremely rapid, and activity in the final common path under these conditions appears to obey the constraints laid out in the standard model. These data also tell us that these choice circuits of the final common path can operate on "goods" of a very simple kind (inasmuch as "red" and "green" options can be considered economic "goods"). But this is only one example, and we simply do not know if this example tells us about how we choose between stock funds.

We also know, however, from the work of Rangel and colleagues (2009), that activity in the ventromedial prefrontal cortex of humans can appear to encode selected options before actions can be chosen. What we do not know is whether this reflects the action of a second independent choice system or the convergence of a frontal area that has yet to cascade through the identified fronto-parietal choice network. Both of these are possibilities.

My own guess is that we will find that both hypotheses are correct to some degree. Our psychological sense that we sometimes make decisions long before we act may well reflect a kind of choice-set reduction performed by the frontal cortex. (This is a point to which we will return in Chapter 15.) We already know that the final common path cannot efficiently choose when there are more than six to eight options before it. We also know that when humans face large choice sets, they often (somewhat arbitrarily) exclude some of those options from serious consideration. This is a process often called *choice-set editing*. It may well be that fronto-cortical valuation circuits that are poorly developed in the monkey brain can effectively control what objects are placed in the final common path for winner-take-all decision making. This would allow both choice-set editing and, when that editing was particularly extreme, a kind of decision making outside of the winner-take-all neoclassical circuits of the final common path. For the moment, however, such hypotheses are pure speculation.

So is the standard model the right model for understanding action-free choices? The Horwitz experiments mentioned above tell us that this is a model that can easily be extended to simple action-free decision making, but how far we can push that conclusion is unclear, especially in humans. For me, this is one of the most important questions that remain to be resolved in the study of the neural architecture for choice. However, in the interest of simplicity (and in the absence of any clear hypotheses about where in the brain an action-free choice circuit might reside), the standard model necessarily retains the form presented above. For now, at least, that is how Occam's razor cuts in any model of the choice architecture.

Conclusions

The defining feature of the standard model is that it employs a two-stage architecture for choice, a valuation stage and a choice circuit. The choice circuit resides in the final common pathway for action and takes as its input a stochastic subjective expected value signal closely allied in concept to the random utility term in McFadden's (2005; Gul and Pesendorfer, 2006) economic model. This signal is represented in the choice circuit as a normalized firing rate with Poisson variance. Normalization takes the form specified by Heeger (1993), and variance takes the form first identified by Tolhurst, Movshon, and Dean (1983) in visual cortex. The stochasticity of choice is adjusted by modulation of the inter-neuronal correlation. This biological modulation of the inter-neuronal correlation was first observed by Krug and Parker (2004); it is used to implement an adjustable stochastic choice function that captures some features of the trembling hand of Selten (1975). The noise structure of the signal in this architecture places a limit on set size. As set size grows, so do error rates. This is a behavioral phenomenon first documented clearly by Iyengar and Lepper (2000) and also Deshazo and Fermo (2002). Actual choice is implemented by either a winner-take-all or a threshold value mechanism. A single circuit operating in one of two modes achieves both forms of choice, a possibility first proposed by Wang and colleagues (Liu and Wang, 2008; Lo and Wang, 2006).

Perhaps the most striking features of the model are its clear inter-disciplinary linkages. It incorporates findings from all three parent disciplines in a single formal structure. With this interdisciplinary model in hand, we turn next to the valuation circuits of the brain that provide the raw materials from which this circuit is hypothesized to produce choice.

Section 3

Valuation

The previous section of this book described what is known about the process of choice at a neurobiological level. It argued that we actually know quite a good deal about how choice operates at theoretic, psychological, and mechanistic levels of analysis. It even suggested that the intersection of constraints from the three parent disciplines of neuroeconomics has yielded new insights at each level of analysis.

This section of the book sets out to describe what is known about the process of valuation. We begin with a survey of the important constraints of standard economic theory and examine the compatibility of key logical objects like "marginal utilities" with the neurobiological mechanisms for sensory encoding. Next, we turn to psychological and neurobiological studies of learning. What emerges here is a surprisingly complete picture of some forms of learning and from this picture a set of important constraints on theory at all levels. After that, we turn to a broad portrait of the final common pathway for valuation and examine the clear failures of that mechanism, which opens important avenues for behavioral economic studies in the neuraxis.

Together with the preceding section, this section completes an overview of the neuroeconomics of both choice and valuation—they lay out the foundational constraints on "because" theories within the emerging discipline.

12

The Problem of Value

Précis

From a neoclassical point of view, choice *is* value. That is because the only way a purely economic scientist could infer what things are worth to people is by observing their choices. Sometimes those choices make sense—they are normatively rational—and by themselves give us a completely coherent picture of what the most parsimonious model of valuation would look like. But sometimes those choices are badly irrational, and no unitary concept of underlying value can, in principle, be constructed simply from choice. That has been both the greatest strength (because it provides a surgical clarity when choices are rational) and the greatest weakness (because irrational choices are common enough that they cannot simply be dismissed) of the neoclassical economic program.

In the pages that follow we will explore the relationship between the notion of value that characterizes traditional neoclassical economic theory and the more dynamic offspring of those theories that seek to account for apparently irrational choices by positing a richer mechanism for valuation. In this first chapter on valuation we explore the important *ex ante* biological and theoretical constraints on value representation that must shape any neuroeconomic analysis.

The most important thing this *ex ante* analysis will reveal is the significance of understanding what are known as "reference points." Soft-*as if* theories of choice have tended to avoid the notion that the utility of an option, as inferred from choice, reflects both the properties of that option and the properties of some "reference point" against which the value of that option is measured. This is because Soft theories that include reference dependence are much more complicated (they rest on much more *restrictive* assumptions) than are those that do not (theories such as Soft-GARP or Soft-EU). Longstanding neurobiological constraints, however, make it clear that the hardware requirements for a reference point-free model (such as Hard-EU) cannot, in principle, be met. As we will see in the coming pages, traditional models such as Soft-EU turn out to be fundamentally incompatible with the basic structure of the human brain. In their place, we will be forced by the biological evidence to turn to reference-based models. To get to those conclusions, however, we have to begin by examining how the vertebrate nervous system encodes the properties of our external world, whether those properties be the taste of a sweet beverage, the feel of an expensive cloth, or the sound of a well-loved song.

Psychophysics: "How Much"?

All sensory encoding that we know of is reference dependent. Nowhere in the nervous system are the objective values of consumable rewards encoded. This has been a core lesson from both neurobiological studies of sensory encoding and psychophysical studies of perception. To illustrate this point, consider what happens in the visual system of the brain as we move from a windowless classroom to a sunny park bench. Sitting in a classroom we see a friend wearing blue jeans, a green shirt, and a white cap. The physical stimuli that give rise to this perceptual experience are $\sim 10^{17}$ photons/second with a mean wavelength of 450 nm streaming off every square centimeter of the blue jeans, $\sim 10^{17}$ 550-nm photons/second streaming off every square centimeter of the green shirt, and $\sim 10^{17}$ photons/second of many wavelengths being reflected off of every square centimeter of the white cap.

Next, we step outside into the bright sun with that friend and are briefly blinded by the glare. About 30 seconds later we sit down on a park bench and look at the friend. He looks the same: blue jeans, a green shirt, and a white cap. Now, however, in bright sun, this identical perceptual experience is being produced by $\sim 10^{23}$ 450-nm photons/second/cm^2 streaming off of the blue jeans, $\sim 10^{23}$ 550-nm photons/second/cm^2

streaming off the green shirt, and $\sim10^{23}$ photons/second/cm^2 of many wavelengths being reflected off the white cap. On a typical day this is a *six-order-of-magnitude* shift in the objective reality, which has been accompanied by no significant change in the subjective experience. Why? The answer should be obvious from an evolutionary point of view. What has changed as we step out of the building is the sun, the nature of the *illuminant*. But of course as animals living on earth, changes in the illuminant located 93,000,000 miles away are not really all that important; what we need to know about to survive are the objects immediately around us. To extract the properties of those objects accurately we have to, essentially, subtract the changing effects of the sun as we move under clouds, into shadow, or out into direct sun.

The Drifting Reference Point Makes Absolute Value Unrecoverable

Psychophysicists and visual scientists have studied this process of illuminant subtraction in tremendous detail, and we now know quite a bit about how it works. In fact, it turns out that the first stage of this adaptation to the intensity of the illuminant occurs at the transducer itself, in the rods and cones of the retina. These cells employ a biochemical mechanism to compute a time-dependent average of light intensity (Burns and Baylor, 2001). This average is used to set a baseline (or reference) intensity level. Changes of light intensity up or down from that baseline level are all that is encoded by the rods and cones of the retina as they communicate with the rest of the nervous system. Let me be clear about what I am saying here: *Information about the objective intensity of incident light is* **irretrievably** *lost at the transducer.* This is information that we know with certainty cannot be recovered elsewhere in the nervous system. There are places in the brain where we extract extremely limited information about light intensity, but this information has almost no influence on what we store about the appearance of the outside world. Instead, light intensity is encoded and stored in a reference-dependent way, and the level of the biophysically computed reference point that defines what is darker and what is brighter drifts as a function of average light intensity over time. All of this happens biochemically at the very first stage of stimulus encoding—inside the transducing cells themselves. Every first-year neuroscience student knows this fact.

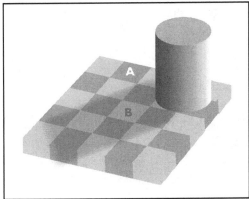

Adelson, 1995

FIGURE 12.1   Ted Edelson's Lighter/Darker Square Illusion.

We can see this kind of phenomenon operating even under more local conditions. In the visual illusion shown in Figure 12.1, both the A and the B squares are reflecting identical numbers of photons to your eyes. We perceive them as different because of a kind of spatial reference dependence invoked in the visual system by the differently shaded squares that surround them.

This encoding strategy of employing a "baseline" reflects an under-lying process of optimization, a kind of trade-off first clearly explained by Horace Barlow (Barlow, 1961a, 1961b; see also Attneave, 1954). Barlow recognized that we gain a selective advantage from knowing about the outside world—knowing, for example, where food and predators can be found. But the more we want to know about the world, the larger the number of hungry neurons that we need to keep inside our heads. If we encode and store a linear representation of light intensity across all possible intensities from all possible photons, then we need many neurons (each of which has a limited dynamic range of finite precision) to achieve this encoding. But if we store more compressed reference-dependent versions of light intensity, then we use fewer of these hungry neurons, fewer neurons that we need to feed every day. Of course, the fewer neurons we have, the less we can store. The more we store, the more it costs; the less we store, the less we know. It was Barlow who first clearly recognized the existence of this trade-off, and it was his intuition that feeding a lot of hungry neurons just to learn things about the brightness of an object 93,000,000 miles away was probably a bad evolutionary investment.

In vision, the adapting baseline (or reference point) is a particularly striking feature of the encoding system because light intensities vary across such a broad range in the natural world. A six-order-of-magnitude change in illumination frequently occurs within seconds as we move from shade into direct sun. Is this huge adaptive range, the ability to shift the reference point by six orders of magnitude, a feature of all of our sensory systems? The answer is largely "yes." The same adaptive baseline feature characterizes all of our sensory systems. In audition, for example, the sensitivity of our hearing varies with background noise. If we move from a quiet room to a rock and roll concert, sound intensities can increase by an astonishing 8 to 10 orders of magnitude (Bacchus, 2006; Robinson and McAlpine, 2008). Our ears respond to this challenge by shifting the reference point in much the same way that we encountered in vision, although through a completely distinct mechanism. This is also the case in olfaction. A rose in the hand may smell sweet in a bedroom, but its odor will be undetectably hidden if we stand in a field of identical flowers. Our sense of touch also behaves this way (Mountcastle, 2005). In the morning when we first dress we feel our clothes. Ten minutes later we not only fail to notice the textures of the fabrics that wrap us, but the nerve endings in our skin have ceased reporting the very existence of these textures to the central nervous system.

This is true for even the most primitive consumable rewards we encounter. Consider the receptor cells embedded in our tongues that allow us to taste salt, an essential nutrient for which large segments of the human race pay handsomely. How salty something tastes depends on the membrane voltages of these salt-specific receptor cells. The more salt that enters sodium-specific ion channels in these cells, the more depolarized these neurons become, the more neurotransmitter they release, and the saltier that food item "tastes." The exact degree of depolarization, the "saltiness" of the food, depends on the amount of sodium in the blood, in the surrounding tissue, and in the oral cavity. In fact, at extremely high and low internal salt levels, the same objective concentration of salt placed on the tongue could yield neural responses of opposite sign (Bertino, Beauchamp, and Engelman, 1982, 1986; Contretras and Frank, 1979). Eat salty foods long enough and they taste less salty or even not salty—this is not just an illusion, it is a feature of our transduction architecture.

The key point is that the human nervous system does not *ever* encode the objective properties of anything, let alone the objective properties of our primary rewards. Drifting reference points make absolute stimulus magnitude unrecoverable, *in principle*. Of course that reflects, as Barlow pointed out, an optimization under constraint. By encoding stimulus intensity relative to a variable baseline, we are able to detect *changes* in the current state of the world accurately, and with many fewer neurons than if we encoded objective properties of the world. As we will see in a few pages, this imposes a striking constraint on Hard (and I believe Soft) economic models.

The key point of this section is that all sensory encoding is reference dependent: nowhere in the nervous system are the objective values of consumable rewards encoded. This means that models that require the encoding of objective stimulus magnitudes cannot accurately describe how humans behave. That is a simple and irrefutable fact.

Encoding Functions Transform Even Relative Value Measurements

Not only do we know that our sensory systems employ reference-dependent encoding schemes, but since the pioneering work of Weber (1834) and Fechner (1860) we have also known that information above and below the reference point is not linearly related to variations in true intensity, a point discussed in some detail in Chapter 4. Fechner argued that all sensory signals were logarithmically transformed either at the transducer or at some point between the transducer and perceptual experience. He argued that the strength of the perceptual experience associated with increasingly bright visual stimuli presented against a dark background increased only as the logarithm of luminance. Subsequently, Stevens (e.g., 1961) showed that Fechner's law was quantitatively incorrect, although his general conclusion, that the objective properties of the real world are not linearly related to subjective experience, was correct. Instead of employing a universal logarithmic compression in all sensory systems, Stevens showed that the intensity of a perceptual experience grows as a power law, the exact rate of growth of the percept being dependent on stimulus type.

Stevens (1957, 1970, 1975) showed, for example, that the experience of warmth on the skin could be well described by the equation:

Perceived warmth of a large patch of skin $=$ (Temp of that skin)$^{0.7}$

To take another example, he found that:

Perceived intensity of an electrical shock $=$ (Electrical current)$^{3.5}$

When I described those experiments in Chapter 4, however, I did not mention that each of these measurements was made at a fixed baseline (the critical point made above), under conditions in which the reference point for that sensory system was held constant.

I then went on in that chapter to tell the following story:

> Consider a little-read neurological and psychological paper from the 1960s (Borg et al., 1967). Two human neurological patients are undergoing surgery. As part of that surgery, the main nerves from the tongues of those patients will be exposed while they are awake and alert. So their surgeons ask them to participate in an experiment. The surgeons will pour sugar solutions of different concentrations on their tongues (while holding the long-term average sweetness constant) and record the activity in the nerves. The surgeons note that although variable, the mean firing rates as a function of sugar concentration increase as a power function having an exponent of about 0.6.
>
> Next, the surgeons adopt Stevens' bisection method and ask the subjects to perform ratings that allow them to construct perceptual intensity curves. The surgeons find that the perceptual curves also describe power functions, again with an exponent of 0.6. They therefore hypothesize that the percept of these subjects is simply a linear report of activity in the nerve.
>
> ...
>
> I want to be careful, now, not to overinterpret this set of trivial observations, so let me say only this: suppose that we were studying an imaginary creature called NewMan whom we knew employed a tongue transducer that encoded sugar concentration in firing rate as a power function with exponent 0.6. The simplest possible creature of this kind would directly experience that firing rate as a

percept. Such a creature would make choices in a way that simply maximized the expected value of tongue firing rates. (He would be choosing so as to maximize the average number of action potentials in the nerve when he obtained his chosen sugar solution to drink.)

This imaginary creature would still be showing risk aversion over sugar solutions, but that risk aversion would arise at the level of the tongue. Evolution, as it were, would have put risk aversion there, rather than in some more complicated structure. And of course not all of the NewMan's risk-averse behavior arises in its tongue. But it is without a doubt interesting that for this creature, under at least some limited conditions, a partial reduction between the neurobiology of sucrose transduction, the psychology of signal detection, and the economics of random utility theory would be entirely plausible

To summarize this section, I want to make two points.

First, all sensory systems encode the properties of the outside world with regard to a drifting reference point, or baseline. The actual value of this reference point, however, is not stored. Indeed, in most cases it is not explicitly encoded by any element of the vertebrate nervous system. Nowhere in the nervous system are the objective values of consumable rewards encoded. Therefore, if we find that a particular class of economic theories of choice requires knowledge of the objective properties of choice objects, we must conclude that that theory is problematic. Models requiring the encoding of objective stimulus magnitudes cannot, in principle, accurately describe how humans behave.

Second, nearly all sensory systems also recode magnitude above or below the baseline using some kind of transforming function. Most of these transformations are compressive (or concave in the domain of gains). This may be important, because most theories of utility suggest that the subjective values of objects should be compressive monotonic transforms of their objective values.

Economics: Marginal Utilities and the Question of "How Good"?

Imagine an animal exploring a novel environment from a nest on a day when both (1) its blood concentration is dilute (and thus its need for water is low) and (2) its blood sugar level is low (and thus its need for food is high). The animal travels west one kilometer from the nest and emerges from the undergrowth into an open clearing at the shores of a large lake. Not very thirsty, the animal bends down to sample the water and finds it brackish and unpalatable. Let us assume for argument that the next day the same animal leaves its nest in the same metabolic state and travels one kilometer to the east, where it discovers a grove of trees that yield a dry but nutritious fruit, a grove of dried apricot trees. It samples the fruit and finds it sweet and highly palatable.

What has the animal actually learned about the value of going west and the value of going east? It has had a weakly negative experience, in the psychological sense, when going west and a very positive experience when going east. Do these subjective properties of its experience influence what it has learned? Do the stored representations derived from these experiences encode the actual objective values of going west and east, or do they encode the subjective experiences? That is a critical question about what the animal has learned, because it determines what it does when it wakes up thirsty. When it wakes up thirsty it should, in a normative sense, go west towards the brackish lake, despite the fact that its previous visit west was a negative experience. This is a problem economists have been aware of for centuries, a problem that has been elegantly solved with a logical object called a *marginal utility*.

In the neoclassical (or for that matter the classical) economic framework, we can approach the decision problem this animal faces by

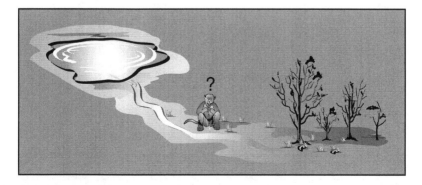

FIGURE 12.2

viewing it as having two kinds of "wealth": a *water wealth* and a *sugar wealth*. This is the total store of water and sugar held by the animal at any one time. For our purposes, we can think of the concentration of the animal's blood (the *osmolality* of the blood) as a measure of the animal's water wealth and the concentration of sugar in the animal's blood as a measure of its sugar wealth.[1]

When we offer the animal a piece of fruit or a drink of water, it is critical, in the traditional neoclassical approach, to realize that what we really offer it is an *increment* in its total sugar or water wealth. What is the subjective value of a piece of fruit to the animal? The answer to that question, for a traditional economist, depends on its current wealth level. To see this, examine the cartoon utility curve for blood sugar in Figure 12.3.

If we ask the animal to choose west or east on a day when it is hungry but not thirsty, that is a day when it has a low blood sugar level.

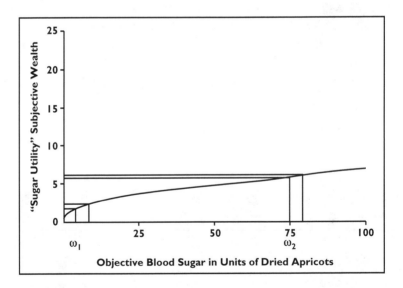

FIGURE 12.3

---

1. Real sugar wealth would have to include fat stores, glycogen stores, and perhaps even cached food. One could include those easily in what follows with no loss to generality.

Its total sugar wealth that day is marked on the x-axis of the graph as ω_1. One piece of fruit increments the animal along the x-axis (increases its *total* sugar utility) by one dried apricot. Note that in this low wealth state, the curve relating subjective and objective value is steep; one apricot increases total subjective sugar wealth by quite a lot. Thus, if the animal starts from ω_1, that one piece of fruit increments its total subjective wealth significantly. As I have drawn the curve here, that is an increment of about 1 util (in these arbitrary units).

On the second choice day that we examine the animal, it has a high blood sugar level, as indicated on the graph by ω_2. Up at this level of the graph, where the utility curve is rather flat, a piece of fruit increases the animal's sugar wealth by only 0.2 utils. It is the increment in utility (the *marginal utility*) provided by the fruit that is important, and *the magnitude of this increment depends on wealth*. The wealthier the chooser is, the lower the marginal utility provided by the same gain. This is a phenomenon known in economic circles as a *diminishing marginal utility*.

The key idea here is that the animal makes a choice about whether to go west or east based on its assessment of the increase in utility that would be provided by the lake or the fruit trees. To do that, it makes an objective estimate of how the water and the fruit would change its objective wealth and then asks how those objective changes in its wealth would increment its aggregate utility. It is critical that the animal have access to all of these objective values, because it is the only way that it can compute marginal utilities as its wealth levels change. If it had access to only the subjective experiences of the first and second days described above, it could never compute the new marginal utilities when it finds itself unexpectedly hungry.

This approach implicitly fully segregates what the animal should learn about its options experientially (their objective values) from the variables that should guide its choice (their marginal utilities). The animal learns the true objective value of the fruit or the water. What drives its behavior when it chooses is the *marginal* value of the fruit or water. This beautiful approach requires that the animal learn the objective values of the objects among which it will choose. One problem with such a formulation, from the perspective of a Hard-theory, is that we know the nervous system never encodes the objective value of anything. Is there also a problem with this approach at the behavioral level?

Context and Choice: When Even Behavioral Data Spoil a Perfectly Good Theory

In 1981, Tversky and Kahneman read a group of human subjects the following story: "Imagine that the U.S. is preparing for the outbreak of an unusual Asian disease, which is expected to kill 600 people. Two alternative programs to combat the disease have been proposed." Then half the subjects were asked to choose between the following two options:

> If Program A is adopted, 200 people will be saved. If Program B is adopted, there is a 1/3 probability that 600 people will be saved and a 2/3 probability that no people will be saved.

Under these conditions 72% of the subjects picked A. Then, Tversky and Kahneman offered a second group of subjects two different options:

> If Program C is adopted 400 people will die. If Program D is adopted there is a 1/3 probability that nobody will die, and a 2/3 probability that 600 people will die.

Framed this way, 78% of their subjects now picked D, even though options A and C are numerically identical (as are B and D).

In the landmark paper where Tversky and Kahneman (1981) first presented this observation, they argued that understanding this finding was critical to understanding choice. The objective values of options A and B are identical to the objective values of options C and D, yet these two sets of options present very different subjective experiences. In option A, we consider the positive psychological experience of saving 200 people; in option C we confront the subjectively distasteful prospect of 400 deaths. What Tversky and Kahneman argued was that these differences affected the decisions their subjects made in a way that could not be predicted from a model that employed marginal utilities and a wealth level. In our terms, they argued that the objective values of these options were not what were guiding human choice, but rather some notion of value that was represented relative to the framework of the story being told to the subjects.

I should hasten to point out that many features of the "Asian disease story" experiment have limited its impact in economic circles. First, all of the subjects knew that this was a make-believe problem; we have no reason to think that they were as serious and thoughtful when answering this question in the lab as they might have been if they had to make this choice when real lives were at stake. It may also be that the subjects saw the wording of the problems as guiding them to a specific correct solution, and the subjects simply gave that correct solution rather than thinking through what they would do if confronted with this situation. It may even be that subjects simply did not understand the options; they may not have been *able* to realize that A and C were two ways to say exactly the same thing. But, if Tversky and Kahneman were right, then choice does not depend simply on wealth and objective value.

Consider another example: Two subjects enter a casino with $400 each and sit down to play craps. This game is about as perfect an example of a set of economic lotteries as one can find in the real world. Craps offers several types of bets. One, called the *odds bet,* is risk neutral.[2] If you have a 1-in-3 chance of winning this bet, you win $3 for every $1 you bet. Others, called the *hard-way bets,* offer payoffs as high as 20:1, but do so with as little as a 1-in-36 chance of winning. Only a very risk-seeking chooser would take these bets. As the game begins we see the two players, Milton and Oskar, wagering primarily on the odds bets. An hour later Milton is up $200 and Oskar is down $200. Once that happens, as anyone who has seriously visited casinos knows, Oskar will begin taking hard-way bets that Milton would never touch. What we observe is that the more Oskar loses (up to a point), the more risk-seeking he becomes. The opposite is true of Milton: the more he wins, the more (again, up to a point) he focuses on risk-neutral odds bets (Kahneman, Slovic and Tversky, 1982).

So how can we explain that widely observed difference in behavior? If we draw a standard utility curve for both gamblers (Fig. 12.4 and Fig. 12.5) and mark their identical starting wealth levels on those curves, then we see that for any reasonable kind of utility function there should not be anything different about how Oskar and Milton view the next throw of the dice.[3] After Oskar has lost $200, and Milton has won $200,

---

2. More precisely: It is a bet that would always be acceptable to a risk-neutral chooser.

3. I am neglecting two old neoclassical saws about why this behavior might be observed, explanations that have always struck me as silly. The first explanation is that Oskar's utility function, just by luck, happens to have a kink in it at this morning's wealth level (Friedman and Savage, 1948). This kink makes him behave oddly about losses, but only because he happens to be at exactly that particular wealth level today. This explanation

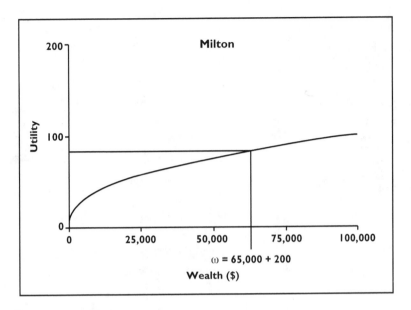

FIGURE 12.4

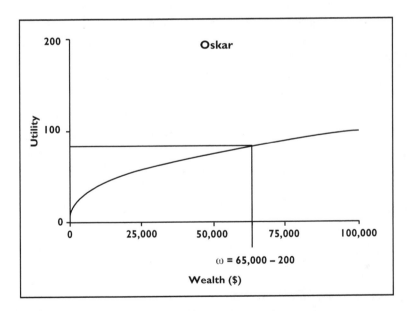

FIGURE 12.5

286

they do move to different points on their lifetime wealth curves, but these points are only trivially different and neither can be seen as risk-preferring at any point. For this reason, according to the standard neoclassical theory these two must be basically the same in their behavior after an hour at the casino, but what we observe is that they behave very differently.

Behavioral Reference Dependency

Kahneman and Tversky (1979) attempted to explain these two classes of behavioral phenomena, the importance of framing stories and the differences between loss-related and gain-related behavior, with something they (borrowing from earlier neoclassical writers) called *reference dependency*. Kahneman and Tversky's conviction was that the wealth-based marginal utility approach we have examined so far fails to capture several features of observed human choice. They felt that a reference-dependent utility function could resolve this problem.

To account for Oskar's penchant for high-risk bets when he was losing, they made the following proposal: Rather than computing marginal utilities against wealth as in the standard theory, *utilities* (not marginal utilities) could be computed directly as deviations from a baseline level of wealth, and then choices could be based on direct comparisons of these utilities[4] rather than on comparisons of marginal utilities. Their idea

---

works fine in principle, but once one realizes that risk-seeking behavior in losses is pervasive everywhere and at all wealth levels, let alone at casinos, this explanation begins to sound like someone bailing a sinking ship. The second explanation one hears is that Oskar simply gets more utility, in the form of pleasure, from highly risky bets than does Milton. Again, this is a silly explanation because it lacks the generality, the applicability to all human behavior about losses, for which the many observations such as these force us to search.

4. Using the word "utility" in this way is an atrocity for a hard-core neoclassicist like me. Utility has a clear technical meaning: it is the thing we maximize by our choices when those choices are technically rational. Reference-based theories can produce situations in which we simply cannot tell what choosers are trying to maximize, and so under those conditions the concept of utility can become very fuzzy. Tversky and Kahneman recognized this and were careful not to use the word "utility" in the way I am using it here. The right word is probably "subjective value," but I use "utility" here to maintain the flow of this explanation. I beg patience from those whom this offends.

was to begin with something like the chooser's *status quo*, how much wealth he thinks he has. Each gamble is then represented as the chance of winning or losing utilities relative to that status quo-like reference point.

Confronting Reference Dependence in Hard Theories

What I hope is becoming clear is that there are some interesting parallels between the notions of reference dependence in Kahneman and Tversky's formulation and the notion of reference dependence in neurobiology. The traditional neoclassical approach proposes that when we make choices, we know the actual values, in objective terms, of the options before us. We then combine these values with our lifetime wealth estimates to compute marginal utilities. The advantage of this approach is that it keeps our choices perfectly consistent. At a neurobiological level, however, we have clear evidence that we cannot know the actual values of the options before us. As we have seen, due to the constraint imposed by the cost of neurons, we have only a reference-based knowledge of the outside world because reference-based encoding is metabolically cheaper than objective encoding. Yet, problematically, Kahneman and Tversky found evidence for reference-point–based decision making in humans. That evidence was the existence of profoundly inconsistent choice behavior.

The core points we have encountered so far in this chapter are: (1) we know from neuroscience that the objective values of objects in the outside world are basically never encoded in the nervous system; (2) standard neoclassical approaches that predict rational behavior use as inputs the objective values of the objects we encounter and our current wealth levels; and (3) observed choice behavior seems to violate the predictions of standard neoclassical theory in a way that suggests we make our choices based upon increments and decrements in utility from some kind of reference point.

For a biological entity to actually perform the calculations at the heart of neoclassical theories such as expected utility, it would need to know (to have stored in its brain) two things: (1) its *total wealth* with regard to anything offered in the environment and (2) the *objective value* of anything offered in the environment. Choosers are presumed, in Hard-EU or in Hard-REU, to make decisions algorithmically between options by comparing the marginal subjective values of those options. To represent those marginal subjective values, they must store their wealth and the objective value of the offered good. Then these two quantities must be combined in the way specified by their subjective value (utility) function. Let me stress again what this means: first, it means that animals must know their wealth status at all times. That seems reasonable; we know that animals can sense such things as blood sugar and blood osmolality. Second, and this is more important, it means that regardless of how good or bad the dried apricot tastes, what the animal must learn and store is the objective value of the dried apricot. We must achieve a complete mechanistic disassociation between the expected marginal utilities that drive choice and the objective values that animals store. At a psychological level, this means that upon tasting a disgustingly sweet dried apricot, an animal that is glutted and nauseated from eating in a dried cherry orchard must accurately store the positive sugar value of that apricot in exactly the same way as if it were initially starving.

In the previous section of this book, I argued that the choice circuitry located in the fronto-parietal network encoded the subjective values of actions. Hard-EU predicts that these circuits reflect, to put it into the terms I am using here, the *marginal subjective values*[5] of the options on offer. If that is exactly correct, then *when animals learn about their environment, what they have to store in the valuation circuits of their brains are the objective values, not the subjective values, of those options.* I cannot stress enough how major a constraint this bit of theory imposes on the neural architecture. If Hard-EU is a *because* theory, then it predicts that the values humans and animals store when they learn about their environment are uninfluenced by the thirst or hunger of the animal. Thus, the fact that we know objective value is never encoded in the vertebrate nervous system effectively disposes of Hard-EU (and all of the related members of this class like Hard-REU) as a serious theory.

---

5. More accurately, the expected marginal subjective values.

Minimizing the Damage: Neoclassical Approaches to Reference Dependence

So what do we do? How can a neoclassical economist searching for the simplest theory commensurate with the available data deal with these findings? To be honest, the dominant response of the economic profession has been to ignore such findings. This stems in part from the fact that under many conditions wealth-based theories and reference-based theories make identical predictions *at the behavioral level*. If, for example, we consider only choice situations that deal with unanticipated gains under conditions in which the reference point or wealth levels are fixed, the two classes of theories are not really very different in their predictions. The two theories differ behaviorally when we begin to talk about comparing losses and gains relative to some shifting reference point.

Recently, however, a small group of neoclassically trained economists have begun to take reference dependency seriously. Matthew Rabin and Botond Kőszegi of Berkeley, for example, have begun to argue that incorporating reference dependency into the corpus of neoclassical theory is critical. As they put it in a recent paper:

> [W]hile an unexpected monetary windfall in the lab may be assessed as a gain, a salary of $50,000 to an employee who expected $60,000 will not be assessed as a large gain relative to status-quo wealth, but rather as a loss relative to expectations of wealth. And in nondurable consumption—where there is no object with which the person can be endowed—a status-quo-based theory cannot capture the role of reference dependence at all: it would predict, for instance, that a person who misses a concert she expected to attend would feel no differently than somebody who never expected to see the concert. (Kőszegi and Rabin, 2006)

Kőszegi and Rabin argue that these are major failings, at a behavioral level, that neoclassical axiomatic economics must address. With that in mind, these scholars have begun to argue, neoclassically, for a set of axioms to define a reference-based theory of utility. They have argued for a theory in which the reference point is defined as one's rational expectations about current and future wealth. This allows them to adopt reference-based utility functions of the type proposed by Kahneman and

Tversky, but on more rigorous neoclassical grounds and with a mechanism for specifying the reference point itself.

Their core idea is that the reference point is a kind of a guess made by each chooser about his or her life-long aggregate wealth level. It is a quantity that needs to encode the value of any currently held rewards and all future rewards decremented by that subject's *discount factor*, the rate at which (for that individual) future gains decrease in their desirability when compared to currently held gains.[6] Formally, they argue that the reference point at any moment in time can be thought of as:

$$\text{Reference Point} = u_t + \gamma^1 u_{t+1} + \gamma^2 u_{t+2} + \gamma^3 u_{t+3} + \gamma^4 u_{t+4} \cdots$$

where γ, the discount parameter, captures the fact that each of us prefers (derives more utility from) sooner rather than later rewards, u_t is the utility of all the stuff we already have, and the subsequent u's are the utilities we expect to gain at each time point in the future. In reality, future utilities are not certain; they are expected utilities, so we should really say that

$$\text{Reference Point} = u_t + \gamma^1 Eu_{t+1} + \gamma^2 Eu_{t+2} + \gamma^3 Eu_{t+3} + \gamma^4 Eu_{t+4} \cdots$$

Interestingly, their theoretical treatment makes several predictions. As Kőszegi and Rabin put it:

> [The theory] shows that a consumer's willingness to pay a given price for shoes depends on the probability with which she expected to buy them and the price she expected to pay. On the one hand, an increase in the likelihood of buying increases a consumer's sense of loss of shoes if she does not buy, creating an "attachment effect" that increases her willingness to pay. Hence, the greater the likelihood she thought prices would be low enough to induce purchase, the greater is her willingness to buy at higher prices. On the other hand, holding the probability of getting the shoes fixed, a decrease in the price a consumer expected to pay makes paying a higher price feel like more of a loss, creating a "comparison effect" that lowers her willingness to pay the high price. Hence, the lower

---

6. This discount factor is, in practice, exceedingly important. It accounts for the fact that real human choosers are "temporally myopic" and means that in practice humans compute the reference point quite locally in time.

the prices she expected among those prices that induce purchase, the lower is her willingness to buy at higher prices.

This reveals the not-so-hidden cost we must pay for accepting a reference-based theory: we must incorporate into our theory an acknowledgement that people really do behave irrationally, in the sense defined by Soft-GARP or Soft-EU. The fact that a consumer will pay more for shoes she expected to buy than for shoes she did not expect to buy, or that an animal would prefer inferior fruit it expected to eat over superior fruit it did not expect to eat, is exactly the kind of irrational behavior that we might hope the pressures of evolution would preclude. What observations tell us, however, is that these behaviors do occur. The neuroscience of sensory encoding tells us that these behaviors are an inescapable product of the fundamental structure of our brains. Having faced this uncomfortable fact, what we have to do next is better understand what having a reference point means for neuroeconomics.

What It Means to Have a Reference Point in a Hard Theory

The reason that Kahneman, Tversky, Rabin, and Kőszegi proposed a reference-based theory of choice was that, as behavioral scientists, they had observed that human risk attitudes were different when making choices about gains versus when making choices about losses. That was a dissonant observation, because in the traditional neoclassical approach there are no explicit differences between *gains* and *losses* – there is nothing in the neoclassical utility function that explicitly segregates the marginal utilities of losses from the marginal utilities of gains. By anchoring the utility function to something like the status quo, Kahneman, Tversky, Rabin, and Kőszegi changed this key feature of the theory: now the utility function could effectively segregate gains and losses that traditional theories could not.

To understand this key difference, let us return to the example of Milton and Oskar playing craps in a casino. If we assume that the reference points for both gamblers are anchored to the wealth level they had when they entered the casino, then the same $20 bet could, in fact, look very different to these two individuals after an hour at the casino. For Oskar, who is $200 below his reference point because of his losses, a very risky bet might look quite good (because of the curvature of the utility function in the loss domain), while that same bet might look insanely bad to Milton, who is measuring utilities in the gain domain. It is important to understand that this difference can arise only because the utility curve (or more precisely the "value function") changes radically at the reference point, as shown in Figure 12.6. If, as in traditional theories, there is no reference point, then there can be no radical difference between losses and gains. For this reason a reference point can prove a very powerful explanatory tool, but it comes with significant theoretical and empirical problems.

Historically, the most important of these problems was that Kahneman and Tversky provided almost no information about how the

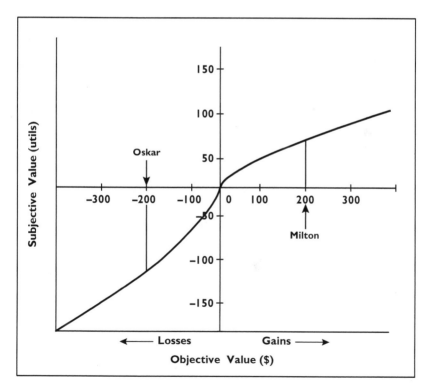

FIGURE 12.6   A reference-dependent value function.

reference point was to be determined. They proposed a theory of choice based on a reference point without providing a theory of the reference point itself. It was clear from a number of experiments they did that one could not simply use current wealth as a proxy for the reference point, as one might initially expect (Kahneman and Tversky, 1979). We can see that fact in the story of Oskar and Milton. If Oskar and Milton updated their reference points after each bet, they would always behave identically (at least as long as they had about the same total lifetime wealth). Their risk attitudes would diverge only if their reference points lagged somewhat behind their recent losses and gains in wealth. If, for example, Oskar and Milton use their wealth levels from an hour ago as their reference point, then the theory predicts their behavior. But that points again to problems with the notion of the reference point. Kőszegi and Rabin addressed this problem by beginning to work towards an axiomatic form of reference-based utility theory and including in that theory a foundation for the reference point.

A second, and more serious, problem with the reference point-based approach is that it means human choosers are really "supposed" to be irrational, in a sense. If we think of technical rationality as meaning that choosers do not switch their preferences around depending on trivial features of the way we ask them questions, then the reference point approach actually *forces* choosers to behave irrationally in ways that really do not make any sense. I am stating that as a drawback here because none of the social scientists advocating for a reference-based theory have given a reason *why* choosers should behave in this way. There is no serious doubt that choosers do behave this way, but there is no *why* in these behavioral proposals that justifies this odd behavior; the theory just describes a computation that can reproduce this odd behavior. What we can see from this neuroeconomic analysis, however, is that these local irrationalities arise *because evolution is trading off the costs of accurate sensory encoding against the costs of irrational decision making.* Where these two functions cross is effectively an equilibrium between these two mechanisms.

So what does this mean for neuroeconomics? To answer that question, let us examine what we might call *Hard-reference point theory.*[7]

---

7. Or, more precisely, Hard-reference-dependent-REU.

Hard-reference point theory would have to propose, like Hard-EU, that we take the objective values of the options before us as inputs to the nervous system. The external world is always our starting point, but after that starting point the theories immediately diverge. Hard-EU requires that we encode and store the objective values of all of the options we encounter. Hard-reference point theory imposes no such severe encoding constraints. The critical feature of reference-based theories is that we do not compute marginal utilities from a stored representation of objective value and wealth each time we make a choice. Instead, reference-based theories permit us to transform objective values into subjective values at any point (or at many points) as we move from the external world to the choice mechanism discussed in the preceding section of this book. In their most extreme form, Hard-reference-based theories allow us to transform the objective properties of objects in the world about which we make choices into subjective representations *at the sensory transducers.* Transformation from objective values to subjective values can happen as early as the first stage of computation in this class of theories. Then subjective (but not marginal) values form the stuff of memory directly. In this formulation, the choice mechanism operates not on objective values and wealth but rather on stored subjective values directly. For an economist, the key insight is that Hard-reference-based theories impose much *weaker constraints* on the neural architecture than Hard-EU does. For a neuroscientist or a psychologist, the key insight is that any system that irreversibly transforms objective stimulus properties into subjective perceptual properties anywhere along the chain from transducer to memory to choice is a kind of reference-based theory of decision. To take one example of a reference-based theory, *Hard-prospect theory* is a theory in which objective values need never be stored and a theory in which the subjectivization of value can occur long before the encoding of value in memory.

This is an incredibly important point. The critical difference between any Hard economic theory with a reference point and any Hard economic theory without a reference point is the constraint imposed on the value encoding and storage mechanisms. All traditional wealth-based theories (such as Hard-EU) *require* that objective values be encoded and stored when choosers learn about their options. While this is also possible within the framework of Hard reference-based theories, *it is not a required property of such theories.* The mechanistically simplest reference-based choice architecture need *never* encode objective value internally. It can instead perform an initial objective-to-subjective value transformation as early as at the primary sensors (and perform subsequent additional transformations at any time) and then simply store subjective values.

The drawback to such a system is that it will produce irrational choices. The degree of these irrationalities will, of course, depend on the precise objective-to-subjective transformations that it employs. But a critical point is that such a theory produces these irrationalities for a reason. These irrationalities arise *because* the system employs objective-to-subjective transformations to minimize the cost of the encoding mechanism. For all of the reasons we discussed in the beginning of this chapter, the cost of objective encoding systems that can span eight or ten orders of magnitude is very high. If we want to reduce that cost, we must adopt a reference-based system for choice. This is an inescapable trade-off in any Hard economic theory. Reference points, in Hard theories, are an optimization under constraint.

In essence, what I am trying to do here is to use the concept of a Hard theory to re-ask the "why do we see evidence of the reference point" question. If we began with the constraint that learning and encoding the values of options is costly, and that to minimize these costs we transform inputs with a reference-based function, then reference-based choice would emerge as the "most rational" way to choose given that constraint. Neuroscience has spent the better part of the past half-century demonstrating that all of our sensations, and much of our memory, perform referenced-based subjectivizations of the sensory inputs that guide our actions. Neuroscientific theory even tells us what constraints encoding information in this way satisfies optimally (e.g., Schwartz and Simoncelli, 2001). That is a global neuroscientific truth that we now know cannot be irrelevant to choice theory.

Let us return one more time to the story of sweetness perception from Chapter 4:

> Two human neurological patients are undergoing surgery. As part of that surgery, the main nerves from the tongues of those patients will be exposed while they are awake and alert....The surgeons will pour sugar solutions of different concentrations on their tongues....

The surgeons note that although variable, the mean firing rates as a function of sugar concentration increase as a power function having an exponent of about 0.6. Next, the surgeons…ask the subjects to perform ratings that allow them to construct perceptual intensity curves. What the surgeons find is that the perceptual curves also describe power functions, again with an exponent of 0.6.

If we think about that story, there are two ways to put it together. In a purely neoclassical vein, we can think about the signal coming through the gustatory nerves as encoding (in $X^{0.6}$ transforming units) the objective value of the sugar solution. When we ask subjects how much they would pay to consume a specific concentration of sugar, we can think of the subjects as taking a stored estimate of that concentration data (after inverting the power-law transformation of the encoder), placing it on their sugar utility function at their current sugar wealth level, and then computing the marginal utility of that increment of sugar wealth. So far so good.

What the preceding neurobiological stories about sensory systems reveal, however, is that signals from the tongue about sugar concentration are not just compressed by a power function; they are also referenced to a baseline level that is not stored. Increases in sugar concentration above that baseline lead to compressed increases (strictly convex increases) in "sweetness." Decreases lead to reductions in firing rate in the sensory nerve, the quantitative details of which are currently unknown.

If our memories about the sweetness of sugar solutions are built from these compressed and reference-dependent measurements (and there is really nothing else from which they can be built), then this marginal utility story does not really make sense. Under these conditions—and they are the standard conditions that prevail in the nervous system—what is represented is not the objective value of the sugar solution, but rather a reference-based representation that is *compressively transformed into a utility-like signal with regard to the reference point*. One great advantage of this is that it explains both why things are reference dependent and why the curvature of the utility function is anchored to the reference point. We employ a reference-dependent mechanism because it increases the efficiency of our sensory and memory encoding systems. The cost is that it imposes some violations of rationality under some conditions.

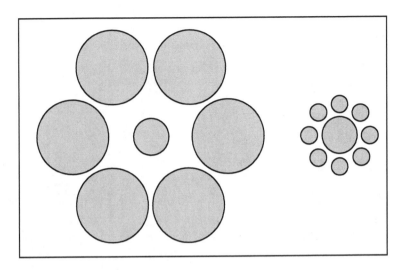

FIGURE 12.7

Amos Tversky argued years ago that the systematic errors we make in choices were something like optical illusions. He would often show the figure above.

In this figure, the central circles on the left and on the right are of identical size, but that is not what we perceive. The baseline for size estimation drifts down in the left figure and up in the right figure. The result is that the central circle on the left appears larger than the central circle on the right. Tversky argued that these kinds of visuospatial reference points in sensory systems were much like the framing effects in choice that had led him and Kahneman to postulate the reference point. What I hope I made clear in this chapter is that Tversky's metaphor is not really a metaphor at all.

13

The Basics of Dopamine: How We Learn and Store Value

Précis

Today neurobiologists and psychologists, perhaps unlike many economists, know a tremendous amount about how humans and animals *learn* the values of their actions. This knowledge grows, in large part, from studies of the neurotransmitter dopamine and the neurons that employ it. Our knowledge of the brain's mechanisms for valuation now extends far beyond the biophysics of dopaminergic synapses in the striatum, but the discovery that dopaminergic neurons encode a *reward prediction error* (RPE) was the key that made most of our modern studies of neural valuation circuitry possible. In this chapter, we (1) review the anatomy of the neural circuits associated with dopamine and valuation, (2) encounter theories of reinforcement learning from psychology and computer science that predate dopaminergic studies of valuation, (3) examine experimental work that forged a relationship between dopamine and these pre-existing computational theories, and (4) reductively follow these insights all the way down to the behavior of ion channels. When we finish, it will be clear that a neuroeconomic theory of valuation sweeps effectively from cell membranes to utility theory, and that con-straints derived from each interlocking level of analysis provide useful tools for better understanding how we decide.

The core insights we will encounter in this chapter are not new. Most neuroscientists have suspected for decades that dopamine plays some role in the processing of rewards (Wise, 2008; Wise and Rompre, 1989).

The most common hypothesis about the function of dopamine in the 1980s and 1990s, for example, was that the firing rates of these cells carried a utility-like signal—that these neurons were the "pleasure center" of the human and animal brain. There were, however, many problems with this theory that made it persistently unclear exactly what it was that dopamine (and the neural circuits with which it is intimately involved) did. While we have known for decades that humans and animals will work to activate their dopamine neurons artificially (for example, by taking dopaminergic drugs such as cocaine), there has also been strong evidence that natural rewards such as food or sex did not reliably activate these neurons. More than two decades ago, scholars, including Chris Fibiger and Anthony Phillips (1986), demonstrated that when a rat was placed in a novel environment, its dopamine neurons were active whenever food and water were first encountered, but that activity died out over hours. After a few days in the environment, the dopamine neurons were almost always silent, even as the animal happily ate, drank, and mated.

Such observations led, in time, to a kind of dopamine ennui. There were many reasons to believe that dopamine played some role in what psychologists called *motivated behavior*, but the "dopamine-is-reward" story simply did not add up. Most scholars recognized this fact; many simply stopped studying dopamine. During the 1990s, however, two small schools of thought rose up in the face of these challenges. The first of these schools argued that dopamine encoded the *salience* of external world events (Horvitz, 2000; Redgrave et al., 1999). Rather than coding reward *per se*, dopaminergic firing rates were proposed to encode how strongly events in the world deviated from expectations, whether those expectations were positive or negative. In this view, dopamine neurons were a kind of attention-getting signal: *That thing just encountered in the environment is better or worse than expected!* This explained why the dopamine neurons responded so strongly when a rat entered a novel environment and encountered food and water, but were later silent. Initially the discovery of food in a small bowl was a surprise (at least to a rat), but after days of finding food in that bowl, the salience of that observation diminished.

The second school that arose from these observations was developed by Michigan's Kent Berridge (Berridge et al., 2009; Kringelbach and

Berridge, 2009). Berridge proposed what is often called the "wanting" hypothesis of dopamine, which was driven by two key problems with the salience hypothesis. First, the salience hypothesis proposed that dopamine signaled all deviations from expectation, be those deviations positive or negative. The hypothesis suggested that dopamine neurons were as activated by adverse events as they were by positive events, but if that were true, then why would humans and animals work to activate these neurons? Some scholars had responded that human drug use was about the experience of salience, not the experience of reward, but that comes very close to saying that animals and humans prefer to experience negative events rather than to experience neutral events. The second problem with the salience hypothesis is that it separates dopamine pretty strongly from notions of reward. Things that have nothing to do with rewards can be salient, even though the core insights about dopamine all center on something related to rewards. Accordingly, Berridge hypothesized that dopamine encoded the experience of "wanting" a reward, which he distinguished from the experience of "liking" a reward.

Against this backdrop, the primate neurophysiologist Wolfram Schultz, then working at the University of Fribourg, began to record the activity of single dopamine neurons in the brains of monkeys while those monkeys participated in a Pavlovian conditioning task. When monkeys sit quietly, dopamine neurons fire at a fixed rate of about three to five spikes per second. This is their baseline rate; so regular is this rate that a number of scholars had even proposed these neurons as a kind of internal clock for timekeeping in animals (Metell et al., 2003).

In Schultz's experiment (Mirenowicz and Schultz, 1994; Schultz, Dayan and Montague, 1997), while these neurons were ticking away, the thirsty monkeys in which they were located sat in front of a water spout, as depicted in Figure 13.1. At unpredictable intervals, a tone was produced by a speaker and a drop of juice was provided by the spout. At first, the dopamine neurons continued to tick away at 3 to 5 Hz when the tone was played, but they responded with a much higher-frequency burst of action potentials when the water was delivered. With time, however, the neurons diminished their response to the water and increased their response to the (temporally unpredictable) tone. In time, the neurons came to be unaffected by the water delivery (they remained at their baseline rate) but were found to be highly activated whenever the

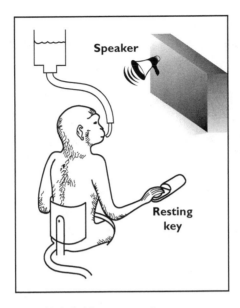

FIGURE 13.1   Cartoon of Schultz' famous experiment.

tone occurred. If, however, at any time Schultz delivered a drop of water not signaled by the tone, then the dopamine neurons still responded to this unpredictable reward with a burst of action potentials. This indicated that it was not that the water itself had lost the ability to activate the dopamine neurons, but rather that the water the monkey had learned to expect had ceased to activate the neurons. Finally, Schultz observed that if the tone was played and the later water reward omitted, the neurons responded to this event by reducing their firing rates below baseline.

These data, and others like them from the dopamine-like[1] system of the honeybee (Montague, Dayan, and Sejnowski 1995, 1996), led young neurobiologists Read Montague and Peter Dayan (then post-docs with Terry Sejnowski at the Salk Institute) to realize that the patterns of activity

---

1. Honeybees employ a close chemical homologue of dopamine called *octopamine*. The fact that the same basic system occurs in species separated by something like 500 million years of evolution suggests how strongly evolution has conserved this mechanism.

Schultz had observed were similar to those predicted by a theory of learning that had recently emerged from computer science. This led them to collaborate with Schultz and to reanalyze his data. They found, to everyone's surprise, that the firing rates of the dopamine neurons were quite precisely predicted by this pre-existing theory of learning (Schultz, Montague, and Dayan, 1997).

What followed were a series of interacting theoretic and empirical studies of dopamine neurons that continue to this day. In a typical group of those studies, a series of single-neuron recordings are used in an effort to verify the predictions of a particular theory of learning, and gaps between theory and experiment are identified. This is then followed by a set of extensions to the theory that allows it to predict more behavioral effects as well as allowing it to account for the novel experimental findings with neurons. These theoretic advances are then followed by further empirical studies, and the cycle repeats. So far, there have been about four of these iterations, and that in only a decade.

This rapid pace of interacting theory and experiment has had a number of effects, some good and some bad. The first is that the theory has become quite mathematically precise, and it has become precise so quickly that many casual observers of the dopamine literature remain unfamiliar with the current (and admittedly quite technical) models of what it is that dopamine is believed to do. Many of these casual observers, scholars who might read one or two important experimental papers from this literature each year, may even be led to conclude that the current theory is being continuously falsified. The rapid cycle of theoretical and empirical advance has unavoidably fostered confusion about the role of dopamine in learning.

The second effect is that there are now too few people who really understand the existing theory. One sees evidence of this all the time at conferences. A bright young scholar presents an empirical result and then declares that it falsifies the "dopamine theory of learning" even though an admittedly difficult-to-read theoretical paper predicted just this observation five years earlier.

The third and most significant effect of these cycles of theory and experiment is an effect on the core community of people who study dopamine activity for a living, among whom there is now almost complete unanimity in the conviction that dopamine neurons participate in reinforcement learning. Indeed, most people in the dopamine community believe that of all of the beautiful computational theories of brain function in existence, the one theory that best accounts for what we see in any brain system is the dopamine theory of learning.

Obviously, I consider myself a member of this latter community and my conviction, like that of most of my colleagues, is that the dopamine story is now largely understood at a basic level. This chapter will make that case in detail. But before we begin, I do want to point out that there is not quite complete unanimity on the functional role of these dopamine neurons. What I will present in the pages that follow is only a theory; it is the consensus theory at this point, but it is still hotly debated by gifted scholars including Berridge and Sheffield University's Peter Redgrave (e.g., Redgrave and Gurney, 2006).

As we move forward, though, I think it is essential to distinguish two kinds of criticisms of the dopamine theory of learning that are often confused. The first class of criticism arises when a scholar argues that some well-predicted phenomenon, such as the burst of action potentials produced by dopamine neurons in response to the tone in Schultz's experiment, is unexplained by theory. This comes from relying on outdated models to define what is "predicted" by the dopamine theory of learning. A scholar might quite accurately note that the Rescorla-Wagner model of learning from the 1970s does not predict the tone-related burst of action potentials observed in the neurons—but, unknown to him, a more advanced form of that same theory that emerged in the early 1980s precisely predicts this burst. This class of criticism arises when people do not take theory seriously enough, and I hope that the pages that follow will do much to reduce these spurious critiques. The second class of criticism identifies real gaps between theory and experiment that have yet to be plugged. We will encounter several of these gaps in the pages that follow. It may seem obvious that these two kinds of criticism are different, but in practice they are hopelessly confused even in the best academic journals. This no doubt reflects a failure of theorists to communicate clearly, and it is a failure we must overcome if we are to move forward. To move towards that end, we now begin a serious examination of the basics of the dopamine systems of the primate midbrain.

The Anatomy of Both Dopamine and Valuation

Dopaminergic Neurons of the Midbrain

It has been widely known since the 1920s and 1930s that vertebrate neurons communicate with one another chemically—that neurons employ neurotransmitters to send signals across the synapse. Prior to the 1950s, however, it was widely assumed that all neurons employed a single neurochemical to achieve this communication, the neurotransmitter acetylcholine. In the late 1950s and early 1960s, a group of Scandinavian neurochemists, including Bengt Falck and Åke Hillarp at the University of Lund, as well as Kjell Fuxe and Annica Dahlstrom at the Karolinska Institute and Arvid Carlsson in Goteborg, demonstrated conclusively that this widely held belief was incorrect (for more background, see Carlsson, 2000). They showed that highly localized clusters of cell bodies synthesized compounds such as dopamine and serotonin, that these cells sent those compounds down their axons, and that these cells released those compounds from their terminals in response to depolarization. What they demonstrated was a set of anatomically discrete and chemically specific systems for neurotransmission.

Their studies revealed, among other things, that clusters of dopamine-containing neurons could be found in over a dozen locations in the mammalian brain. Of these nuclei, however, only three sent axons along a long-distance trajectory that could influence brain activity in many areas. These long-distance projections had their origin in what are known as the A8, A9, and A10 cell groups, and all of them lie within the midbrain (Fig. 13.2).

This was a striking observation because it suggested a functional specialization. The idea that specific clusters of cell bodies with highly specific projection pathways passed through the axonal fields of the brain suggested that these cells might have highly specific functions. In the 1960s that was an exciting and controversial idea; now it has been incorporated into the corpus of classical neurobiology.

In any case, the original A8 and A10 cell groups are located, respectively, in dorsal and ventral portions of the ventral tegmental area (VTA). Just anterior to these two groups is the A9 cluster located in the substantia nigra pars compacta (SNc). Lying in these three clusters, all of

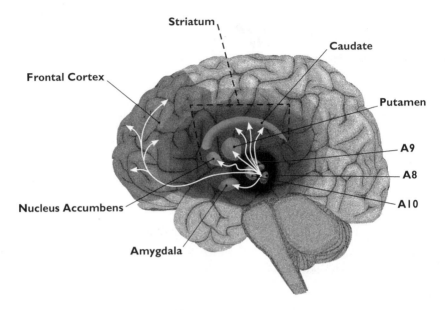

FIGURE 13.2   The A8, A9 and A10 cell groups.

these dopamine neurons are unusually large cells for neurons. The size of the cell bodies no doubt reflects the fact that the biosynthetic machinery of the cells must be able to support their unusually long axons, which make unusually large numbers of synapses. In fact, many of these neurons release dopamine not only at discrete synapses but also into the general intracellular spaces along their trajectories using a specialization called the *en passant* synapse (Cooper, Bloom, and Roth, 2003).

Early studies of these neurons seemed to suggest an unusually high degree of spatial segregation by cell group. The A9 cluster in the substantia nigra seemed to make connections exclusively to the caudate and putamen, the principal nuclei of the dorsal striatum. The A8 and A10 group axons appeared to travel more ventrally, making contact with the ventral striatum and the fronto-cortical regions beyond. Subsequent studies have challenged this dogma to some degree: there does seem to be some intermixing of the three cell groups, although a topography remains (Haber et al., 2000; Williams and Goldman-Rakic, 1998).

However, studies of the activity of these cells in awake behaving monkeys stress homogeneity. Recordings from both the VTA and SNc seem to tell the same story. While knowing that one is recording from a dopamine neuron may be difficult (e.g., Margolis et al., 2006), all cells that look like dopamine neurons in the core of the VTA and SNc regions seem to respond in the same way during conditioning or learning tasks.[2] Even the structure of the axons found in these areas seems to support this notion that activity is homogenous across this population. It is now known, for example, that the axons of adjacent neurons are actually electrically coupled to one another in this system (Grace and Bunney, 1983; Vandecasteele et al., 2005). Modeling studies suggest that this coupling makes it more difficult for individual neurons to fire alone, enforcing highly synchronous firing across the population (Komendantov and Canavier, 2002).

A final note is that dopamine neurons have long-duration action potentials. A dopamine action potential might take as long as two to three milliseconds, compared to as little as 0.1 millisecond in some other systems. This is relevant because it places a very low limit on the maximal firing rates that these neurons can produce (e.g., Bayer, Lau, and Glimcher, 2007).

What emerges from these many studies is the idea that the dopamine neurons are well suited to serve as a kind of specialized low-bandwidth channel for broadcasting the same information to large territories in the basal ganglia and frontal cortex. The large size of the cell bodies, the fact that the cells are electrically coupled, and the fact that they fire at low rates and distribute dopamine homogenously throughout a huge innervation territory: all these unusual things mean that they cannot say much to the rest of the brain, but what they say must be widely heard.[3]

---

2. As I write the final revisions to this chapter, a new group of putatively dopaminergic neurons has been identified physiologically in the far dorsolateral substantia nigra (Matsumoto and Hikosaka, 2009a). What is interesting about these neurons is that they have physiological properties very different from those of all other dopaminergic neurons studied to date. If there is indeed a second group of physiologically distinct dopaminergic neurons, a conclusion still highly controversial, then yet another exciting round of advances in theory may not be far off.

3. The very latest data do suggest some very significant differences between the time courses of the dopamine levels produced in the dorsal striatum and in the ventral striatum. Paul Phillips and his colleagues (Zhang et al., 2009) have produced beautiful data suggesting a specialization of dopamine transmitter release mechanisms in these two areas that may play an important role in further refining existing theory.

The Frontal Cortex

It is also important to recognize that the dopamine neurons lie embedded in a large and well-described circuit, the details of which will prove important for understanding valuation. This circuit involves two principal subdivisions of the mammalian brain: the frontal cortex and the basal ganglia.

The frontal cortex is the cortical tissue lying anterior to the central sulcus, marked in black in Figure 13.3. Along the anterior bank of this sulcus lies the motor cortex, the final common output pathway for control of the skeletal musculature. While all mammals have frontal cortices, it is very important to note that the size of the frontal cortex, as a fraction of brain volume, changes enormously as one moves from animals such as rats or hedgehogs to animals such as monkeys and lemurs, and changes even more as one moves to humans. It should be clear from Figure 13.3 that primates as a group have evolved an enormous frontal cortex, and that the human frontal cortex is simply gigantic. It has to be stressed that the metabolic cost of this additional tissue is also gigantic: more than 20% of what humans eat goes to feed our brains (and the brain accounts for only about 4% of our bodies by weight), and much of that fuel drives the frontal cortex. An animal without a huge frontal cortex can survive by eating much less.

Recall from Chapter 7 that the cortex can be divided into discrete functional maps that can be identified on both cytoarchitectural and functional grounds. The same is true for the frontal cortex, although here the functional properties associated with each of the anatomically distinct sub-maps remain largely unknown. The recent evolutionary growth of the frontal cortex in the primate line could have arisen along either of two developmental strategies with regard to this specialization: each of the pre-existing sub-maps in less complicated species could simply have been increased in size, or new sub-maps could have been added as the size of the cortical sheet increased frontally. Studies by anatomists indicate that *both* of these processes have likely occurred during evolution (Bailey and von Bonin, 1951; Brodmann, 1909; von Bonin and Bailey, 1947; von Economo, 1929). Monkeys and humans have larger maps than do rats, but, and this is perhaps more important, monkeys have maps that rats do not have, and humans have maps that monkeys and rats do not have.

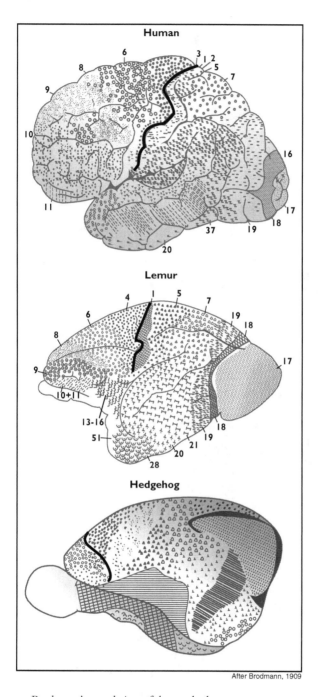

FIGURE 13.3   Brodmann's parcelation of the cerebral cortex.

This limits the conclusions we can draw about the human brain from studies of animals with much smaller cortices. It seems likely, for example, that the orbitofrontal cortex of the human is unique. Areas in our brains homologous to the orbitofrontal cortex of the rat likely lie at the very back edges of our much larger frontal cortex. Rat and human orbitofrontal cortexes are almost certainly *not* the same thing, a fact often overlooked in casual discussions of brain function.

In all of these species, however, the outputs of the frontal cortical areas fall into two broad categories: intra-cortical connections that connect frontocortical areas to one another, and cortico-basal ganglia connections that send the output of these frontal circuits to the basal ganglia circuits that contain the cell bodies of the dopamine neurons.

The Basal Ganglia

The outputs of the frontal cortex pass in a topographic manner to the two main input nuclei of the basal ganglia complex, the caudate and the putamen, which are collectively known as the striatum. Structurally, the caudate and putamen (and the ventral-most parts of the putamen, known as the ventral striatum) are a single nucleus that has separate names because, during infant brain development, a dense band of axons punches a series of holes through the striatum to connect the overlying cortex with the underlying brainstem and spinal cord, dividing the striatum into the caudate dorso-medially and the putamen ventro-laterally. Neurochemical and anatomical studies indicate that the caudate–putamen–ventral striatum can, indeed, be viewed as a single structure at the organizational level (Holt, Graybiel, and Saper, 1997) (Fig. 13.5). Essentially the same cell types and patterns of connectivity occur throughout these nuclei. However, in a general way there is an organizational gradient that does arise in the dorso-ventral extent of this large compound nucleus: as one moves ventrally from the dorsal caudate towards the ventral striatum, there is a gradual shift in some of the architectural and neurochemical features of the structure.

These two input nuclei project principally to two output nuclei, the globus pallidus and the substantia nigra pars reticulata. These nuclei then, in turn, provide two basic outputs. The first and largest of these outputs returns information to the frontal cortex via a thalamic relay.

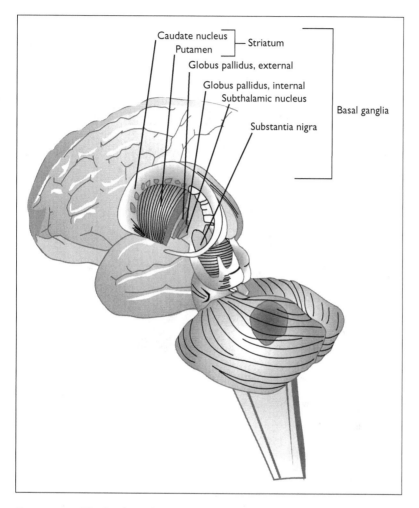

Caudate nucleus ⎤
Putamen ⎦— Striatum
Globus pallidus, external
Globus pallidus, internal
Subthalamic nucleus
Substantia nigra

Basal ganglia

FIGURE 13.4   The Basal ganglia.

Interestingly, this relay back to the cortex maintains a powerful topographic sorting (Kelly and Strick, 2003, 2004). The medial and posterior parts of the cortex that are concerned with planning skeletomuscular movements send their outputs to a specific sub-area of the putamen, which sends signals back to this same area of the cortex via the globus pallidus and the ventrolateral thalamus. In all, five principal sub-domains of the frontal cortex project to five sub-domains of the basal ganglia, which in turn project back via the output nuclei to the cortical regions

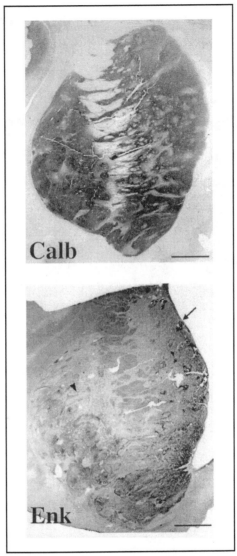

FIGURE 13.5 Cross-section through the caudate-putamen stained for calbindin and enkephalin.

of origin.[4] Together these connections thus form a kind of long feedback loop that ultimately generates behavioral output though the skeleto-muscular and eye movement control pathways that form two of the five subdomains of the massive frontal-basal ganglia system (Fig. 13.6).

The second principal class of output from the basal ganglia targets the midbrain dopamine neurons and also forms a feedback loop. These outputs pass to the dendrites of the dopamine cells, where they combine with inputs from the brainstem that likely carry signals about rewards being currently consumed. In this way, the dopamine signals reflect some combination of outputs from the cortex and from places such as the tongue. The combined signals are then broadcast, by the dopamine neurons, throughout the basal ganglia and the frontal cortex.

Before moving on to theoretical issues that will help us to understand the functional implications of these anatomical findings, I should stress that I have presented here only the most rudimentary features of these anatomical circuits. The basal ganglia, for example, involve nearly a dozen nuclei with very complicated (and well-described) circuitry.

For an overview of the basal ganglia, the reader is referred to Graybiel (2002) and Hikosaka et al. (2000). Many of the components I have not even mentioned play critical roles in human behavior and disease. What I have described is the absolute minimum circuit knowledge that is required for making sense of dopamine's role in learning and valuation.

The Theory of Reinforcement Learning

From Pavlov to Rescorla-Wagner

The second set of ideas required for making sense of dopamine and learning come from psychology and computer science. That tradition goes back quite far but has its modern origins in the work of Ivan Pavlov and B. F. Skinner. Pavlov observed, in his famous experiment on the

---

4. It has recently been proposed on anatomical grounds that rather than seeing these five domains as fully separate, one could perhaps more accurately view them as serially interconnected. It has been argued that they form a kind of "information spiral" that begins with areas critical for more abstract valuation and ends with areas central in movement control (Haber et al., 2000).

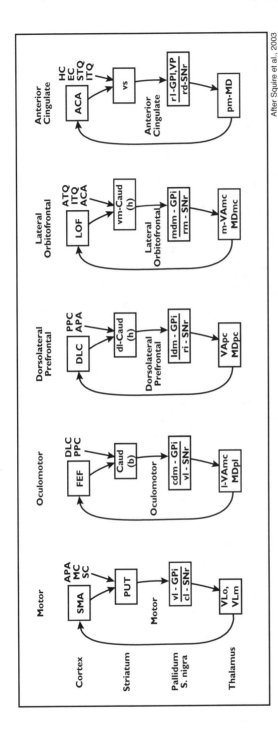

FIGURE 13.6 Hypothetical parallel segregated circuits connecting the basal ganglia, thalamus, and cerebral cortex. The five circuits are named according to the primary cortical target of the output from the basal ganglia: motor, oculomotor, dorsolateral prefrontal, lateral orbitofrontal, and anterior cingulate. ACA, anterior cingulate area; APA, arcuate premotor area; CAUD, caudate; b, body; h, head; DLC, dorsolateral prefrontal cortex; EC, entorhinal cortex; FEF, frontal eye fields; GPi, internal segment of globus pallidus; HC, hippocampal cortex; ITG, inferior temporal gyrus; LOF, lateral orbitofrontal cortex; MC, motor cortex; MDpl, mediulis dorsalis pars paralarnellaris; MDmc, medialis dorsalis pars magnocellularis; MDpc, medialis dorsalis pars parvocellularis; PPC, posterior parietal cortex; PUT, putamen; Sc, somatosensory cortex; SMA, supplementary motor area; SNr, substantia nigra pars reticulate; STG, superior temporal gyrus; VAmc, ventralis anterior pars magnocellularis; Vapc, ventralis anterior pars parvocellularis; VLm, ventralis lateralis pars medialis; VLo, ventralis lateralis pars oralis; VP, ventral pallidum; VS, ventral striatum; cl, caudolateral; cdm, caudal dorsomedial; dl, dorsolateral; l, lateral; ldm, lateral dorsomedial; m, medial; mdm, medial dorsomedial; pm, posteromedial; rd, rostrodorsal; rl, rostrolateral; rm, rostromedial; vm, ventromedial; vl, ventrolateral.

salivating dog, that if one rings a bell and follows that bell with food, dogs become conditioned to salivate after the bell is rung (Pavlov, 1927). This process, where an *unconditioned response* comes to be elicited by a *conditioned stimulus*, is one of the core empirical regularities around which psychological theories of learning have been built. Pavlov hypothesized that this behavioral regularity emerges because a pre-existing anatomical connection between the sight of food and activation of the salivary glands comes to be connected to bell-detecting neurons by experience. In the language of classical psychology, the *associative strength* of the linkage between the percept of the ringing bell and the salivary glands is strengthened by repeated exposure.

This very general idea was first mathematically formalized when American psychologists Robert Bush and Frederick Mosteller (1951) proposed, essentially, that the probability of Pavlov's dog expressing the salivary response on sequential trials could be computed through an iterative equation where

$$A_{next\_trial} = A_{last\_trial} + \alpha(R_{current\_trial} - A_{last\_trial})$$

In this equation, A_{next_trial} is the probability that the salivation will occur on the next trial (or more formally, the associative strength of the connection between bell and salivation). To compute A_{next_trial}, one begins with the value of A on the previous trial and adds to it a correction based on the animal's experience during the most recent trial. This correction, or *error term*, is the difference between what the animal actually experienced (in this case the reward of meat powder expressed as $R_{current\_trial}$) and what he expected (simply what A was on the previous trial). The difference between what was obtained and what was expected is multiplied by α, a number ranging from 0 to 1, which is known as the *learning rate*. When $\alpha = 1$, A is always immediately updated so that it equals R from the last trial. When α is 0.5, only half of the error is corrected and the value of A converges in half-steps towards R. When the value of α is small, say around 0.1, then A is only very slowly incremented towards the value of R.

From Bush and Mosteller's point of view, α could be seen as an empirical parameter that showed just how fast the animal's probability of responding grew with repeated experience. Learning is not instantaneous, and this parameter allowed Bush and Mosteller to capture that fact. From a more engineering-oriented point of view, α allows us to build animals that can survive in a world where rewards are unpredictable. Consider what happens when the bell is rung and the probability that Pavlov will bring the food is only 0.5. Under these conditions, an α of 1 would cause the associative strength to see-saw up and down between 1 and 0. If, in contrast, α were a very small number, the system would converge slowly towards an A of about 0.5, the actual probability that the food will be delivered.

The most important point here is that A reflects an estimate of the probability of reward in this example. Assuming that we want that estimate to be accurate, and that we have plenty of time to work out what that probability is, and that the real-world probability never changes, we want α to be very, very small. Many economists will recognize this as a feature of the Bellman equation from dynamic linear programming, to which the Bush and Mosteller equation is related.[5]

So in a sense the Bush and Mosteller equation computes an average of previous rewards across all previous trials. In this average, the most recent rewards have the greatest impact, while rewards far in the past have only a weak impact. If, to take a concrete example of this, we set α to 0.5, then the equation takes the most recent reward, uses it to compute the error term, and multiplies that term by 0.5. Half of the new value of A is thus constructed from this most recent observation. That means that the sum of all previous error terms (those from all trials further in the past) has to count for the other half of our estimate. If we look at that older half of the estimate, half of that half comes from what we observed one trial ago (thus 0.25 of our total estimate) and half (0.25 of our estimate) from the sum of all trials before that one. To put this another way, the iterative equation reflects, on each iteration, a weighted sum of previous rewards. When the learning rate (α) is 0.5, the weighting rule effectively being carried out is

$$A_{now} = 0.5R_{now} + 0.25R_{t-1} + 0.125R_{t-2} + 0.0625R_{t-3} + \ldots$$

5. One might here have the intuition, which can be proven correct, that in an equation of this kind A must converge (under some conditions) to the true expected value of the stimulus. The normative features of this approach have been well developed by Rich Sutton and Andy Barto in their 1998 book.

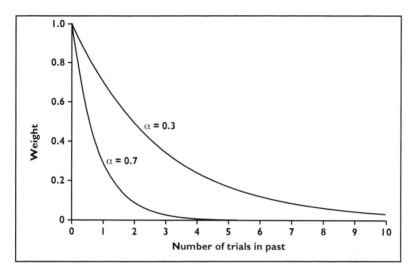

FIGURE 13.7   The weighting rule for 2 alphas.

The weighting rule, one cannot help but notice, is an exponential series, the rate at which the weight declines being controlled by α.

When α is high, that exponential function declines rapidly and puts all of the weight on the most recent experiences of the animal. When α is low, it declines slowly and averages together many observations. We can capture this most easily by rewriting the equation above as

$$A_{now} = \alpha^1 R_{now} + \alpha^2 R_{t-1} + \alpha^3 R_{t-2} + \alpha^4 R_{t-3} + \ldots$$

Economists will immediately recognize this as a kind of "backwards" discount function where α is, in essence, a kind of forgetting rate. It captures the speed with which we discount, or forget, old rewards.

Rescorla-Wagner and Expected Value

The Bush and Mosteller equation is important because it was the first use of this kind of iterative error-based rule and it forms the basis of all modern approaches to this problem. This is a fact often obscured by what is known as the "Rescorla-Wagner model" of classical conditioning (1972). The Rescorla-Wagner model was a very famous effort to extend the Bush and Mosteller approach (1951) to the study of what happens to associative strength when two cues predict the same event. Consider what happens when a tone and a bell both precede the food, or what happens when a dog learns that a bell precedes the food and then a tone is introduced with the bell. What associative strength does the bell acquire under these conditions? Those were pressing questions for psychologists that Robert Rescorla and Alan Wagner largely answered in the 1970s with their innovative extension of the Bush and Mosteller rule. Their findings were so influential in that community that the basic Bush and Mosteller rule is now often mistakenly attributed to Rescorla and Wagner.

The next important point to make is that these early psychological theories were, in essence, about associative strengths between classically conditioned stimuli and conditioned automatic responses. These models were about learning, but not about choice and not really about value. In the world of dynamic programming, however, these basic equations were easily extended to include a notion of value. To make that clear, consider an animal trying to learn the value of pressing a lever when pressing that lever yields four pellets of food with a probability of 0.5. Returning to the Bush and Mosteller (or Rescorla-Wagner) equation,

$$A_{next\_trial} = A_{last\_trial} + \alpha(Number\_of\_Pellets_{current\_trial} - A_{last\_trial})$$

Since on half of all trials the animal is rewarded and on half he is not, and since all rewards have a value of four, we know exactly what this equation will do. If α has a value of one, A will bounce up and down between zero and four; if α is infinitely small, A will converge to two. That is striking because two is the expected value of pressing the lever. So in an environment that does not change, when α is small, this equation converges to the expected value of the action:

$$EV_{next\_trial} = EV_{last\_trial} + \alpha(Number\_of\_Pellets_{current\_trial} - EV_{last\_trial})$$

or

$$EV_{now} = \alpha^1 Pellets_{now} + \alpha^2 Pellets_{t-1} + \alpha^3 Pellets_{t-2} + \alpha^4 Pellets_{t-3} + \dots$$

These are identical equations, the upper one being a recursive form suited to trial-by-trial computation and the lower one being, in essence, an unrolled version of the upper one.

Today, the Bush and Mosteller (or Rescorla-Wagner) equation forms the core of how most people think about learning values. The equation provides a way for us to learn expected values. If we face a stable environment and have lots of time, we can even show that this equation is guaranteed to converge to expected value (for more on this point, see Sutton and Barto, 1991, 1998).

Two key issues then remain before we can return to dopamine: How does this relate to utility, and how does this relate to reference points?

Utility and Reference Points

The Bush and Mosteller equation converges to expected value if we take as an input the objective value of each reward. How is the Bush and Mosteller equation related to utility? It should be obvious that the Bush and Mosteller equation will converge to the true expected utility of an action if we use utility, rather than true value, as its input:

$$EU_{next\_trial} = EU_{last\_trial} + \alpha(U(Pellets_{current\_trial}) - EU_{last\_trial})$$

To understand this fact, let us assume that the utility of pellets grows as a power function of the number of pellets, $Pellets^{0.6}$ for example; we could simply replace $U(Pellets)$ with $(Pellets^{0.6})$. Then the Bush and Mosteller equation would converge to the expected utility of four pellets delivered with a probability of 0.5 (which is about 2.3 in arbitrary units).

Consider again an animal trying to learn the value of approaching a dispenser that provides a sugar solution. We know that the firing rate carried by the sensory nerves from the tongue is a power function of sugar concentration. What would happen if we used the output of that nerve as the input to a reinforcement learning system organized around the Bush and Mosteller equation? Under those conditions,

$$Q_{next\_trial} = Q_{last\_trial} + \alpha((SugarConc^{0.6}) - Q_{last\_trial})$$

where $Q_{next trial}$ is the learned value of the dispenser. We would be learning the expected utility, not the expected value, of approaching the sugar water dispenser. What I hope this makes clear is something that has often been overlooked. Given that all of our sensory systems perform transformations (including non-invertible reference point subtraction) at the very first stages of encoding, no reinforcement learning system could ever learn the objective values of our actions. We could only ever learn the subjective values of those actions.

This is an observation with profound implications for understanding reference points. We will develop this point in more detail in a moment, but consider a fully stationary world (a world where nothing ever changes) that lasts forever. At any given moment in time, we can compute the expected utility of all of our future actions based on all of our past rewards. That is precisely the computation that, in a nutshell, underlies Q_{next_trial}. In a very real sense, then, we can think of Q_{next_trial} as being our rational expectation of what rewards, in units of subjective value, we expect from a future action. Q_{next_trial} is thus, at least to a first approximation, a kind of reference point with regard to a given action. Whether we get more reward than we expect or less than we expect when we actually perform that action is captured in the equation by the term

$$(SugarConc^{0.6}) - Q_{last\_trial}$$

a term which is known as the *reward prediction error* (RPE). It is important to note that this is a kind of reference-dependent representation of expected subjective value sitting at the heart of standard models of learning.

Sutton and Barto: The Temporal Difference Model

The story of reinforcement learning I have described up to this point is a story from psychology and, to a lesser extent, from dynamic programming. That story changed abruptly in the 1990s when computer scientists Rich Sutton and Andy Barto (1991) began to think seriously about these pre-existing theories and noticed two key problems with them:

1. The theories all treated time as passing in unitary fixed epochs usually called *trials*. In Bush and Mosteller (and Rescorla–Wagner), for example, trials pass one after another, and updates to the values of actions occur only between trials. In the real world, time is more continuous, and Sutton and Barto realized that a coherent theory of learning would have to reflect this. Different events in a trial might mean different

things, might indicate different things about value; at the very least, time within a trial had to be more completely represented.

2. The second key problem was that these theories dealt in only a rudimentary way with how to link sequential cues (for example, a tone followed by a bell) with a later event of positive or negative value. The theories were good at learning that a tone or a lever predicted a reward, but not so good at learning that a light that perfectly predicted the appearance of a lever meant that the later appearance of the lever told you nothing new.

Their work also identified two smaller problems with existing theory:

1. The Bush and Mosteller formulation looks like it could compute the true expected value (or utility) of a stimulus in an unchanging world, but we know very little about how it would behave with regard to optimality when the world is constantly changing. Sutton and Barto asked how models such as Bush and Mosteller's could be related to a more normative theory of learning.

2. Sutton and Barto, being computer scientists, also asked how real-world systems might be adjusted to approximate the ideal behavior of perfectly normative systems. They examined the impact of optimism biases and other features of that type in simulated reinforcement learning systems.

To address all of these issues, Sutton and Barto developed what has come to be known as temporal difference (TD) learning. That model is presented in detail in their lovely book on reinforcement learning. Here, I only briefly summarize the most important advances that they achieved.

Sutton and Barto began by arguing that, in essence, the Bush and Mosteller approach stated backwards the problem that learning systems were trying to solve. Bush and Mosteller has shown how we can learn the values of *previous* events, but Sutton and Barto argued that the goal of a learning system should really be to predict the value of future events. Of course predictions have to be based on previous experience, so these two ideas are closely related, but TD learning was designed with a clear goal in mind: *Predict the value of the future.*

That is an important distinction because it changes how we have to think about the RPE. In Bush and Mosteller-class models, RPE is the difference between a weighted average of past rewards and the reward you just experienced. When those are the same, there is no "error" and the system does not learn. Sutton and Barto, by contrast, argued that the RPE term should be viewed as the difference between one's rational expectations of all future rewards and any information (be it an actual reward or a signal that a reward is coming up) that leads you to revise your expectations. If, for example, we predict that we will receive one reward every minute for the next 10 minutes and a visual cue indicates that instead of these 10 rewards we will receive one reward every minute for 11 minutes, then an RPE exists *when the visual cue arrives*, not 11 minutes later when the extra (and at that point fully expected) reward actually arrives. This is a key difference between TD-class models and Bush and Mosteller-class models.

To accomplish the goal of building a theory that both could deal with a more continuous notion of time and would build a rational (or near-rational) expectation of future rewards, Sutton and Barto switched away from simple trial-based representations of time to a representation of time as a series of discrete moments that together make up a kind of *super-trial*. They then imagined learning as a process that occurred not just at the end of each super-trial but at each of these discrete moments.

To understand how they did this, consider a (common) Bush and Mosteller-like version of TD learning in which each trial can be thought of as made up of 20 moments. What we are trying to do is build a prediction about what rewards can be expected in each of those 20 moments. The sum of those predictions is our total expectation of reward. We can represent this 20-moment expectation as a set of 20 learned values, one for each of the 20 moments. This is the first critical difference between TD-class and Rescorla-Wagner-class models. The second difference lies in how these 20 predictions are generated. In TD, the prediction at each moment indicates not only the reward that is expected *at that moment* but also the sum of (discounted) rewards available in each of the subsequent moments.

To understand this, consider the value estimate, V_1, that we attach to the first moment in this 20-moment trial. It needs to encode the value of any rewards expected at that moment, the value of any reward expected at the next moment decremented by the *discount factor*, the value of the next moment further decremented by the discount factor, and so on. Formally, that value function at time tick number one is

$$V_1 = r_1 + \gamma^1 r_{t+1} + \gamma^2 r_{t+2} + \gamma^3 r_{t+3} + \gamma^4 r_{t+4} + \ldots + \gamma^{19} r_{t+19}$$

where γ, the discount parameter, captures the fact that each of us prefers (derives more utility from) sooner rather than later rewards. The size of γ depends on the individual. Since this is a reinforcement learning system, it also automatically takes probability into account as it builds these estimates of r at each time tick. This means that the r's shown here are really expected rewards or average rewards observed at that time tick. If we were to imagine that these expected rewards were coded neurally after transformation to utility (as described in the previous chapter), then the above equation would reduce to

$$V_1 = E[u_1 + \gamma^1 u_{t+1} + \gamma^2 u_{t+2} + \gamma^3 u_{t+3} + \gamma^4 u_{t+4} + \ldots + \gamma^{19} u_{t+19}]$$

where E indicates that this is expected, or average, reward and u indicates that this discounted expectation is in units of utility.[6] What should be immediately striking about this equation is that it is basically identical to the Rabin and Kőszegi definition of the reference point we encountered in Chapter 12, although in that case this reference point was being used to guide choice rather than learning. In the TD model, therefore, learning occurs whenever the stream of obtained rewards will in the future deviate, or has now deviated, from expectations. In the language of neoclassical economics, learning occurs whenever we experience utility shocks.

TD learning, however, goes farther at an algorithmic level than the Rabin- Kőszegi definition of a reference point for choosing among utility shocks because it shows how these long-run expectations could be updated. TD accomplishes that by taking the difference between the old prediction and the current prediction (much like Bush and Mosteller) to generate a *prediction error*. This prediction error is then multiplied by a learning rate and added to the estimated value of the current time tick.

---

6. Or if we want to be fully cardinal, in units of *subjective value*.

Two kinds of events can thus lead to a positive prediction error: the receipt of an unexpected reward, or gaining information that allows one to predict a later (and previously unexpected) reward.

To make this important feature clear, consider a situation in which an animal sits for 20 moments, and at any unpredictable moment a reward might be delivered with a probability of 0.01. Whenever a reward is delivered it is almost completely unpredictable, which leads to a large RPE at the moment the reward is delivered. This necessarily leads to an increment in the value of that moment. On subsequent trials, however, it is usually the case that no reward is received (since the probability is so low), and thus on subsequent trials the value of that moment is repeatedly decremented. If learning rates are low, the result of this process of increment and decrement is that the value of that moment will fluctuate close to zero. Of course this is, under these conditions, true of all of the 20 moments in this imaginary trial.

Next, consider what happens when we present a tone at moment five followed by a reward at moment 15. The first time this happens, the tone conveys no information about future reward, no reward is expected, and so we have no prediction error to drive learning. At the 15th moment, in contrast, we receive an unexpected reward, so a prediction error occurs that drives learning in that moment. Now the goal of TD is, effectively, to reach a point at which the reward delivered in the 15th moment is unsurprising. The goal of the system is to produce no prediction error at moment 15 when the reward is delivered. Why is the later reward unsurprising? It is unsurprising because of the tone. So the goal of TD is to shift the prediction error from the reward to the tone.

TD accomplishes this goal by attributing each obtained reward not just to the *value function* for the current moment in time but also to a few of the preceding moments in time. (Exactly how many is a free parameter of the model.) In this way, gradually over time, the unexpected increment in value associated with the reward effectively propagates backwards in time to the tone. It stops there simply because there is nothing prior to the tone that predicts the future reward. If there had been a light fixed in time before that tone, then the prediction would have propagated backwards to that earlier light. In exactly this way, TD uses patterns of stimuli and experienced rewards to build an expectation about future rewards.

The question that this raises is: How rational is an expectation built in this way? Can TD really build accurate models of the value of the world? This is, of course, a normative question. The answer to this question is probably "no" in real life, but Sutton and Barto do provide a clear link to normative theory when they explain this issue. They point out that if we allow rewards to propagate far enough backwards in time, the TD model becomes equivalent to an ideal dynamic programming solution—it does become normative. The drawback to this ideal solution, however, is that it takes a subject infinite time to build her representation of the set of value functions for the environment. The speed with which experienced rewards propagate backwards in time thus reflects a trade-off between speed of learning and accuracy of learning. This is an insight that seems a critical step towards understanding all normative theories of learning.

Finally, Sutton and Barto embed in TD a number of "tricks" that make learning more efficient. To take one of the best examples, many versions of TD set the value of a novel stimulus not to 0, as in the example above, but to some small positive number. This amounts to embedding the assumption that any novel event is positive to some degree. That may seem a slightly dangerous assumption, but Sutton and Barto (1998) as well as others (Brafman and Tennenholtz, 2003) have shown that this presumption can be used to drive a kind of exploration that results in faster and more efficient learning under many conditions.

Partial Summary of Reinforcement Learning Theory

TD has several very interesting features that represent the state of the art in contemporary learning theory. TD begins with the assumption that animals wish to build predictive models of the gains and losses that they can expect to encounter. TD provides a mechanism, rooted in optimal dynamic programming, for deriving these expectations. This mechanism is not strictly normative, but it can approximate the normative solution under some sets of constraints. Finally, TD allows one to explore the effects of shifting prior assumptions about the world, or even shifting the average value of time (Niv et al., 2007). But none of these interesting features mean anything to a Hard theory unless TD can be shown to be related to the actual mechanisms for learning in the mammalian brain.

The Theory and Physiology of Dopamine

The insight that dopamine activity was related to RPEs had its origin in the classic studies of Schultz and colleagues mentioned at the beginning of this chapter. In the mid 1990s, Schultz recorded the activity of single dopamine neurons while monkeys were classically conditioned. In that experiment, thirsty monkeys sat quietly under one of two conditions. In the first condition the monkeys received, at unpredictable times, a squirt of water into their mouths.

Schultz found that under these conditions the neurons responded to the water with a burst of action potentials immediately after any unpredicted water was delivered (Fig. 13.8). In the second condition, the same monkey sat while a visual stimulus was delivered followed by a squirt of water (Fig. 13.9). The first time this happened to the monkey, the neurons responded as before: they generated a burst of action potentials after the water delivery but were mostly silent after the preceding the visual stimulus. With repetition, however, two things happened. First, the magnitude of the response to the water declined until, after dozens of trials, the water came to evoke no response in the neurons. Second, and with exactly the same time course, the dopamine neurons began responding to the visual stimulus. As the response to the reward itself diminished, the response to the visual stimulus grew.

When Read Montague and Peter Dayan saw this, they realized that it was not simply the reward prediction defined by Bush and Mosteller-class models such as Rescorla-Wagner (which would have been interesting

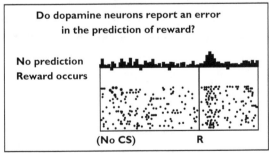

Adapted from Schultz et al., 1997

FIGURE 13.8

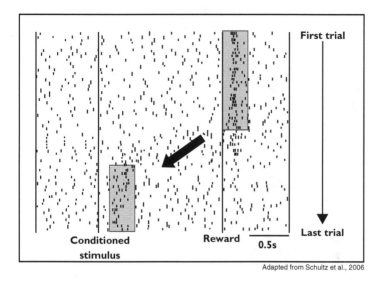

Adapted from Schultz et al., 2006

FIGURE 13.9

enough in its own right), it was *exactly* the RPE signal predicted by a TD-class model. Recall that a TD model generates an RPE whenever the subject's expected reward changes. For a TD-class model, this means that once an unpredictable visual cue comes to predict a reward, it is the unexpected visual cue that tells you that the world is better than you expected. The key insight here is that the early burst of action potentials after the visual cue is what suggested to Montague and Dayan that Schultz was looking at a TD-class system.

Two Dopamine Responses, One Theory

This is a point about which there has been much confusion, so I want to spend a moment here to clarify this important issue. Many scientists who are familiar only with Bush and Mosteller-class models (like the Rescorla-Wagner model) have looked at Schultz's data and been struck by these two different responses—one at the reward delivery, which happens only early in the session, and a second at the visual cue, which happens only late in the session. The Bush and Mosteller algorithm predicts only the responses synchronized to the reward itself, so these scholars often conclude that dopamine neurons are doing two different things, only one of which is predicted by theory. If, however, one considers the TD-class of models (which were defined more than a decade before these neurons were studied), then this statement is erroneous. Sutton and Barto's insight in the early 1980s was that reinforcement learning systems should use the RPE signal to drive learning whenever something changes one's expectations about upcoming rewards. Once a monkey has learned that a tone indicates a reward is forthcoming, then hearing the tone at an unexpected time is as much a positive RPE (a positive utility shock) as is an unexpected reward itself. The point here is that *the early and late bursts observed in the Schultz experiment are really the same thing in TD-class models.* This means that there is no need to posit that dopamine neurons are doing two things during these trials: they are just encoding RPEs, pure and simple, in a way well predicted by theory.

Negative RPEs

Schultz went on to extend these findings. In the same paper mentioned above, Schultz also examined what happens when an expected reward is omitted, when the animal experiences what we can call a *negative RPE* (Fig. 13.10). To examine that, Schultz first trained his monkeys to anticipate a reward after a visual cue as described above and then, on rare trials, simply omitted the water reward at the end of the trial. Under these conditions, Schultz found that the neurons responded to the omitted reward with a decrement in their firing rates from baseline levels.

That also makes sense from the point of view of a TD-class—and in this case a Bush and Mosteller-class—RPE. In this case, an unexpected visual cue predicted a reward. The neurons produced a burst of action potentials in response to this prediction error. Then the predicted reward was omitted. This yields a negative prediction error, and indeed the neurons respond after the omitted reward with a decrease in firing rates. One interesting feature of this neuronal response, however, is that the neurons do not respond with much of a decrease. The presentation of an unexpected reward may increase firing rates to 20 or 30 Hz from their 3- to 5-Hz baseline. Omitting the same reward briefly decreases firing rates to 0 Hz, but this is a decrease of only 3 to 5 Hz in total rate.

If one were to assume that firing rates above and below baseline were linearly related to the RPE in TD-class models, then one would have to conclude that primates should be less influenced, in their

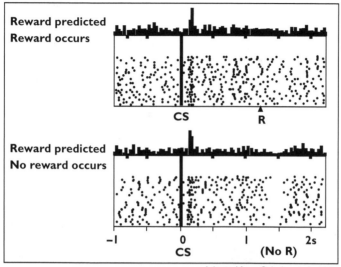

Adapted from Schultz et al., 1997

FIGURE 13.10

valuations, by negative prediction errors than by positive prediction errors, but we know that both human and non-human primates are much more sensitive to losses below expectation than to gains above expectation (Chen et al., 2006; Kahneman and Tversky 1981, 1986; Lakshminarayanan et al., 2008; Santos and Lakshminarayanan, 2008). Thus, Schultz's finding that positive utility shocks shift dopamine firing rates more than do negative utility shocks suggests either that the relationship between this firing rate and actual learning is strongly nonlinear about the zero point, or that dopamine codes positive and negative utility shocks in tandem with a second system specialized for the negative component. This latter possibility was first raised by Daw and colleagues (2002), who specifically proposed that two systems might work together to encode RPEs, one for coding positive and one for coding negative RPEs, a point to which we will turn later in this chapter.

Relating TD Models and Normative Theory to Dopamine Firing Rates

The TD-class models, however, predict much more than simply that some neurons must respond positively to positive utility shocks and negatively to negative utility shocks. These iterative computations also tell us about how these neurons should, in a more normative sense, combine recent rewards in their reward prediction. Recall from earlier in this chapter that saying a system recursively estimates value by computing

$$EV_{next\_trial} = EV_{last\_trial} + \alpha(Number\_of\_Pellets_{current\_trial} - EV_{last\_trial})$$

is the same as saying that the computation of value averages recent rewards using an exponential weighting function

$$EV_{now} = \alpha^1 Pellets_{t-1} + \alpha^2 Pellets_{t-2} + \alpha^3 Pellets_{t-3} + \alpha^4 Pellets_{t-4} + ...$$

where α, the learning rate, is a number between one and zero. If, for example, α has a value of 0.5, then

$$EV_{now} = 0.5Pellets_{t-1} + 0.25Pellets_{t-2} + 0.125Pellets_{t-3} + 0.0625Pellets_{t-4} + ...$$

Now, if the dopamine neurons really do encode the RPE, they encode the difference between expected and obtained rewards. In a simple conditioning or choice task, that means that they encode something like

$$RPE = R_{obtained} - [0.5Pellets_{t-1} + 0.25Pellets_{t-2} + 0.125Pellets_{t-3}$$
$$+0.0625Pellets_{t-4} + ...]$$

The normative definition of the TD model presented by Sutton and Barto (1998) tells us little about the value α should take under any specific set of conditions (here I arbitrarily made it 0.5), but we know that the decay rate for the weights in the bracketed part of the equation above should decline exponentially for any stationary environment. We also know something else: when the prediction equals the obtained reward, the prediction error should equal zero. That means that the actual value of $R_{obtained}$ should be exactly equal to the sum of the exponentially declining weights in the bracketed part of the equation.

Bayer and Glimcher (2005) tested these predictions by recording from dopamine neurons while monkeys engaged in a learning and choice task. In their experiment, monkeys had to precisely time when in a trial they would make a response for a reward. One particular response time would yield the most reward, but that best time shifted unexpectedly (with a roughly flat hazard function) across large blocks of trials. On each trial, then, the monkey could, at least in principle, cumulate information from previous trials to make a reward prediction. Then the monkey made his movement and received his actual reward. The difference between these two should have been the RPE and should thus be correlated with dopamine firing rates.

To test that prediction, Bayer and Glimcher simply performed a linear regression between the history of rewards given to the monkey and the firing rates of dopamine neurons. The linear regression asks, in essence: What is the weighting function that combines information about these previous rewards in a way that best predicts dopamine firing rates? If dopamine neurons are an iteratively computed RPE system, then increasing reward on the current trial should increase firing rates. Increasing rewards on trials before that should decrease firing rates, and should do so with an exponentially declining weight. Finally, the regression should indicate that the sum of old weights should be equal (and opposite in sign) to the weight attached to the current reward. In fact, this is exactly what Bayer and Glimcher found (Fig. 13.11).

The dopamine firing rates could be well described as computing an exponentially weighted sum of previous rewards and subtracting from

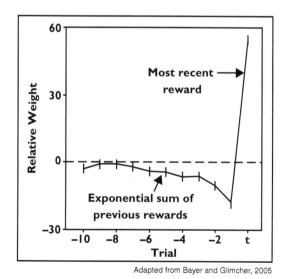

Adapted from Bayer and Glimcher, 2005

FIGURE 13.11   The Bayer and Glimcher weighting function.

that value the magnitude of the most recent reward. Further, they found as predicted that the integral of the declining exponential weights were equal to the weight attributed to the most recent reward. It is important to note that this was not required by the regression in any way. Any possible weighting function could have come out of this analysis, but the observed weighting function was exactly that predicted by the normatively anchored theory from which the TD model was derived.

A second observation Bayer and Glimcher made, however, was that the weighting functions for positive and negative utility shocks were quite different. Comparatively speaking, the dopamine neurons seemed fairly insensitive to negative shocks. Although Bayer, Lau, and Glimcher (2007) later demonstrated that with a sufficiently complex nonlinearity it was possible to extract positive and negative RPEs from dopamine firing rates, their data raise again the possibility that negative RPEs might well be coded by another system.

Dopamine Neurons and the Probability of Reward

Following on these observations, Schultz and colleagues observed yet another interesting feature of the dopamine neurons well described by the TD model. In a widely read paper, Schultz and colleagues (Fiorillo et al., 2003) demonstrated that dopamine neurons in classical conditioning tasks seem to show a "ramp" of activity between cue and reward whenever the rewards are delivered probabilistically.

Recall from our earlier discussion of TD-class models that these systems essentially propagate responsibility for rewards backwards in time. This is how responses to unexpected rewards move through time and attach to earlier stimuli that predict those later rewards. Of course, the theory predicts that both negative and positive utility shocks should both propagate backwards in trial time in the same way.

Now, with that in mind, consider what happens when a monkey sees a visual cue and receives a 1-milliliter water reward one second after the tone with a probability of 0.5. The value of the tone is thus 0.5 milliliter (or more accurately 0.5 times the utility of 1 milliliter). On half of all trials the monkey gets a reward, a positive utility shock of 0.5, and on half it gets no reward, a negative utility shock of 0.5. One would imagine that these two RPE signals would work their way backwards in trial time to

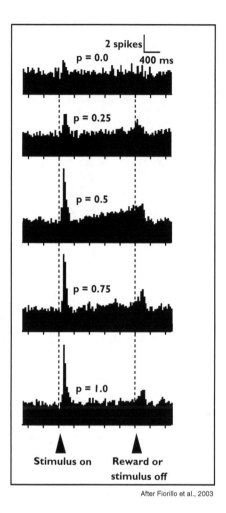

After Fiorillo et al., 2003

FIGURE 13.12   Schultz's ramp.

the visual cue. Averaging across many trials, one would expect to see these two propagating signals cancel one another out. However, what if the dopamine neurons responded more strongly to positive than to negative shocks (as Bayer and Glimcher [2005] showed that they did)? Under that set of conditions, the TD-class models would predict that average activity would show the much larger positive shock propagating backwards in time as a ramp—exactly what Schultz observed (Fig. 13.12).

This observation of the "ramp" has been quite controversial and has led to a lot of confusion. In his initial reports, Schultz said two things about the ramp: that the magnitude and shape of the ramp carried information about the history of previous rewards, and that this was a novel feature suggesting that the neurons encoded "uncertainty" in a way not predicted by theory. The first of these observations is unarguably true. The second is true only if we assume that positive and negative RPEs are coded as precise mirror images of one another. If instead, as the Bayer and Glimcher (2005) data indicate, negative and positive RPEs are encoded differentially in the dopamine neurons, then the ramp is not only predicted by existing theory, *it is required*. This is a point first made by Yael Niv and colleagues (Niv, Duff, and Dayan, 2005).

Utility Transformations and Dopamine Neurons

Throughout the most recent parts of this discussion of the dopamine neurons, I have focused on the idea that these cells encode a prediction error from which something like the expected value of an action or a tone can be computed. Let us return now to the earlier observation that if the inputs to the dopamine neurons were transformed to subjective values, then a TD-like system would converge towards something more like expected utility than like expected value. This is a terribly important point in light of the issues raised in Chapter 12. If dopamine firing rates both encode a reference point and converge to a subjective rather than an objective value, then this has significant implications for theories of choice. So do these neurons embed subjective or objective value in their firing rates?

This is a controversial issue that has only just begun to be addressed. In the Bayer and Glimcher (2005; Bayer, Lau, and Glimcher, 2007) studies, for example, a linear mapping between milliliters of juice and RPE was assumed. Schultz and his colleagues (Tobler et al., 2005), however, have begun to examine this issue. In one recent experiment, they systematically varied the magnitude of the largest reward in a choice set. They found that dopamine firing rates were a compressive function of reward magnitude (and perhaps also reflected a shifting reference point, although this is much more controversial). Without going into their findings in detail, the data do suggest the existence of a compressive transform upstream of the dopamine neurons. Combined with the fact that we know that objective values are basically never represented in the nervous system, this indicates pretty clearly that what the dopamine neurons do (if they are in fact a TD-class RPE encoder, as we believe) is allow us to learn and store the subjective values (the utilities, if you like) of actions and events in the outside world.

Caplin and Dean

So how sure are we that dopamine neurons encode an RPE? It is certainly the case that the average firing rates of dopamine neurons under a variety of conditions conform to the predictions of the TD model, but just as the TD-class succeeded the Bush and Mosteller class, we have every reason to believe that future models will improve on the predictions of TD. So can there ever be a way to say conclusively that the activity of dopamine neurons meets some absolute criteria of necessity and sufficiency with regard to learning?

To begin to answer that question, Andrew Caplin and Mark Dean (2007), economists at NYU and Brown University respectively, took a leaf from the standard neoclassical approach and turned it towards the study of RPE models. Just as Houthakker had shown that saying someone maximized a monotonic utility function was the same as saying he or she obeyed the axioms of GARP, Caplin and Dean asked whether there was a compact testable axiomatic way to state the current "dopamine hypothesis."

After careful study, Caplin and Dean were able to show that all classes of existing RPE-based models could be reduced to three axiomatic statements. Any RPE system, whether a Bush and Mosteller-class model or a TD-class model, must meet three axiomatic criteria. Saying that an observed system violated one or more of these axioms, they showed, was the same as saying that it could not, in principle, serve as an RPE system. Thus, what was important about Caplin and Dean's axiomatization of the class of all RPE models is that it provided a clear way to test this entire class of hypotheses.

In a subsequent experiment, Caplin, Dean, Glimcher, and Rutledge (2010) then performed an empirical test of the axioms on brain activations (measured with functional magnetic resonance imaging) in areas receiving strong dopaminergic inputs. They found that activations in the insula violated two of the axioms of RPE theory. This was an unambiguous indication that the activity in the insula (at least as measured by BOLD) could not, in principle, serve as an RPE signal for learning. In contrast, activity in the ventral striatum obeyed all three axioms and thus met the criteria of both necessity and sufficiency for serving as an RPE system. Finally, activity in the medial prefrontal cortex and the amygdala yielded an intermediate result. Activations in these areas seemed to weakly violate one of the axioms, raising the possibility that future theories of these areas would have to consider the option that RPEs either were not present or were only a part of the activation pattern here.

This Caplin and colleagues (2010) paper was important because it was, in a real sense, the final proof that some areas activated by dopamine, the ventral striatum in particular, can serve as an RPE encoder. The argument that this activation "only looks like" an RPE signal can now be entirely dismissed. The pattern of activity that the ventral striatum shows is both necessary and sufficient for use in an RPE system. That does not mean that it has to be such a system, but it draws us closer to that conclusion.

The Biophysics of Dopamine

Up to this point, the kinds of neuroscientific facts and theories that have gone into Hard economic theories have been at the reductive level of action potentials or above. There have been a few small exceptions, for example my comments on the role of thermal noise in behavioral stochasticity. When it comes to understanding how we learn value, however, it becomes important to understand how the biophysical mechanisms of information storage, which are now fairly well understood, constrain Hard theories.

Although not often discussed in neuroeconomic circles, the standard model of dopamine as an RPE encoder rests on very specific cellular mechanisms that describe both how dopamine would actually produce stored representations of value, and how these value representations would be accessed. This underlying theory is important for two reasons. First, it imposes additional constraints that extend all the way to behavior.

Second, the existence of this well-defined biophysical mechanism for storing the values of actions provides additional support for the hypothesis that a reference-dependent utility shock-driven learning system lies at the heart of human valuation. To these ends we begin with a cursory overview of the general cellular mechanism for learning and memory.

Long-Term Potentiation

In the 1940s and 1950s, one of the fathers of modern neuroscience, Donald Hebb (1949), proposed that some mechanism altered the strength of connections between pairs of neurons and that it was this adjustable connection strength that was the physical manifestation of memory. Hebb's initial goal in making this cellular-level proposal was to explain how conditioned reflexes operated at the biophysical level. You will recall that Pavlov had first demonstrated these reflexes in dogs exposed to bells followed by food. After many repetitions of this bell–food pairing, Pavlov found that simply ringing the bell elicited salivation in the trained dogs. This was the observation that drove the Bush and Mosteller model at roughly the same time that Hebb was searching for a biological mechanism for learning.

Hebb proposed what turned out to be the first of several closely related biophysical mechanisms for learning that operate by changing synaptic strengths. To understand Hebb's proposal, consider a pre-existing neural pathway (iconically diagrammed in Figure 13.13 as a single neuron labeled "bell") that connects the neural circuits for bell sensing with the neural circuits for salivation. Further, imagine that the strength of this excitatory connection between this "bell-sensing circuit" and the "salivation circuit" is low at the beginning of Pavlov's experiment. The fact that this synapse is weak is why the bell does not initially elicit salivation.

Parallel to this neuron and also impinging on the salivation neuron (which we can think of it as "standing for" a larger neural circuit) is a third neuron activated by the detection of food. The connection between this "food-detecting circuit" and the "salivation circuit" is also hypothesized to be pre-existing, but in this case strongly excitatory. This pre-existing strong synaptic connection accounts for the pre-experimental ability of food to elicit salivation.

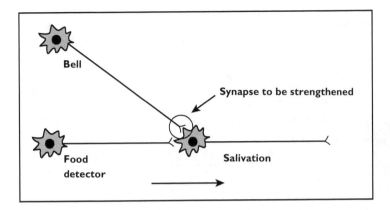

FIGURE 13.13   Hebb's classic circuit.

Hebb's goal, when thinking about such a circuit, was to describe a self-regulating mechanism that would strengthen the bell-to-salivation synapse during the classical conditioning process. To achieve that goal, Hebb made a simple proposal:

> When an axon of cell A is near enough to excite a cell B and repeatedly or persistently takes part in firing it, a growth process of metabolic change takes place in one or both cells such that A's efficacy, as one of the cells firing B, is increased.

This is sometimes rephrased as "cells that fire together wire together." Hebb proposed that whenever a presynaptic and a postsynaptic cell are active at the same time, the synapses connecting those cells are strengthened. Consider how this works in Pavlov's experiment. Before conditioning, the "bell cell" may fire often (whenever bells ring), but not at times when the other inputs to the salivation cell are active, and not at times when pre-existing strong inputs to the salivation cell are active. This means that the bell-to-salivary synapse is not active when the salivary cell tends to be firing. That changes during conditioning: the bell cell is activated and food is presented at essentially the same time. This means that the pre-existing strong synapses between the food and salivary neurons are depolarizing the cell at the same time that the bell cell is firing. If cells that fire together wire together, then both of these synapses strengthen, and in time the bell comes to elicit the salivation independently. In essence, this is a mechanism for encoding correlations; more formally, this is a mechanism that implements the replicator equation from evolutionary game theory, an application that will be familiar to many economists (Loewenstein, 2008; Loewenstein et al., 2009).

At the time that Hebb was proposing this rule for synaptic modification at the biophysical level, more traditional psychologists working at a higher level of abstraction were modeling how connection strengths grow as a function of RPEs. In some sense it must have been clear to these two groups that these two phenomena, described at very different levels of analysis, must have been related, but a full reductive synthesis of these approaches was still years off.

That reductive synthesis began to take shape when Tim Bliss and Terje Lomo (1973) discovered, in the rabbit hippocampus, unambiguous evidence for the physical instantiation of Hebb's mechanism. Bliss and Lomo demonstrated that cells that fire together really do wire together. More precisely, what they and subsequent researchers demonstrated was that at the time of any synaptic activity, the level of depolarization in the postsynaptic neuron (for many but not all synaptic types) regulates synaptic strength in a long-lasting way, a phenomena they called long-term potentiation (LTP).[7] A description of the precise biochemical mechanism of LTP (well known to every first-year neuroscience student) lies outside the scope of this presentation, but the core idea here is critical for understanding how Hebb's idea and the ideas of Bush and Mosteller go together. LTP is a process that strengthens a synaptic connection whenever a synapse is active at the same time that its target neuron is in a state of depolarization. Not all neurons have the ability to produce LTP, but many do. Neurons with this ability are found basically throughout the brain, and at particularly high densities in the striatum and frontal cortex. Finally, I need to stress that this process is quantitative in a cardinal way: *the level of depolarization as a function of time in the postsynaptic neuron controls the magnitude of the increment in synaptic strength.*

---

7. Subsequent studies have revealed a complementary process for the long-term reduction of synaptic strength known as long-term depression (LTD).

Dopamine and the Three-Factor Rule

Subsequent biophysical studies have demonstrated several other mechanisms for altering synaptic strength that are closely related to both the theoretical proposal of Hebb and the biophysical mechanism of Bliss and Lomo. Jeffery Wickens (1993; Wickens and Kotter, 1995) proposed the most relevant of these for our discussion, which is often known as the three-factor rule. What Wickens proposed was that some synapses might be strengthened whenever presynaptic and postsynaptic activity co-occurred with dopamine, and these same synapses would be weakened when presynaptic and postsynaptic activity occurred in the absence of dopamine.

Subsequent studies using a wide range of cellular and sub-cellular techniques have now provided impressive evidence in support of this proposal (for a review of this literature, see Reynolds and Wickens, 2002). When dopamine is present, active synapses appear to be strengthened in the basal ganglia, in the cortex, and in the amygdala.

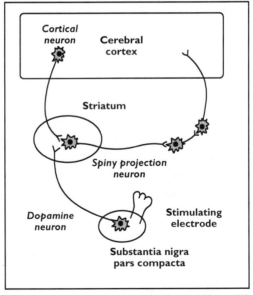

Adapted from Reynolds & Wickens, 2002.

FIGURE 13.14

Dopamine and Reinforcement Learning

Why is this important if we are thinking about models of reinforcement learning? Suppose we had the ability to regulate the synaptic strengths of a large group of cells as a function of the RPE. To be specific, imagine that an animal experiences a large positive RPE: he just earned an unexpected reward. The TD model tells us that under these conditions we want to increment the value attributed to all actions or sensations that have just occurred. Under these conditions, we know that the dopamine neurons release dopamine throughout the frontocortical–basal ganglia loops, and do so in a highly homogenous manner. That means we can think of any neuron equipped with dopamine receptors as "primed" for synaptic strengthening. When this happens, any segment of the frontocortical–basal ganglia loop that is already active will have its synapses strengthened.

To see how this would play out in behavior, consider that neurons of the dorsal striatum form maps of all possible movements into the extra-personal space. Each time we make one of those movements, the neurons associated with that movement are active for a brief period, and that activity persists after the movement is complete (Lau and Glimcher, 2007, 2008). If any movement is followed by an RPE, then the entire topographic map is transiently bathed in the global RPE signal carried by dopamine into this area (Fig. 13.15). What would this combination of events produce? A permanent increment in synaptic strength only among those neurons associated with recently produced movements. What would that synapse come to encode after repeated exposure to dopamine? It would come to encode the subjective value of the movement.

It is critical to understand here that essentially everything in this story is a pre-existing observation of properties of the nervous system. We know that neurons in the striatum are active after movements as required by (the eligibility traces of) TD models. We know that a blanket dopaminergic RPE is broadcast throughout the frontocortical–basal ganglia circuit. We know that dopamine produces LTP in these areas when correlated with underlying activity. In fact, we even know that after conditioning, synaptically driven action potential rates in these areas encode the subjective values of actions (Lau and Glimcher, 2005, 2007, 2008; Samejima et al., 2005). So all of these biophysical components exist,

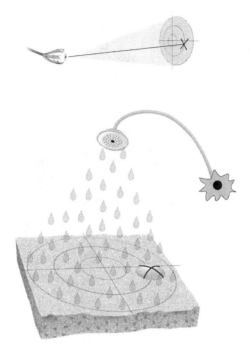

FIGURE 13.15

and in a configuration that could implement TD-class models of learning.

We even can begin to see how the RPE coded by the dopamine neurons could be produced. We know that neurons in the striatum encode, in their firing rates, the learned subjective values of actions. We also know that these neurons send outputs to the dopaminergic nuclei—a reward prediction. We also know that the dopaminergic neurons receive fairly direct inputs from sensory areas that can detect and encode the subjective magnitudes of consumed rewards. The subjective value of sugar solutions encoded by the tongue, for example, have an almost direct pathway through which these signals can reach the dopaminergic nuclei. Given that this is true, constructing an RPE signal at the dopamine neurons simply requires that excitatory and inhibitory synapses take the difference between predicted and experienced reward in the voltage of the dopamine neurons themselves.

Conclusions

It is important to acknowledge that this story is far from complete. We do not know, for example, how negative RPEs are encoded or whether they give rise to the complement of LTD (*long-term depression*).[8] We do not really know how the forward prediction of discounted future rewards is encoded in the striatal and frontal circuits. But the broad outlines here are surprisingly clear at a number of levels.

At the level of biochemistry, we can describe how synapses are modified by experience. At the level of neural circuits, we can show how these observed properties would give rise to a subjective value-encoding scheme. At the level of psychological and computer scientific theory, we can show how these circuits would implement near-normative learned representations of value. At the level of economics, we can begin to see how these processes are related to the reference-dependent computations that seem to underlie human choice.

---

8. Although Wickens (1993; Wickens et al., 1996) has suggested that this depression might occur whenever presynaptic and postsynaptic neurons are co-activated in the absence of any dopamine.

14

Locating and Constructing Subjective Value in the Front of the Brain

Précis

The core argument presented in the second section of this book was that choice occurs when a discrete group of fronto-parietal networks select one of two or more options for physical execution. The existing data indicate that these fronto-parietal networks serve as a "final common path" for choice. This final common path seems to represent relative expected subjective value in a stochastic way.

We know that the outputs of these tightly inter-coordinated fronto-parietal areas are then fed to movement control circuits for the computationally intensive (although economically uninteresting) process of movement generation. We know that these circuits are organized around the kinematic structure of actual movements—that is, they topographically map movements and not goods. But we also know that these circuits converge in the same way, and apparently at the same speed, whether a monkey must choose between two goods (for example, a red option over a green option; e.g., Horwitz et al., 2004) or between two movements (for example, a 10 degree rightward over a 10 degree leftward movement; e.g., Platt and Glimcher, 1999). This suggests that structures antecedent to the fronto-parietal networks must map goods into an action-based or movement-based representation as choice occurs (at least for the cases so far studied). It suggests, in other words, that these antecedent structures interactively participate in the fronto-parietal choice process, at least to some degree.

Completely unaddressed in the section of this book dedicated to the choice process were the issues of how subjective values are generated, how subjective values are stored, and which options are fed forward to these fronto-parietal networks for selection. The logical arguments and data presented in Chapters 12 and 13, however, offered some constraints on how these valuation circuits must work.

Chapter 12 made it clear that we must learn and store the subjective values of our options, not their objective values. This placed important constraints on the Hard-economic theories that can be used to describe human decision making. Our pre-existing understanding of sensory encoding in the vertebrate nervous system makes it clear that much technical irrationality observed in choice behavior must arise from the way that sensory experience, the root of subjective value, is encoded. The shifting baselines, or reference points, of all sensory encoding systems require that vertebrates produce some degree of irrationality in their choices—some violations of axioms such as transitivity are unavoidable in systems that operate using these informationally efficient techniques for encoding the properties of the outside world.

The studies of value learning and dopamine presented in Chapter 13 provide additional insights into how subjective values must be learned and stored. We know that RPE-based systems can be used to learn and store expected utility-like representations of value (Caplin and Dean, 2009), but the very structure of the dopamine system highlights the reference dependence of learning itself. The dopamine system takes as an input a reference-dependent signal, a signal that has been observed by physiologists, of exactly the kind postulated in economics by Kőszegi and Rabin (2006, 2007, 2009) for use in choice.

Given this suite of observations, the next critical questions for understanding expected subjective value all focus on how this quantity is represented and constructed. How and where do we construct and store the expected subjective values that guide choice? In this chapter I hope to make it clear that everything we know today suggests a few clear answers to this question, although our understanding of the constructive process by which expected subjective value is generated is in its infancy. First and foremost, our available data now indicate that the expected subjective values of actions reside principally in the frontal cortex and the striatum. These areas, working in concert with other areas, including the amygdala and the insular cortex, appear to be the physical seat of valuation. There is no doubt that many different sub-regions in these areas contribute to this overall process, but all of our data suggest that the medial prefrontal cortex (MPFC) and the striatum are central areas in this constructive process. These areas appear to be a funnel. All of the expected subjective values that guide choice seem to be represented in these areas, and it is variability in the inputs to these areas that almost certainly regulates the moment-to-moment valuations that guide choice. Second, we also know that these areas must not represent relative expected subjective value in the same way as do the fronto-parietal choice networks. If these areas stored and represented *relative value within a choice set* (as neurons in area LIP do), then we would have no way to compare two objects we know well but that we have never before compared. We must be able to store and represent the fact that $10,000 is better than $1,000 even if we have only previously compared $10,000 to $1,000,000. This simple observation points out that valuation areas must store a more absolute kind of expected subjective value than we encountered in the fronto-parietal choice networks. This is a representation that must (at least to some extent) support comparisons between all of the objects we have ever encountered, and so must store the values of all of these objects within a single common framework.

In the pages that follow, we will encounter both of these important issues in detail, but before we do that I want to make one thing abundantly clear: I believe that understanding how subjective value is constructed and how options are selected for arbitration in the choice circuits (a point taken up in Chapter 15) will be the great frontier for neuroeconomics in the decades to come. We have only the crudest understanding of how circuits in the dorsolateral prefrontal cortex (DLPFC), the orbitofrontal cortex (OFC), the amygdala, and the insula (to name just a few) work together to construct the changing subjective valuations that guide our choice. When we understand that mechanism, we will truly understand preferences, both when they are rational and when they are not. About this constructive process we have very little information today, but the information we have will provide the framework from which that future understanding of preferences will be built. It is to that framework that we now proceed.

The Medial Prefrontal Cortex and the Striatum: A Seat for Subjective Value

What are the sources of the relative expected subjective values that seem to guide choice in the fronto-parietal networks? Existing fMRI data show there are a small number of areas that are actively correlated with subjective value under essentially all reward and choice conditions that have ever been studied. The ventral striatum and the MPFC show up in dozens, if not hundreds, of studies under essentially all choice (and non-choice valuation) conditions as coding something like subjective value.

In fact, the very first fMRI studies of monetary gains and losses in humans began by identifying these areas as critical to valuation. In a set of almost simultaneous studies conducted at the turn of the millennium, Rebecca Elliot, Mauricio Delgado, and Brian Knutson all began to demonstrate that activity in the ventral striatum was correlated with the experience or expectation of gains and losses. Delgado and colleagues (2000), for example, showed that activity in the ventral striatum was correlated with both monetary rewards and monetary punishments. Elliot and her colleagues showed that activity in this area correlates with the magnitude of cumulative rewards (Elliot et al., 2000), and Knutson showed that activity in this area correlates with the anticipation of reward (Knutson, 2001a, 2001b, 2003). Subsequent studies have clearly borne out these initial correlations; the expectation of monetary reward (Breiter et al., 2001), the expectation of primary rewards (O'Doherty et al., 2002), the receipt of monetary rewards (Elliott et al., 2003), monetary expected values (Knutson et al., 2005), behavioral preference rankings among rewards (O'Doherty et al., 2006), potential gain magnitude and loss magnitude as scaled by subject-specific levels of loss aversion (Tom et al., 2007), and discounted reward value at delays ranging from minutes to six months (Kable and Glimcher, 2007) are all correlated with activity in the ventral striatum.[1] Single-unit recording studies in the dorsal striata of

---

1. However, I should note that Rangel and colleagues (Hare et al., 2008) have argued that these signals in the ventral striatum could be simply RPE signals, not subjective value signals *per se*. The logic of their argument is clear and clever. If a subject expects nothing and receives a reward, then the RPE and the subjective value of the reward are identical. This is a fact that can make it very difficult to discriminate subjective value and RPEs in many experimental designs. Further, the observation that the ventral striatum

monkeys, both in the caudate (Lau and Glimcher, 2007) and the putamen (Samejima et al., 2005), tell a similar story. Neurons in these areas have been identified that clearly code action values, a point detailed in Chapter 13. All of these data suggest that whenever rewards are received or preferences are expressed, activity in the striatum encodes the magnitudes of those rewards or preferences.

A similar story seems to hold in the MPFC, particularly in more ventral sub-regions of that area. Activity here has been shown to be correlated with monetary reward magnitude (Knutson et al., 2001a, 2001b, 2003), preference ordering among primary rewards (McClure et al., 2004), the expected value of a lottery (Knutson et al., 2005), the subject-specific valuation of gains and losses (Tom et al., 2007), subject-specific discounted reward value (Kable and Glimcher, 2007), and willingness to pay (Plassman et al., 2007). Activity in this area appears to be correlated with subjective valuations under all of these conditions.

This has led a number of scholars to propose that mean activity in the MPFC and the striatum encodes expected subjective value. Different neuronal subpopulations in these areas must encode different options, which suggests that these areas must therefore employ a topographic encoding scheme that segregates the populations that encode the expected subjective values of various actions or goods. The details of this encoding scheme, which probably lies beneath the resolution of fMRI, are only just beginning to be understood, and the encoding schemes

---

receives dense dopaminergic projections from the ventral tegmental area makes it nearly certain that activity in this area should track RPEs, in addition to whatever else it may track. For these reasons, and others, these authors have argued that only the MPFC contains a generalized expected subjective value signal. While this is a sophisticated and compelling argument that reveals a deep understanding of RPEs, it is also not a view well aligned with either evolutionary data or single-unit monkey physiology data at this time. The monkey physiology data gathered in the caudate (Lau and Glimcher, 2008) and putamen (Samejima et al., 2005) all show unambiguous evidence for subjective value encoding (as well as RPE encoding) in the dorsal two thirds of the striatum. We do not yet know if that is true of the ventral-most part of the striatum, but previous physiological studies of these areas suggest continuity (or at the most gradual change) in representational features across these three areas (e.g., Holt, Graybiel, and Saper, 1997). We also know that animals without frontal cortices (such as reptiles) can learn and represent subjective values, a finding that clearly suggests a role for the striatum in subjective value representation throughout the vertebrate line.

employed by the two areas are almost certainly different. (There are, for example, hints that the striatum employs an action-based encoding scheme and that the frontal cortex employs a more goods-based encoding scheme. If this is the case, then the frontal-to-striatal projections would serve as the critical mapping system that connects goods with actions. There are also hints that different classes of rewards may map to different subregions in the MPFC [e.g., Chib, Rangel, et al., 2009].) The current evidence seems to make it clear that these two areas serve as the final common representation of subjective value for use by the choice mechanism. Two studies make this point particularly clearly, one about inter-temporal choice conducted by Kable and Glimcher and a second about loss aversion conducted by Tom, Fox, Trepel, and Poldrack.

Kable and Glimcher

Given the opportunity to choose between $20 now and $20 in a week, essentially all humans prefer the immediate reward. In contrast, if a human is asked to choose between $20 now and $100 in a week, nearly all humans choose $100 in a week. The point at which each individual human switches, whether he or she chooses the delayed reward when it is worth $30, $50, or $70, varies from person to person and can be thought of as reflecting the impulsivity, or patience, of that individual.

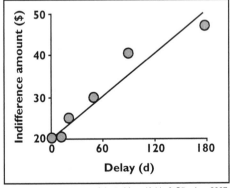

Adapted from Kable & Glimcher, 2007.

Figure 14.1   Indifference points as function delay.

To quantify that impulsivity, behavioral economists typically select a single delay, for example a week, and determine for each subject the amount of money that must be offered at that delay to make the subject precisely indifferent between an immediate and a delayed reward, as in the example above. Figure 14.1 shows a series of such indifference points as a function of delay for a typical human subject. Notice that for this subject, as we increase delay, the amount we must offer him increases as a linear function of delay. If we ask him to choose between $20 now and $25 in a month, he is indifferent. If instead we search for his indifference point at a delay of 3 months, we find it lies at $40. The indifference points of essentially all humans fall along such straight lines (Laibson, 1997), and it is the slope of these lines that characterizes each individual's degree of impulsivity. Perhaps surprisingly, humans choosing over money and animals choosing over food and water can all be characterized by straight lines when the indifference points are plotted in this way, although the slopes of those lines can vary widely.

For historical reasons, economists often take the reciprocal of these curves, as shown in Figure 14.2, to indicate the rate at which the value of money or food declines as a function of delay. We can think of these new curves as showing us the fraction by which a reward declines as a function of delay, and economists often refer to curves such as these as

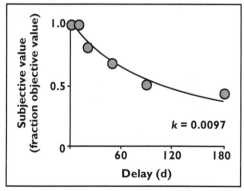

Adapted from Kable & Glimcher, 2007.

FIGURE 14.2

discount functions.[2] If we take the reciprocals of these straight lines, the equation that describes these discount functions is a hyperbola of the form

$$SV = \frac{1}{1 + kD}$$

where SV is subjective value as a function of delay, D is the delay to the reward, and k is a constant capturing the impulsivity of the individual chooser, the reciprocal of the slope of the line.

It is now widely documented that this equation, a hyperbolic discount function, does a good job of capturing the way in which value declines as a function of delay for every vertebrate species that has ever been examined (e.g., Laibson, 1997). Perhaps more importantly, this equation does a better job of capturing the decline in subjective value as a function of delay than does a simple exponential equation in which the value of a gain declines by a fixed percentage at each moment in time. Let me rush to point out that a chooser whose subjective values decline hyperbolically would necessarily violate the axioms of rational choice theory. For our empirical purposes here, however, the most important points to keep in mind are that subjective value declines in a reliable fashion as a function of delay and that different individuals show differing rates of decline—idiosyncratically distinct subjective values.

Kable and Glimcher used these two observations to ask a simple question: Is there a brain area that shows a pattern of activation that idiosyncratically predicts the subjective values each chooser places on all delayed gains as revealed by choice (even if that valuation structure violates the constraints of rationality)? To answer this question, Kable and Glimcher characterized the discount functions (or more precisely the discounted utility functions) of ten human subjects and scanned those subjects while they made choices between immediate and delayed rewards. They used the behavioral characterizations to construct, for

---

2. To be more precise, curves computed in this way actually reflect both the way money grows in subjective value with quantity and the way it declines with delay. In economic terms, these curves reflect both the utility function and the discount function working together, a *discounted utility function*. For the purposes of this discussion of expected subjective value, this is a point that can be neglected at no loss in generality.

each subject, a choice-by-choice estimate of the subjective values that particular subject would have encountered as she considered her choices. They then simply asked whether there was any brain area that showed a pattern of activation that was linearly correlated with this behaviorally derived estimate of subjective value. Importantly, this choice-by-choice estimate was different for each subject, because the subjective values each subject experienced were controlled by his or her unique degree of impulsivity.

Kable and Glimcher found that activity in the MPFC and ventral striatum was tightly correlated with subjective value within each individual subject. Put another way, they found that subjects who were impulsive had impulsive medial prefrontal cortexes and ventral striata, and patient subjects showed patience in these brain areas—exactly the result one would expect if these areas were the site at which subjective value was computed and represented—for all the delays they explored, for all the many different degrees of impulsivity their subjects showed, and for all the monetary values they encountered. The data seemed to indicate that these two areas (and presumably the dorsal striatum as well, based on monkey studies such as Lau and Glimcher [2008]) are the representation of subjective value that guides choice.

While this study provides particularly striking evidence for this hypothesis that these two areas encode subjective value for use by the choice circuits, these findings really serve as a confirmation of the many studies that yielded similar results and that were discussed above. Indeed, even studies of risk and ambiguity by Levy and colleagues (2010) show a similar result. In those studies, whether subjective value is influenced by risky lotteries or ambiguous prospects, activity in the MPFC and striatum seems to encode subjective value.

Tom, Fox, Trepel, and Poldrack

Sabrina Tom, Russell Poldrack, and their colleagues (Tom et al., 2007) provided yet more evidence in support of this conclusion in their studies of losses and gains during economic lotteries. In their experiment, subjects were, in essence, asked whether they would accept a lottery ticket that yielded a 50% chance of winning $X and a 50% chance of losing $Y. What they found, replicating earlier work by Kahneman and

Tversky (1979), was that the average subject will accept such a lottery only if X is about twice the size of Y. This is the phenomenon of loss aversion discussed in Chapter 5, a phenomenon that I argued can be logically considered only if we assume that gains and losses are computed from some pre-existing reference point.

Of course, Tom and colleagues found that each individual was different; some subjects were more loss averse than others. Subsequently, they simply sought to find what brain areas showed activations correlated with the subjective values of gains and what brain areas showed activations correlated with the subjective values of losses. They found that the same areas were sensitive to gains and losses. Activation in the MPFC was positively and linearly correlated with gains, while deactivations in this same area were linearly correlated with losses. It was, in essence, as if activations and deactivations in this area were correlated with the subjective values of gains and losses. The same was true for much of the striatum.

The Tom result is important for two reasons. First, it provides additional evidence that subjective values, *either losses or gains*, are represented in a unitary fashion in these two critical brain areas. Second, and perhaps more importantly, their data suggest that activity in these areas reflects shifts from a fixed baseline activity—a unique zero point. Gains reflect shifts upwards in activity from baseline and losses reflect shifts downwards from that baseline. Shifts downwards are greater, for the same magnitude of gain or loss, than shifts up. Further, the degree of this loss/gain asymmetry is predicted by the degree of loss aversion measured behaviorally in that individual. That is an astonishing point because it means that the baseline level of activation measured by the scanner—the unique zero point—*is* the physical instantiation of the reference point proposed by Kőszegi and Rabin in economics for choice and by Sutton and Barto in computer science for learning. Not only does the observation of the reference point in the central circuit for valuation make it clear that reference points are an unavoidable part of the human mechanism for valuation, but this finding also provides us with an empirical tool for rendering the reference point directly *observable*.

Summary: Striatum and Medial Prefrontal Cortex

The first lesson we learn from studies of purely neurobiological valuation is that there exists in the human brain a central representation of subjective value in the striatum and MPFC. The exact boundaries of the representation in these regions remain under dispute, but it is now clear that if one wants to measure expected subjective values, one can do so using a brain scanner or an electrode in these general areas. Further, we can now say with some confidence that these areas employ a reference-dependent mechanism for subjective value encoding and that this reference point can also be directly observed using a brain scanner. But what are the inputs to these areas that give rise to this valuation signal, and what form must these inputs to the last stage of the valuation circuit take? We turn next to that question, beginning with studies of the OFC, an important input to the medial areas, where human and monkey studies have begun to reveal some key encoding principles.

Constructing Value

There can be little doubt at this point in time that a suite of fronto-cortical areas contribute to the constructed representation of expected subjective value observed in the MPFC and the ventral striatum. Each of these contributory areas appears to use slightly different mechanisms for computing subjective value, but we know that in some way the outputs of these valuation mechanisms must be combined in the medial prefrontal and ventral striatal representations. Indeed, the medial prefrontal and ventral striatal representations may even differ subtly in their contributions to the valuation signals we observe in the fronto-parietal choice networks.

Clear evidence that multiple systems contribute to the valuation process comes from a number of sources, but perhaps the most compelling data arise from the rodent studies of Bernard Balleine and his colleagues (for a review of these findings, see Balleine et al., 2008). Balleine and colleagues have shown that after very extensive training, animals choosing between two actions become surprisingly insensitive to additional manipulations of reward value. They behave as if their estimates of subjective value have become fixed, a behavioral process sometimes called "habitization". Put more formally, heavily over-trained animals behave as if, during the course of training, learning rates have shifted from a relatively high value (allowing a rapid response to changes in reward values) to a very low value (allowing only a slow response to changes). What is really interesting about these findings, however, is that lesions of the dorsolateral striatum of the rat (corresponding roughly to the monkey and human caudate nucleus), but not of the dorsomedial striatum, disrupt this shift. After dorsolateral striatal lesions, rodents behave as if they are incapable of habitization, as if their learning rates become fixed at a high value irrespective of experience.

These data point out that multiple systems contribute, in ways we are only just beginning to understand, to the representation of value we see in the central valuation areas, at least in the rodent. Several groups of scholars, including Nathaniel Daw and Peter Dayan (e.g., Dayan and Daw, 2008), have extended these insights from the rodent and have developed evidence that suggests the existence of at least as many as four distinct human systems, each with slightly different properties, that contribute to value learning (Dayan, 2008). How do these several interacting systems work? The answer is that we simply do not know, but growing evidence has identified at least five anatomical brain areas that contribute to the constructed representation of value we observe in the MPFC and the ventral striatum. These areas are the OFC, the DLPFC, the amygdala, the insula, and the anterior cingulate cortex (ACC), as depicted in Figure 14.3.

Not only do we know that these five areas contribute to our stable representation of value, but we also have reason to suspect that they play

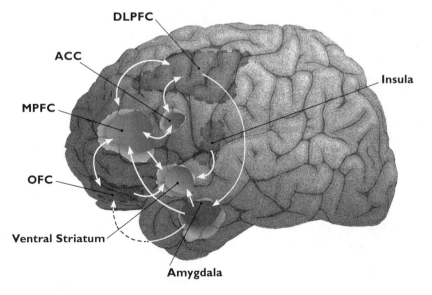

FIGURE 14.3

some role in storing those values over long periods of time. That imposes some serious constraints on how they represent expected subjective value. Recall that it is relative expected subjective value that is represented in the fronto-parietal networks. We know that a more absolute representation of subjective value must arise elsewhere in the nervous system: both humans and animals would be incapable of efficiently choosing between pairs of well-known objects that have never been compared directly by that subject if a more absolute form of subjective value were not stored somewhere. Current empirical evidence gathered in the OFC of the monkey may begin to explain how these more absolute representations of value arise, and may constrain theories of where they reside. We therefore turn next to the OFC.

Orbitofrontal Cortex

We have known for some time that the medial orbitofrontal region plays a key role in valuation. The pioneering work of António Damásio and his colleagues on decision making in patients with orbitofrontal lesions (Bechara et al., 1995) made it clear that individuals without this area show an altered sensitivity to risk in their choices among symbolically communicated monetary rewards. Subsequent studies by Hsu and colleagues (2005) demonstrated that subjects with lesions in this area seem to show nearly perfect risk neutrality. These individuals appear to be almost completely insensitive to monetary risk, their subjective valuations for monetary lotteries being guided only by expected value.

Brain scanning data from this area are more limited than data from the more dorsal areas of the frontal cortex because gathering accurate fMRI signals in this region can be technically challenging. O'Doherty and colleagues, however, have largely overcome this limitation and have gathered compelling data suggesting that activity in this area does encode something about subjective value (Glascher, Hampton, and O'Doherty, 2009; also Plassmann, O'Doherty, and Rangel, 2008). Their data suggest that activity in this region may provide a more abstract representation of subjective value than we have observed in the fronto-parietal decision networks. Here the values of abstract goals may be represented independent of the actions that yield those goals.

The most compelling data in this regard, however, come from studies, conducted by Schultz and his colleagues (Tremblay and Schultz, 1999) and by Camillo Padoa-Schioppa and John Assad (2006, 2008; Padoa-Schioppa, 2009), of single neurons in the OFC of the monkey.[3] Both of these groups have demonstrated that neurons in this area have firing rates correlated with the subjective values of options offered in a choice set.

Tremblay and Schultz demonstrated that neurons located more laterally in this area seem to encode the subjective values of offered food and water rewards. In their experiments, monkeys were presented with blocks of trials in which the values of two possible rewards were held constant. At the end of each block, these values were changed. What Tremblay and Schultz found under these blocked conditions was that the small number of neurons they sampled appeared to encode a signal that looked like *relative* subjective value.

In a much larger study, however, Padoa-Schioppa and Assad examined neurons located more medially in this area and came to a slightly different conclusion. Like Tremblay and Schultz, they found that neurons in this area seemed to encode the subjective values of the rewards offered to the monkeys. Like Glascher, Hampton, and O'Doherty (2009), they found that the neurons did not encode the subjective values of movements *per se*, but rather the subjective values of the rewards (the goods) themselves. A particular neuron might encode the subjective value of an apple juice reward, irrespective of the movement required to obtain that reward. But most interesting was their finding that the neurons appeared to encode a more absolute form of subjective value than had been seen in the fronto-parietal choice network.

In the Padoa-Schioppa and Assad experiments, the monkeys were offered choices between two options *that changed on every trial.* Under these conditions, they found that the representation of option A, for example, was unaffected by the value of option B. If the neuron responded with ten action potentials to an offer of 0.5 milliliters of apple juice, it did so regardless of what reward was offered as option B, be it strawberry or pear juice at large or small volumes. This is exactly the kind of absolute

---

3. It is tremendously important to note that comparing data between human and monkey in the frontal cortex can be quite challenging. When we speak of the OFC in humans, we refer primarily to Brodmann's (1909) area 11. Orbitofrontal regions in the monkey, however, may best correspond to all of areas 10, 11, and 13 in the human, based on Walker's (1940) classic analysis.

representation of subjective value that we expect to find in subjective value storage areas on theoretical grounds.

To better understand this point, we need to return to the general theory of cortex embodied in the Schwartz-Simoncelli equation, discussed in Chapter 10. Recall that Schwartz and Simoncelli (2001) argued that the role of cortical normalization is to maximize the joint information encoded in a cortical network. Normalization occurs, they argued, to ensure that each neuron carries as much information as possible about its subject, in the information theoretic sense.

To understand this point, consider the visual cortex of an animal living in an environment where every point in the visual world was uncorrelated, a world of colored television snow. In such a world, neurons at every point in the V1 topographic map would carry fully independent information, *because the information that they were encoding in the outside world was fully independent*. In such a setting, no cortical normalization would be required to maximize the information content of the cortical architecture. Of course, that is not what the real world looks like. In the real world, adjacent patches of visual space tend to look alike, and the degree of this correlation falls off as a complex function of spatial distance and spatial frequency, which are quite specific features of the visual world in which we live. This means two things. First, it means that if you know something about a single point in the visual world, you can make educated guesses about the properties of its near neighbors. Second, it means that if you want to minimize redundancy in the information carried by adjacent neurons, you need to effectively subtract the activity of these nearby neurons with some kind of normalization. In this regard, the Schwartz-Simoncelli equation tells us how to take a description of the statistical properties of a set of visual images and use them to derive the normalization scheme that maximizes joint information in just such a neuronal population.

A byproduct of this insight is that it tells us how to minimize the size of cortex for any specific encoding problem. If a piece of cortex performs no normalization of a visual world that includes at least some local correlations, then it does not maximize joint information—it codes less information than it could if well normalized. To put that another way, it uses more neurons to code the visual image because it employs an inefficient encoding scheme. If we knew in advance how much information we needed to encode, and the statistical structure of the world we wanted to encode, the normalization function would tell us how to achieve that informational content in the most efficient manner possible—how to accomplish it with a minimum number of neurons.

Why is all of this relevant to absolute subjective value coding in the OFC? If the function of the OFC is to store (or represent) the subjective values of all of the choice objects we have ever encountered, the Schwartz-Simoncelli approach tells us how it should do that. Remember that animals in their natural environments really encounter surprisingly few choice objects: there are only so many kinds of food or so many potential mates most animals face. If the function of the OFC is to represent the values of those options, it is important to remember that it does not have to efficiently represent *all* possible options, only that subset of options that the animal actually has encountered or will encounter. To put this in more visual terms, the human visual system does not have to encode information about colored television snow (a statistically uncorrelated visual world), it only has to encode the properties of the real visual world (which includes many structural correlations and is a much smaller set of images than the set of all television snow-based images). In a similar way, the OFC does not need to represent all possible choice options, only the options that occur in the real world of a given chooser. It is thus against that particular set of options that the brain must implement the efficient encoding strategies of the Schwartz-Simoncelli equation.[4]

Seen this way, the differing functions of areas such as LIP in the choice circuit, and the OFC in the subjective value circuit, call for different sizes and different organizations *because* they are both shaped by the sets of options that they must represent. The fronto-parietal choice circuits represent a small choice set for temporally immediate use—for decision making. These areas maximize the information that they carry when they normalize instantaneous subjective value *only across the choice set*. If we were to hypothesize that the OFC, in contrast, represented the set of all possible choices, then an efficient OFC would normalize over that much larger set of choice objects. The result, of course, would be a

---

4. I neglect here for simplicity the fact that the temporal frequency with which a choice object is encountered also has a critical impact on the optimal encoding strategy.

much more absolute representation of subjective value. Small changes in the size, quality, or frequency of a single reward would have little or no effect on the representation because the representation spans a much larger choice space. But it is equally important to point out that this general theory of cortex also tells us that there is no such thing as a truly absolute representation of subjective value. All neural representations are normalized to some degree, a point that has been made repeatedly in the literature on visual encoding since Barlow (1961).

Can these insights from the general theory of cortex help us to understand why the data from Padoa-Schioppa and Assad suggest a more absolute representation of subjective value and the data of Schultz and colleagues suggest a more relative representation? Perhaps. One way to understand this difference may be to consider the time courses over which the cortical normalization occurs and how this might interact with the representation in these areas. In the fronto-parietal choice areas, we know that normalization occurs with a very short timescale. Activity in these areas reflects the value of an option normalized only by the currently available options. In areas with more stable representations, normalization would have to be computed across much longer timescales. In the limit, such an area might compute a normalized representation over the course of a lifespan.

The discrepancy between the Schultz and Padoa-Schioppa data suggest that the OFC may in fact be normalized at an intermediate timescale. In his experiment, Schultz presented monkeys with long blocks of trials in which the rewards were held constant and then suddenly varied. In the Padoa-Schioppa and Assad experiments, the long-term statistical structure of the rewards was held constant by random trial-by-trial variation of rewards. An area that computed its normalization function over a time course of minutes to hours would, it should now be clear, appear to be a relative encoder in the Schultz experiment and an absolute encoder in the Padoa-Schioppa and Assad experiment.[5]

A recent paper by Padoa-Schioppa (2009) seems, in fact, to bear out this hypothesis. In that set of experiments, Padoa-Schioppa examined the dependency of neuronal sensitivity on reward magnitude in the OFC.

---

5. This is a point first made by Padoa-Schioppa and Assad in one of their papers.

He found that how sensitive a neuron was to the magnitude of an offered reward depended on the range of rewards offered *during that experimental session*. As he put it, "Across the population, the neuronal sensitivity (defined as the change in neuronal activity elicited by the increase in one value unit) was inversely proportional to the value range [encountered within that session]." This is exactly the kind of adaptive sensitivity predicted by the Schwartz-Simoncelli equation for an area coding options efficiently *within a single session* of choices.

That observation also ties well to studies of reinforcement learning in this same area by scholars, including Daw and Dayan. Daw and colleagues (2006; and Daw and Shohamy, 2008) proposed that the orbitofrontal region performs a very traditional TD-class reinforcement learning computation to compute and store subjective values over fairly short time courses. Daw has argued that the orbitofrontal region may be specialized for short-term reinforcement learning-like encoding of value; if that is true, we might naturally expect it to normalize value over this intermediate timescale.

To summarize, we now have some evidence that the OFC stores and represents subjective value in a more absolute form than do the fronto-parietal choice networks. The value representation here reflects a normalization of value across more choices and longer timescales than the choice networks, but not across the much longer timescales that describe a lifetime. This then begs a much larger question: Where is value stored across the much larger timescales that characterize a life? The fact that we can make meaningful choices about options we encountered years ago means that we do store, and presumably normalize, value across extremely long timescales. But we simply do not know where value is stored in this way. One obvious candidate would be the long-term memory encoding areas of the medial temporal lobe (e.g., Squire and Kandel, 2009), but to date no one has seriously examined the possibility that value is encoded in these areas.

In any case, it now seems clear that the OFC in both humans and monkeys provides a key input to the central valuation areas of the MPFC and the striatum and may even provide direct outputs to the fronto-parietal choice networks. This is clearly one of the key brain areas from which subjective value is constructed.

The Dorsolateral Prefrontal Cortex

Growing evidence seems to suggest a complementary role for the DLPFC in value construction. Like the orbitofrontal region, this area is heavily interconnected with the central valuation areas but seems to be specialized for evaluating delayed gains in some way. A number of studies have demonstrated that activity is greater in this area when subjects engage in what is often called self-control. One particularly good example of this has recently been provided by Peter Sokol-Hessner, Liz Phelps, and their colleagues (2009). This study asked subjects to select from a set of lotteries specifically designed to assess loss aversion under two conditions. Under the first condition, subjects simply made choices and their degree of loss aversion was measured. Under a second condition, subjects were encouraged to "think like a trader" to "imagine that they were gambling with someone else's money." This second treatment, the authors found, significantly reduced the loss aversion evidenced by these subjects. But perhaps more interestingly, the treatment that led to lower levels of loss aversion was also associated with heightened activity in the DLPFC.

Another study that points in a similar direction, and does so more explicitly, is by Hare, Camerer, and Rangel (2009). In that study, human dieters were asked to place values on the healthiness and tastiness of snacks and then, while in a brain scanner, to make choices among pairs of snacks that varied in both of these subjectively rated dimensions. They found that while activity in the MPFC continued to be correlated with the choices subjects made, activity in the DLPFC was highest when subjects chose a healthy snack that tasted bad over an unhealthy snack that tasted good. In keeping with the notion that the DLPFC participates in some kind of self-control, they interpreted this finding as indicating that when subjects exert self-control, activity in the DLPFC is high.

More causal studies point in a similar direction. Daria Knoch and Ernst Fehr (Knoch et al., 2006) have explored the effects of reversible inactivation of the DLPFC (using repetitive transcranial magnetic stimulation) while human subjects participated in the traditional behavioral economic experiment called the ultimatum game (Guth et al., 1982). In that game, a first player is given $10 to split with a second player. The first player proposes a split and the second player then decides if that split is acceptable. If the second player accepts, the money is divided. If the second player rejects, then neither player gets anything.

If a second player seeks only to maximize her immediate gain in this game, then she does so by accepting any non-zero offer from the first player. If she seeks to maximize long-term gain she may best do so (under a particular set of assumptions) by establishing a reputation for rejecting uneven splits. Interestingly, Knoch and colleagues found that inactivation of the DLPFC caused subjects to be more likely to accept any non-zero offer. This suggests that subjects may be less concerned with fairness and long-term strategies in their responses when the DLPFC is inactivated.

These data begin to hint that the DLPFC may compute and represent subjective values over much longer time courses and in more abstract terms than the orbitofrontal areas. Daw, in particular, has developed this theme. He has suggested that the representation of subjective value in this area is anchored to more complex models of the sequential structure of the world than can be computed using traditional reinforcement learning methods (Daw et al., 2005; Daw and Shohamy, 2008). His hypothesis is that this area essentially looks backwards in time to search for patterns in the world related to rewards and then places values on these temporally complex "world states." Another possibility under active exploration is that activity in this area acts as a kind of brake on impulsivity, a source of self-control that can be viewed as a renewable but limited resource that agents can deploy to maximize their long-term welfare.

Together, all of these studies suggest an interactive relationship between the orbitofrontal and dorsolateral cortices in valuation, although those exact roles clearly remain unclear. Both areas are interconnected and both project to the medial prefrontal areas that appear to serve as a final common path for valuation. Both areas clearly carry valuation signals, although those valuation signals seem to appear under only limited conditions, and seem to influence choice in only some tasks. This is important because it provides one of our first insights into how neural subcomponents interact in the construction of value.

The Amygdala

We have now known for several decades, based on the work of scholars such as Joe Ledoux (2000, 2007) and Elizabeth Phelps (2006), that the amygdala plays a key role in the process of fear conditioning, and much of the available data suggest that lesions to the amygdala disrupt both instinctual and learned fear responses. We also know that when normal subjects experience fear, that psychologically defined state is almost invariably correlated with activation of this nucleus. Single-neuron studies in animals have also supported this attribution of a fear-related function to the amygdala. Neurons in the lateral and medial parts of the nucleus, for example, seem to play key roles in the production of many fear-related behaviors.

Together with the fact that the amygdala is heavily connected to both the ventral striatum and the OFC, these data have led a number of scholars to conclude that activation of the amygdala is equivalent to the psychological state of fear: if you see the amygdala activated, you can conclude that the subject is afraid and is thus placing some kind of negative utility on the current situation. It is important to stress that this is simply not correct. Phelps (2006; also Anderson and Phelps, 2002), who is probably the leading expert on the human amygdala today, has made this point repeatedly. While it is true that activity in the amygdala is positively correlated with fear, the inverse is not necessarily true: just because the amygdala is active does not mean that the subject is afraid.

Single-neuron studies may help explain why amygdalar activation is not equivalent to fear. Salzman and colleagues (Belova, Paton, and Salzman, 2008; Lau and Salzman, 2009; Morrison and Salzman, 2009) have recently shown that neurons in the medial part of the nucleus encode subjective value under a range of circumstances. The firing rates of these neurons are *positively* correlated with subjective value, just as it appears that the firing rates of more lateral neurons may be negatively correlated with subjective value based on the Phelps and Ledoux experiments. Recent fMRI results also seem to bear out this observation: Levy and colleagues (2010) have demonstrated that activity in the amygdala measured when subjects consider risky or ambiguous lotteries is positively correlated with subjective value.

One resolution of this apparent paradox may be that the output of the amygdala does in fact encode negative outcomes more strongly than positive outcomes, but encodes both as a positive correlation with subjective value. Such a signal sent to the central valuation areas would clearly indicate the negative value of an option, but it would do so on the same value scale employed by these other areas.

In summary, it seems clear that the amygdala is well situated to convey information about subjective values, both positive and negative but perhaps more about negative, both to the striatum and the OFC. While we do have good evidence supporting the notion that fear-related mental states are associated with both amygdala activation and changes in decision making, the mechanism by which this is accomplished remains unclear. Still, the amygdala clearly plays a role in valuation, and the near term should see important insights into that role for this brain area.

The Insula and the Anterior Cingulate Cortex

Another area that seems to play some role in value construction is the insular cortex. This is an enormous section of the lateral cortex that has traditionally been associated with visceral sensations of disgust (Augustine, 1996; Singer, 2007; Singer et al., 2009), and thus presumably with some classes of dis-utile events. Recent studies of decision making under conditions of ambiguity suggest that some portions of this cortex may be active and correlated with subjective value when ambiguous lotteries are encountered. Unfortunately, little else is known about the role of the insula in subjective value construction, although it is also well connected with the central valuation areas.

Another area of clear importance is the ACC. The ACC of the primate, which is roughly homologous to all of the frontal cortex in rodents, has long been known to play a role in decision making. Before fMRI was available, electroencephalographic studies indicated that this area was particularly active when subjects made errors in simple decision-making tasks, especially when subjects detected those errors (e.g., Falkenstein, Hohnsbein, Hoormann, and Blanke, 1990, 1991; Gehring et al., 1993). These observations, and others, led to the hypothesis that the ACC serves as a center for conflict resolution. The key idea in this hypothesis was that whenever subjects were near indifference between two widely disparate options, or when differing valuation subsystems produced disparate valuations, the ACC played a key role in establishing the subjective values that guided choice (e.g., Yeung et al., 2004).

More recently, that conclusion has been challenged and an alternative hypothesis has emerged that suggests that the area may encode error likelihood or certainty (Brown and Braver, 2005). Yet another hypothesis arises from single-unit studies in monkeys that suggests individual neurons in this area have firing rates correlated with reward magnitude, reward probability, or some combination of the two (Kennerley and Wallis, 2009a, 2009b; Kennerley et al., 2009).

Again, this is an area well connected with the core valuation areas and clearly involved, likely in a specialized way, in value construction. The details of that role, however, remain obscure at this time.

Conclusions

There is now no serious doubt that many areas contribute specialized input to the core valuation circuits of the MPFC and the striatum. Our current data identifies at least five of these areas, although there are doubtless more. It is also almost necessarily true that future research will identify important subdivisions of these large areas that perform unique functions.

Of particular interest today among these five are the orbitofrontal and dorsolateral prefrontal cortices, which seem to play slightly opposing roles in the valuation process. The orbitofrontal area appears, at this time, specialized for the representation of immediate consumable rewards, while the dorsolateral seems involved in longer-term gains that require what is popularly called self-control. These observations beg the question of how disparate inputs from these two areas are arbitrated in the core medial areas. Answering that question will, without a doubt, be one of the key challenges for neuroeconomics in the years to come.

15

Beyond Neoclassics: Behavioral Neuroeconomics

Précis

The greatest strength of the neoclassical economic program has been its clarity and rigor. When describing a model, a neoclassical theorist almost certainly does not believe that it accurately describes all behavior, but he or she knows exactly what it does describe. The greatest weakness of the neoclassical program is that the clearly stated models it employs have only limited predictive power. Why is that?

One reason is that the neoclassical models we have today are too simple. It has to be true that one cannot model all of human choice behavior with three or four simple mathematical rules. As the neuro-economic studies of mechanism described here have revealed, neoclassical-style models will have to grow in complexity. As that complexity grows, many of the failures of contemporary neoclassical economics will be remediated. But there may be a second, and much more troubling, reason that neoclassical models fail.

The entire neoclassical program begins, irrespective of the specific model or axioms one examines, with the assumption that choice behavior is coherently organized to achieve some goal. In a classic theory such as GARP (Houthakker, 1950) we ask, "What are the characteristics of choice behaviors that are required if that behavior were aimed at maximizing some (or any reasonable) function?" If we observe that preferences are complete and transitive, then that is the same as observing that choosers are acting to maximize *something*—a something we call utility.

In a theory such as expected utility (von Neumann and Morgenstern, 1944) we ask, "What are the characteristics of choice behaviors aimed at maximizing the long-run probabilistic expectations of anything?" (Again, an anything we call utility). In a theory such as "satisficing" (Simon, 1957) we ask, "What are the characteristics of choice behavior aimed at maximizing long-run expectations, given that achieving that maximization will be costly?"

For evolutionarily trained biologists, this is a modeling approach that is naturally attractive. The assumption that behavior is trying to accomplish a coherent goal seems almost implicit in the evolutionary study of behavior. All educated people believe that the process of evolution pushes animals *towards* the maximization of inclusive genetic fitness. Indeed, as I am often fond of quoting John Maynard Smith (1982) as having said about these theories of maximization,

> In human applications this measure is provided by "utility"—
> a somewhat artificial and uncomfortable concept: In biology,
> Darwinian fitness provides a natural and genuinely one-dimensional
> scale [for thinking about maximization].

But how sure can we be that human choice behavior really can be described as coherent, as structured towards achieving some goal? That is a concern here because the neoclassical program is inescapably the study of coherent maximization. Can we assume that there is really anything coherent about human behavior? If the neoclassical models fit, then the answer is "yes." But if they do not fit, if they cannot be made to fit, then the answer may be "no." So how well do these neoclassical models fit behavior?

In answering that question, it is important to remember that the class of neoclassical theories is, at most, about 100 years old and is in a constant state of revision. This book, up until this point, has been a particularly extreme form of that revision. It has been an effort to close the gap between theory and behavior mechanistically but with the elements and sensibilities of the neoclassical toolkit. And I think it is fair to say that this strategy has been more successful than many critics of the neoclassical approach had expected. The reference point seemed mysterious and beyond the range of axiomatic theory 20 years ago. Today we have a mathematical model that serves as the economic basis for understanding the reference point (Kőszegi and Rabin, 2006), a precise explanation of how the reference point arises in systems that learn (Sutton and Barto, 1998), neurobiological evidence that our learning mechanism instantiates that reference point (Bayer and Glimcher, 2005), and even empirical techniques for the direct measurement of the reference point in humans (Fox and Poldrack, 2009). So clearly, many behavioral phenomena that appear to lie outside the assumption of coherent maximization will eventually turn out to be explicable with these types of tools.

Put another way, I have been arguing that neuroeconomics can be a process for enriching (or, if you prefer, complicating) the original neoclassical models with algorithmic constraints. Such a process assumes that the neurobiological architecture is not so very different from the "as if" architectures that Samuelson, Friedman, von Neumann, and others recognized were necessary for the efficient maximization of utility. Like Maynard Smith, I assume that evolution does not merely push us *towards* efficient behavioral maximization, but that evolution often comes very close to achieving maximization.[1] It is important for me to note, though, that even I realize that this kind of neoclassical–algorithmic approach cannot entirely close the gap between neoclassical theory and real behavior. Evolution is slow and random, environments often change quickly, and there must be times when behavior is simply not coherent within a particular environment or domain.

So what happens when humans or animals truly do not maximize *anything* with their behavior? What happens when the complexity of the environment, or the rate of change of the environment, outstrips evolution's rate of optimization? What happens when an organism's response to its environment becomes incoherent? When that occurs, a gap is necessarily introduced between the maximization functions that are the *raison d'être* of the neoclassical approach and the actual mechanisms of behavior. These are gaps that neoclassical theory cannot, and should not, attempt to fill.

---

1. Let me stress for my colleagues in evolutionary biology that I do recognize the importance of such factors as sexual selection and game theoretic "arms races" but also see the evidence of convergent evolution-quantified maximization tests as telling. This is a point taken up in some detail in my book *Decisions, Uncertainty, and the Brain*.

This source of incompleteness in economic theory will have to be filled with the tools of *behavioral economics*, the intellectual school in the economic community that stands in opposition to the neoclassical program. Let me hasten to add, however, that neurobiology can and will play a critical role even as we add these behavioral economic theories to our model of choice. Hybrid models that relate behavioral economics and neuroscience are just as important as their neoclassical brethren, but they will be fundamentally different in many ways.

What are some examples of phenomena that lie outside the reach of the neoclassical approach, and what do these kinds of neuroeconomic theories look like? What do we know, neurobiologically, about the algorithms that give rise to phenomena that require behavioral economic explanations? To begin to answer that question, consider two examples that are particularly well developed today.

The Editing of Choice Sets and the Symbolic Communication of Expectation

The Editing of Choice Sets

We know that the encoding of relative expected subjective value observed in the fronto-parietal networks cannot support efficient choice over large choice sets. This arises from the high intrinsic variance of this system and is a point taken up in detail in Chapter 10. We also know, behaviorally, that when humans face large choice sets, they appear to edit those choice sets down to a smaller size (see Payne, Bettman, and Johnson, 1992, 1993, for a review) and that this editing induces irrationalities, irrevocable failures of maximization. How, then, does the brain deal with these choices? Our current evidence strongly suggests that frontal valuation circuits may be able to perform an editing-like operation that limits the number of options presented to the fronto-parietal circuits for choice. These frontal circuits can likely control what options make it to the choice network. Inasmuch as we can hope to understand the neurobiological roots of that process, we might begin to understand how neuroeconomics contributes to an understanding of choice that goes beyond the boundaries of the neoclassical approach.

The Symbolic Communication of Expectation

We also know that the expected subjective values that emerge from experience differ from the expected subjective values that emerge from symbolic presentations. The use of symbolic information, such as the statement that one will win $100 with a probability of 0.35, produces behavioral decisions that differ in important ways from the decisions that arise when we make our choices based on experience. The most important of these discrepancies emerges when humans face symbolically communicated choices that involve low-probability events. Under these conditions, humans violate the independence axiom in a way that seems to overweight low probabilities. Humans behave irrationally, failing to maximize anything, when very low and very high symbolic probabilities are involved. Expected subjective values constructed from highly symbolic information are an evolutionarily new event, although they are also hugely important features of our human economies, and it may be the novelty of this kind of expectation that is problematic.

This is probably the greatest challenge to the neoclassical approach. Expected utility theory (as opposed to GARP-like utility theories, which do not involve explicit probabilities) is an effort to define a maximization approach for symbolically communicated probabilities. If that is a phenomenon that lies outside the range of human maximization behavior, then we may need to rethink key elements of the neoclassical program. This is a second example of a key extra-neoclassical phenomenon.

To understand how neuroeconomics can, and will, go beyond the neoclassical program, we turn next to a detailed examination of these two phenomena (choice set editing and symbolic communication of expectation). Let me stress that there are many examples of this kind, but these are two of the most important of the apparently extra-neoclassical phenomena, and two of the clearest examples of how behavioral neuro-economics will evolve.

Choice Set Editing in Frontal Areas

As discussed in Chapter 10, the fronto-parietal choice areas employ a normalization scheme for representing the objects of choice that has both advantages and disadvantages. At the level of metabolic cost, representing the relative values of each element in a choice set is extremely efficient because it allows for the accurate representation of choice sets by very small networks of neurons. As long as choice sets remain small, the system yields behavior identical to that produced by a more metabolically expensive system that more closely approximates the absolute values of each element in the choice set. As the size of a choice set grows, however, these systems behave more and more stochastically. By the time choice sets reach sizes of 10 or 15 elements, convergence in these networks seems to be guided more by random fluctuations in firing rates than by subjective value.

In considering this fact, one cannot help but speculate that these limitations on the choice set size may not have affected the maximization behavior of our ancestors too significantly. Animals (or early humans) choosing between a few consumable rewards or a small number of possible sexual partners may have only rarely pushed these networks into regimes where inefficiently stochastic behavior was produced. In our modern society, however, large choice sets are common. American grocery stores often carry upwards of 20,000 different products. The selection of investments for retirement accounts may require that we sort through literally hundreds of options. Just buying a car may involve dozens of alternatives. How does the neural architecture we inherited from those ancestors deal with these kinds of complicated problems?

At a behavioral level, we already have some evidence that humans deal with these kinds of large choice sets in basically two different ways. The first strategy is to approach large choice sets hierarchically, a strategy that effectively limits the number of options at each of several stages in the choice problem. The second strategy is, in essence, to employ an arbitrary rule that restricts, or edits out, a subset of the choice set. The goal of this second strategy is reduce the choice set to a manageable size using a simple heuristic (Payne, Bettman, and Johnson, 1993).

To see these two strategies at work, consider choosing a new four-seat, two-door car. There are about 30 brands of cars available in the United States; each offers about eight models; each model comes in about 10 colors. If one had to choose only a model and color (and of course there are more choices than these), one would face a choice set of about 2,500 elements. We know that humans cannot behaviorally engage choice sets of this size efficiently, and we know that, at a neural level, the choice architecture cannot accurately identify the highest subjective value option in a choice set of this size.

The first strategy for choice sets of this size, hierarchical sorting, segregates the problem into a series of sequential decisions, each of which offers a manageable choice set size. Should I buy a domestically manufactured or a foreign manufactured brand? Of those brands, which should I buy? Of that brand, what model do I prefer? Of that model, what color? An important problem with this strategy is that it is not, under many circumstances, guaranteed to identify the single car that has the highest subjective value for the chooser. Put more formally, this is a strategy that will yield global violations of the axioms of rational choice across the entire choice set, even though each of the hierarchical decisions may respect some limited form of the axioms. This is a strategy that simply does not maximize anything, a point that has been made numerous times by nearly all of the key players in behavioral economics (for example by Payne, Bettman, and Johnson [1993] in their book *The Adaptive Decision Maker*).

The second strategy, choice set editing, typically relies on identifying what are called the *attributes* of the objects of choice. In this strategy, each of the cars in the full choice set is conceived of as possessing a set of attributes. For example, a car might be *red*, *expensive*, *very safe*, *fuel-efficient*, and *inexpensive to maintain*. Each of these properties is an attribute. To a first approximation, we can think of each of the attributes as conferring some degree of utility on the car. Fuel efficiency may be a very important attribute to one chooser but not to another. In choice set editing, what is presumed to occur is that one or two of the most important attributes are used to reduce the effective size of the choice set. For example, one might edit the choice set down by considering only red cars. One edits, selecting a subset of the original choice set based on the attribute of color, for further consideration. The subset is then imagined to be subjected to a more neoclassical-like comparison that achieves maximization, but only within the boundaries of the subset. Like hierarchical choice, editing by attributes leads to choices that are not globally rational, choices that can violate the axioms of rational economic theory. This is also a point that has been carefully made in the literature.

The neuroeconomic implications of these two psychological theories of choice should be clear. The neurobiological data we have gathered so far indicates that a Hard-utility-like theory (with all of the constraints we have encountered so far) can do a good job of explaining how choice works with small choice sets. What happens as choice set size grows? The theory presented up to this point suggests that choice should simply become random as choice set size grows. And of course we know that is not the case. People may not be entirely rational (they may not achieve perfect maximization) in their choices among cars, but they are not as random as the Hard-EU-based theories we have explored up to this point suggest. These psychological choice theories thus suggest behavioral economic-style extensions to our existing Hard-neoclassical theory which may account for the fact that humans perform better on large choice sets than the purely neoclassical neuroeconomic model presented so far would predict. These theories suggest that mechanisms in the frontal cortex and basal ganglia may edit down the size of choice sets before passing options to the fronto-parietal networks for actual decision making. To understand how that might work, we need to turn next to pre-existing psychological and neurobiological studies of visual search.

Searching for Visual Targets

Imagine the subject of a psychological experiment being asked to find the gray T in this display of black Ts.

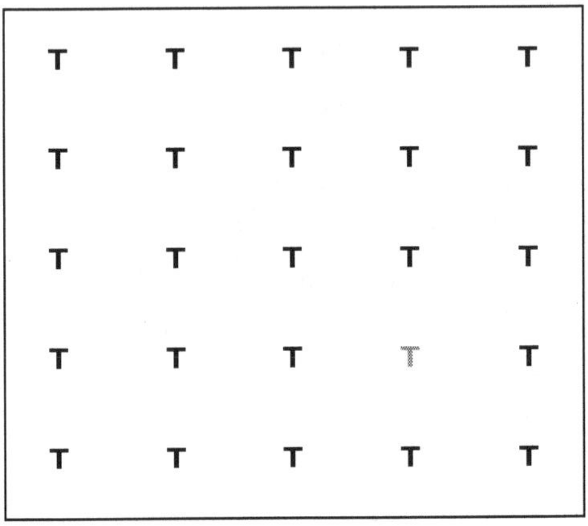

FIGURE 15.1

What is striking is that this is easy. It is a task performed quickly and efficiently by the human visual system. In fact, increasing the number of black Ts in this display has very little impact on how quickly subjects can locate the gray T in the display. The same is true for the second display, in Figure 15.2, if we search for the single black O embedded in a display of many Ts.

Finding the O in a field of Ts is also fast and easy. Increasing the number of Ts has little effect on search time. But interestingly, the problem becomes much harder when we begin to combine the attributes of brightness and form. Now try finding the gray O in this display of black Os and gray Ts, shown in Figure 15.3.

Finding the visual target that is both gray and an O is much more difficult. Further, as the size of the set of non-targets grows under these conditions, the time it takes to find the gray O also grows. In fact, average search times under these conditions are a roughly linear function of the number of non-targets. This has led a number of perceptual psychologists (Treisman, 1982; Wolfe, 1998) to suggest that when searching for a target that is defined by the conjunction of two *visual attributes*, what people do is to serially search, one by one, through each element in the display until they find one that matches the search criteria. This serial search strategy is proposed to occur whenever a parallel search cannot be conducted along the category space of a single attribute—whenever we cannot, for example, simply look in parallel for whatever is gray in the display.

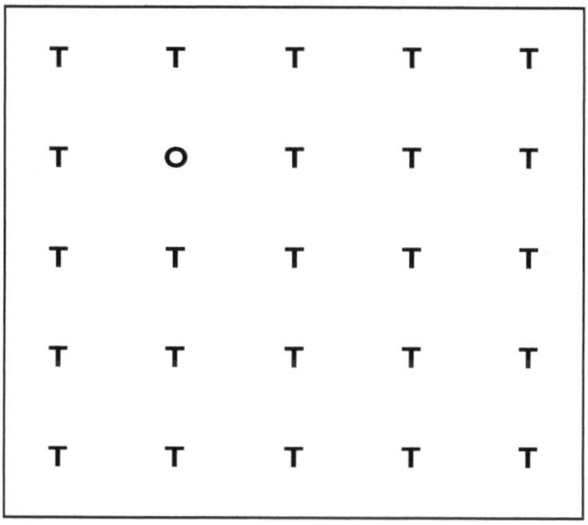

FIGURE 15.2

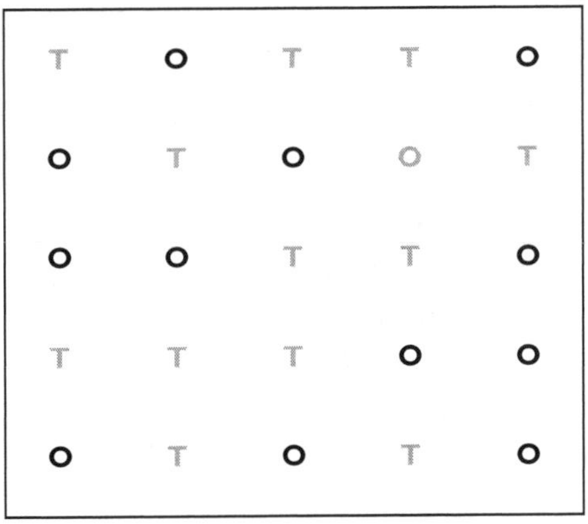

FIGURE 15.3

The basic psychological theory on which this explanation rests posits the existence of a class of predefined attributes such as color, form, and motion. Whenever search within an attribute class can identify the target, that search is fast, parallel, and largely unaffected by set size. Search across attribute classes, however, is proposed to employ a different, slower, and essentially serial mechanism. When this mechanism must be employed, the theory proposes that each stimulus must be examined individually until the target is identified. As soon as the target has been identified, the search process is assumed to terminate. Of course, this theory thus makes very specific predictions about the relationship of mean search times and the variance of those search times to set size, predictions that have been validated by many experiments.[2]

So how does this happen neurally? We do not know the answer to that question for sure, but what we know about the architecture for vision makes some interesting suggestions. Recall, from Chapter 7, what we learned about the basic structure of the primate visual system.

---

2. This particular model is not uncontroversial. There are Bayesian parallel search models that make similar predictions under many conditions, a point I and others have made in the literature. But the value of these models in the present context lies in what they can tell us about choice and neural architectures. I ask forbearance from my colleagues in visual search and attention.

Visual information exits the retina and proceeds, via the thalamus, to the primary visual cortex, also called area V1. The next step in visual processing is a hierarchical decomposition of the image by features, but within topographically organized submaps of the visual world (see Fig. 15.4). Information about the speed and direction of motion, for example, seems to be extracted topographically in area MT, which encodes, in neural firing rates, the speed and direction of visual motion at each point in the visual world. Information about color seems to be largely (but not exclusively) extracted in area V4. Information about the identity of faces seems to be extracted in a map at the anterior end of the temporal lobe. Each of these maps appears to extract and topographically represent a feature, or attribute, of the visual image.

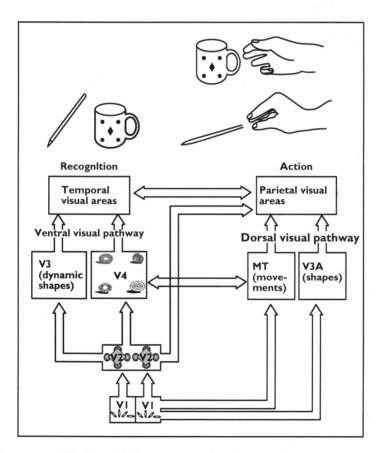

FIGURE 15.4   The hierarchical organization of visual cortex.

With this information in hand, a number of scholars have proposed that when we see a fast parallel search occurring, what we are really seeing is a search occurring *within* a single topographic map. The idea, in essence, is that a winner-take-all operation—like the one we encountered in area LIP—occurs within a single map and yields a single site of activation within that map, identifying the target of interest. The principle, then, is that the attributes that support rapid parallel search are those attributes encoded by the individual hierarchically organized maps of the visual system. In this theory, slow serial search occurs whenever information across two maps must be compared. When this is required, when a conjunction of two or more attributes defines a visual target, then a serial process operates slowly and extracts information about the stimuli across maps, one stimulus at a time.

Cortical Maps and Choice Attributes

So what does this suggest about hierarchical and attribute-based decision making? The suggestion seems fairly clear. Imagine that, like the visual cortex, valuation-related cortex consists of a set of maps that encode the attributes of the choice objects we encounter in life. One map might encode, for example, the visual attractiveness of our choice objects, another might encode the sweetness of foods, another the monetary cost. In fact, the visual maps themselves might participate in this encoding, with maps related to color serving to represent the colors of our choice objects. This suggests that maps for attributes of choice objects might exist just as maps for the attributes of visual stimuli exist.

Now consider a circumstance in which 100 choice objects each vary along five attributes, with each attribute encoded in a separate cortical "map" located frontally. How would the pre-existing architecture support editing or hierarchical choice? It would do so by using within-map winner-take-all computations. If, for example, we had to reduce the choice set by color, we could use the color-attribute map to suppress all non-red cars. What would remain for forwarding to the fronto-parietal choice architecture would be only those cars that are red. If we choose at that point, then our fronto-parietal networks would see only the red cars, and efficient maximization among that limited set would be fairly effortless.

The critical ideas here are as follows: (1) We already know that attributes are encoded in distinct brain maps; (2) We also know that computations within brain maps can be used to quickly and efficiently extract stimuli or objects that share a common value (say red) in attribute space; and (3) We know that the choice operator in the fronto-parietal network does best when it faces small choice sets. Together these three ideas suggest that choice set editing or hierarchical sequencing should reflect the structure of attribute encoding in the brain. That simply has to be the default model for understanding decision making in large choice sets. Finally, it is critical that even Hard-neoclassicists like me acknowledge that models such as this are going to lie outside the neoclassical paradigm as we understand it today.

Choice Set Summary

Large choice sets are problematic. At a behavioral level, the rationality of choices declines as choice set size increases. At a neurobiological level, the structure of variance in the fronto-parietal network limits choice efficiency as set sizes grow. The suggestion from studies of visual search by psychologists and neurobiologists is that editing by attributes (attributes being defined by the structure of cortical representation) may be the way that we overcome this limitation. The advantage of attribute sorting is that we can tailor the actual choice set size to the limits of the choice architecture using well-understood neurobiological mechanisms. The disadvantage is that we violate rationality by incompletely analyzing our choice sets—but of course we already know that humans do just that.

The Symbolic Communication of Expectation

Almost all of the choices and decisions examined in the third section of this book have been between objects whose values were learned through repeated experience. The neural systems that allow us to learn through experience are now fairly well understood, and this understanding will shape our models of valuation and choice among these objects. Dopaminergic systems allow us to learn the values of goods through iterative mechanisms that converge towards a representation of something like the expected utilities of actions. For many economists, however, this is a very incomplete picture of valuation. How are these experience-based iterative valuation systems related to the symbolically derived representations of the subjective values of goods or lotteries we have not previously experienced? If we ask a subject to value a 37% chance of winning a new type of automobile with well-described attributes, how is that related to the kinds of valuation that have been discussed so far in this book? For that matter, how are these iteratively learned valuations related to the subjective values of traditional economic lotteries? This notion that humans can have preferences among choice objects presented symbolically, choice objects with fixed probabilities and monetary values, lies at the heart of economics. Von Neumann, Morgenstern, and Savage invented expected utility theory to extend theories such as WARP and GARP to probabilistic events that they saw as being communicated linguistically. Do the same mechanisms, and theories, work equally well for the symbolic and experiential communication of objects?

In the rest of this chapter, we turn to the similarities and differences between valuations constructed symbolically versus valuations constructed experientially. Expected utility-like theories, in their Hard forms, predict that we encode probabilities and utilities separately and take the product of those quantities to compute the desirability of a choice object. If we change the probability, we change the expected utility (or expected subjective value) of that object without changing the stored utility of the object itself. What studies of dopamine have revealed, however, is that probabilistic expectations learned from experience do not have this property. Probabilistic expectations learned from experience behave mechanistically much more like simple utilities than like expected utilities. If we change the probability that a lever will yield a reward, a monkey or human pressing that lever must relearn the value of pressing that lever from scratch. When we learn the value of an action that yields a probabilistic reward, we learn something much more like the utility of that action (utility in the Hard-theory sense) than something like a true expected utility (expected utility in the Hard-theory sense). In contrast, probabilistic expectations communicated symbolically, probabilities much more like the Hard-expected utilities von Neumann might have envisioned, behave much more erratically (they violate rationality) and set limits on the usefulness of nearly all Hard theories of expected utility (including expected subjective utility). For this reason, as we will see, it may make more sense to use the notion of an *expected* subjective value to uniquely refer to symbolically communicated choice objects, a further break with the Soft economic tradition required by our growing understanding of mechanism. To begin this discussion, we turn to a behavioral experiment that highlights the need for a richer notion of expected utility or expected subjective value that was conducted by Ralph Hertwig and colleagues.

The Value of a Lottery: Learning Versus Being Told

Hertwig, Barron, Weber, and Erev (2004) examined the decisions of Technion University students who were asked to make choices between two lotteries. In a typical example, the students might be asked to choose between one lottery (called "H") that offered a 5% chance of yielding $70 and a second lottery ("L") that offered a certain gain of $3. What made this experiment interesting, however, was that the subjects were broken into two groups before they were presented with these options. The first group was told about these options symbolically. They were simply asked linguistically to choose between "a 5% chance of $70 and a sure $3." The second group learned these probabilities only through experience. Those subjects were shown two buttons on a computer, each of which represented one of the two possible lotteries. They were then told to sample the two lotteries as many times as they liked, by pushing each of the buttons, before making an actual decision. Each time they pushed the "H" button there was a 5% chance it would show a $70 win and a 95% chance it would show a $0 win. Each time they pressed the "L" button it showed a $3 win.

It is critical to understand here that the subjects who experienced these distributions of wins and losses from pressing the button were performing a lottery experiment in just the same way Schultz's monkeys perform an experiment when dopamine neurons are being studied. They sampled these lotteries repeatedly, and we have every reason to believe that their dopamine systems constructed an estimate of the average value of the lotteries upon which their later choice was based. The other students, who learned the probabilities symbolically, were performing the decision experiment in exactly the way Kahneman and

Tversky, or Allais for that matter, would have done it. Unsurprisingly, Hertwig and colleagues found that the behavior of students performing the Kahneman and Tversky-style experiment replicated the standard findings of Kahneman and Tversky. These students weakly violated the independence axiom: they behaved as if they overrepresented low-probability events and underrepresented high-probability events. More formally, Hertwig and colleagues estimated the probability weighting function employed by the students (the function that relates "subjective probability" to objective probability) and found that it took the traditional Kahneman and Tversky form described in Chapter 5 and shown in Figure 15.5.

What was surprising, however, was that the subjects who experienced the probabilities through repetitive sampling behaved quite differently in their choices. They also weakly violated the independence axiom, but under these conditions the subjects *underweighted* low-probability events and *overweighted* high-probability events as shown in Figure 15.6.

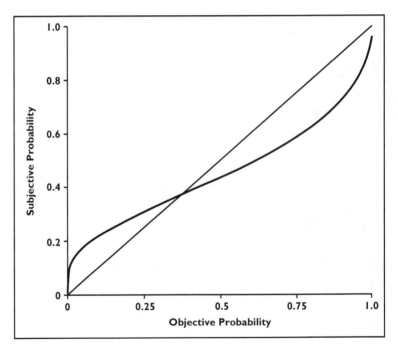

FIGURE 15.5   The probability weighting function for symbolically communicated probabilities.

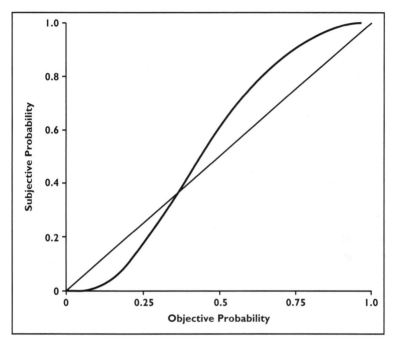

FIGURE 15.6   The probability weighting function for experientially communicated probabilities.

How, as neuroeconomists, can we understand this phenomenon? We need to first recognize that the underweighting of low probabilities observed in the human subjects who learned by experience is also a feature of animal behavior in most traditional conditioning tasks such as the ones employed by Schultz and his colleagues. The choices of animals show that they behave as if they underweight very low probabilities. That turns out not to be surprising, given what we already know theoretically about repetitive experiential learning. In models that employ a reward prediction error term and a learning rate, models such as TD learning and Bush and Mosteller, we recursively compute the average value of an action. The rate at which these systems learn, or the rate at which new events influence the system's estimate of the average value of an action, is controlled by the learning rate term as described in Chapter 13. Put another way, these systems *forget* about old rewards at a rate controlled by the learning rate parameter. If a system of this kind has a very low learning rate, say 0.001, then it forgets almost nothing when it computes the average value of an action. The drawback to such a system, however, is that when the environment changes, it revises its average estimate of value very, very slowly. What we have is a trade-off between how fast we forget and how quickly we update. Empirically, we find that most animals in most experiments adopt learning rates ranging between about 0.2 and 0.8, learning rates at which these systems actually *forget* old rewards quite quickly. In fact, at a learning rate of 0.5, one of these systems will have almost completely forgotten about any event that occurred as recently as 10 trials ago. *That means that if a large reward occurs with low probability, under typical conditions it will have only a very brief influence on average estimates of value.* Under such conditions, low-probability events will thus be underrepresented and high-probability events overrepresented in the long-term average estimate of value that drives behavior. What this means is that *the underweighting of low probabilities and overweighting of high probabilities that Hertwig and colleagues observed (in their experiential learners) is predicted by our neural model of how we learn the values of our actions.* Exactly how badly low probabilities are underweighted and high probabilities are overrepresented is quantitatively predicted by the size of the learning rate: the lower the learning rate, the more accurate the representation of these extreme probabilities.

Hertwig and colleagues recognized this fact and suggested that models of risk and decision should incorporate two independent mechanisms for representing probability: an experiential mechanism and a symbolic mechanism. We can, quite naturally, take that logic a step further given what we know about mechanism. The mechanism we have discussed up to this point is experiential, it is well understood, and it predicts underweighting of low probabilities and overweighting of high probabilities to an extent quantitatively described by the learning rate. The probability-weighting function of Kahneman and Tversky suggests that a second symbolic mechanism exists, likely mediated by the language areas of the brain, for encoding linguistically communicated probability more directly.

In traditional Soft-economic theories this dichotomy poses a significant problem, but the sensitivity of Hard-theories to mechanism, our focus in these *because* theories on why behavior takes the form it does, makes it easy to segregate these two processes. The dopamine-based mechanisms for estimating the subjective values of risky options, these experiential systems, employ a Bush and Mosteller-type iterative calculation. This means that the single value they produce encodes both the probability and magnitude of reward obtained under probabilistic conditions *in a single variable*. We already know that there is no way for these systems to separate probability and magnitude of reward, and we know how these subjective values come to under-represent low-probability events. For this reason, the outputs of these systems really have to be considered utility-like objects rather than expected utility-like objects. These are, in any reasonable mechanistic sense, subjective values, not expected subjective values. While it is true that these variables do embed probability, they do so in a non-invertible way that makes the representation distinct from expected utility-like representations. This suggests that the subjective values learned by reward prediction error-based systems should be considered subjective values even when those values reflect probabilistic events.

The term "expected subjective values," it seems mechanistically clear, should be reserved for the product of symbolically presented probabilities and subjective values of any kind. That allows us to respect the mechanistic distinction Hertwig and colleagues identified as we develop Hard economic theories.

Given that distinction, what do we know about true (symbolic) expected subjective values? Where are the probabilities that control these expectations represented? How do these explicit representations influence subjective value? A number of studies have examined the choices people make when presented with symbolic probabilities in both monetary and consumable rewards (Breiter et al., 2001; Hsu et al., 2005, 2009; Huettel et al., 2005, 2006; Levy et al., 2010; Luhmann et al., 2008; Tom et al., 2007). Essentially all of these studies show activations in the medial prefrontal cortex and ventral striatum that are correlated with expected subjective values. What that tells us is that expected subjective values, in the sense used here, are encoded in these final common areas. There is even evidence that the dorsal striatum may encode expected subjective value (Hsu et al., 2005) in humans under at least some conditions. We know less about the other areas in the frontal cortex involved in the construction of value. Future studies will be required to hone our answers to these questions.

Probability Summary

As Maurice Allais first pointed out, human choosers violate the *independence axiom*, the core feature of most neoclassical models that explicitly incorporate probability into choice. Kahneman and Tversky argued that these violations can be parsimoniously characterized with "probability-weighting functions" that relate symbolic numerical probabilities to decision weights.[3] In the language of probability weighting functions, these behaviors reflect an *overweighting* of low-probability events.

Studies of animal decision making, and subsequent studies of humans learning expected utilities through experience, have revealed a second class of independence axiom violation. In the language of probability weighting functions, these violations reflect *underweighting* of low-probability events. The learning mechanisms that have been described to date suggest that the latter class of independence axiom violations reflect a Bush and Mosteller equation-like computation of the subjective value of choice objects. Rather than seeing these as direct violations of the independence axiom, however, one can characterize them as well-described algorithmic misestimations of the average subjective value. In essence, one can see any subjective value computed in this way (whether it be from probabilistic or determinate outcomes) as simple subjective values free from probability information.

The violations of the independence axiom observed by Allais, Kahneman and Tversky, and so forth remain more problematic. These are choices that reveal inconsistencies in our expected subjective valuations— inconsistencies that many reasonably consider failures of our rationality. As such, these are distortions that probably lie outside the range of neoclassical neuroeconomics and that will call for truly behavioral neuro-economic explanations. It seems plausible that the symbolic communication of probabilistic events, a very recent evolutionary event in the history of our species, reflects true failures of our neural apparatus for maximization.

---

3. Other explanations of these same behavioral phenomena are also possible.

Conclusions

Animals often succeed in achieving clear maxima with the tool of their behavioral choices. Moose foraging in the tundra achieve a nearly perfect intersection of constraints with their foraging decisions (Belovsky, 1984). Birds have been shown to almost perfectly trade off increased flight weight against stored numbers of calories (Metcalfe and Ure, 1995). Prey selection in several species balances handling costs against energy value perfectly (Bres, 2006; Killen et al., 2007; Richman and Loworn, 2009). The list of well-studied cases in which animals achieve maxima in feeding or reproduction grows daily. These are the phenomena for which neoclassically based Hard-theories of choice are ideal tools. Many other phenomena, in contrast, seem to reflect fundamental failures of maximization. How humans subjects face large choice sets or encode symbolically communicated probabilities are just two examples.

The gray area between choices well modeled by neoclassical versus behavioral tools is vast and poorly charted. Advances in neoclassical theory and the incorporation of algorithmic models into the neoclassical corpus broaden the reach of these models. At the same time, a deeper understanding of human choice behavior reveals more and more of the idiosyncrasies that call for behavioral economic explanations. The history of economics, however, tells us how neuroeconomics will have to engage this latter set of choices. Just as neoclassical theory defined the starting point from which behavioral economics begins its explanation, neoclassically anchored models must serve as the starting point from which neuroeconomics will develop as a broadly interdisciplinary field. We have just begun to explore the strengths of our neural architecture for choice and valuation. Understanding the weaknesses of that same system will doubtless follow, although that understanding is today in its infancy.

Section 4

Summary and Conclusions

This final section presents a concise overview of most of what we know about the neural architecture for choice. The first chapter of this section presents in mathematical form a complete encapsulation of the constraints on representation and choice that were developed in the preceding pages. The second and final chapter reviews the most important of these constraints, identifies several large and unanswered questions that face neuroeconomics today, and sounds a cautionary note about the use of neuroeconomic data in welfare economics.

16

Foundations of Neuroeconomic Models

Précis

The goal of neuroeconomics is to produce a single unified model of human decision making that spans the economic, psychological, and neuroscientific levels of analysis. *Because* models, rather than the traditional *as if* models of economics or the nonstructural models of neuroscience and psychology, are what defines the neuroeconomic approach. Hard-theories, *because* theories, describe logical operations that not only predict behavior but also closely approximate the underlying physical and mental processes that give rise to those behaviors.

Two classes of argument have been recently advanced by a group of economists to suggest that contemporary work on these *because* theories is doomed to irrelevance. The first of these economic arguments concedes that our knowledge of psychology and neuroscience may someday permit the generation of linked interdisciplinary hypotheses, but concludes that what we know today about the brain and behavior is hopelessly insufficient for the generation of useful neuroeconomic theories. The second of these arguments suggests that a linked interdisciplinary theory of choice is impossible in principle. It is impossible, these critics argue, because no partial reduction of economics to psychology or neuroscience will ever be achievable. They concede that economics may be of use to neuroscientists but hypothesize that the converse will not be the case.

In contrast, a group of psychologists and neurobiologists have argued that even the phrase "neuroeconomics" is distasteful because of its obvious ties to what Thomas Carlyle (1849) called "the dismal science."

These critics conclude that economics' dependence on compact axiomatic approaches and the widely demonstrated falsification of the most popular axiomatic formulations make it clear that economics can never hope to contribute significantly to our understanding of choice behavior in any way. Trying to use the structural neoclassical economic approach to guide or constrain neurobiological and psychological studies of decision making will inevitably, these critics argue, diminish the power of the mechanistic analyses indigenous to these sciences. Neuroscience and psychology will someday, these critics often conclude, offer economics the boon of a complete and mechanistically correct alternative theory, but economics will never be of use to neuroscientists and psychologists.

The only truly meaningful reply to such criticisms is success. We can prove that interdisciplinary syntheses are possible, and useful, only by achieving at least one such synthesis, and in the preceding pages I have suggested that, contrary to the arguments of single-discipline critics who often know little about the current state of brain science or about the details of contemporary economic debate, a wide range of interdisciplinary syntheses have already been accomplished. To take just a single example from the preceding pages, consider the choices humans and animals make when they sample probabilistic rewards repeatedly, when they learn the value of an action through experience. Traditional neoclassical economic theory employs the axiomatic notion of expected utility to explain these kinds of choice. That theory fails because the independence axiom is violated. Traditional psychological theory proposes that an iterative learning process produces an associative strength related to the notion of utility but is silent on choice. Neurobiological studies of dopamine-based systems describe, in molecular detail, the process by which synaptic strengths are changed by rewards and connect those synapses to movement production via structures in the fronto-parietal networks.

I hope that I have convinced you that the neuroeconomic synthesis suggests that a surprisingly complete model of the learning and choice process can be constructed from these disparate observations. Caplin and Dean have shown us, at an axiomatic level, how systems of this type can be connected to choice. Sutton and Barto have shown us how such a system can account for the relationship between the algorithmic implementation of learning and the idiosyncrasies of choice itself. Studies such as Schultz's have shown us how the details of the neural implementation constrain such models as Sutton and Barto's, and provide scholars such as Caplin and Dean with the very constraints required to shape powerful structural axiomatic models. And this is only one example.

My reply to critics of this interdisciplinary approach is not just that we may *someday* achieve a neuroeconomic synthesis, but rather that the neuroeconomic synthesis is already well under way. The preceding pages have laid out a broad range of constraints, from all three of neuroeconomics' primary parent disciplines, constraints that many scholars working within neuroeconomics believe must shape the class of all future models of how we decide.

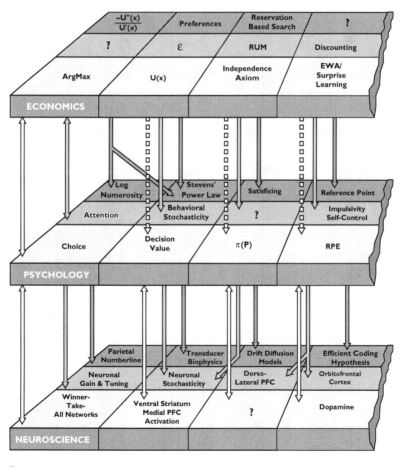

FIGURE 16.1   .

The data and theories of each of neuroeconomics' parent disciplines constrain the sets of models compatible with the observations of that discipline. By reductively linking the disciplines, we permit these constraints to interact. The result is that we are able to identify a much smaller subset of models compatible with the constraints of all three disciplines. In addition to making this largely philosophical point, a second goal of this book has been to describe many of the actual intersecting constraints we know about today. This second goal has been to identify the small subset of decision-making models that are compatible with the consilience of our three parent disciplines.

What are the key constraints we have identified that any reductively linked theory of choice must respect? The first thing we discovered is that the choices we make occur because our brains explicitly represent the economic concept of preferences in the form of cardinalized expected subjective values. These cardinalized subjective values take the form, in the choice circuit, of relative expected subjective values. These relative expected subjective values show an adjustable Poisson-like stochasticity. Choice can occur when one of two things happens: (1) A rapid change in the global state of the choice networks effectively selects, from the current set of options, that option having the highest current relative expected subjective value; or (2) The network state has been set to identify a threshold relative expected subjective value. As soon as the (stochastically varying) value of any one option exceeds that threshold, choice occurs.

We also know that these relative expected subjective values are computed from a more absolute representation of subjective values generated and stored (almost certainly in at least two stages) in the frontal cortex, the basal ganglia, and perhaps also in the medial temporal lobe. When offered a choice set, some or all of these values, combined with linguistic information about probabilities, pass to the fronto-parietal network for actual choice. Exactly how many and which of these options are passed on to the choice network reflects the structure of option representation in these areas.

Regardless of which options are passed to the choice network, however, the values we place on goods about which we have experience, our preferences, are learned by a system we are also beginning to understand. Our sensory systems encode the properties of incoming stimuli, and these incoming data are subjected to iterative Bush and Mosteller-like calculations of value. The properties of the sensory encoding systems, which are shaped by both experience and genetics, define many of the features of subjective values that emerge from that process, the features of our preferences. We know that these preferences reflect a shifting reference point that first appears during sensory encoding. Curvature in the sensory transduction functions, a sensory property that we already understand, accounts for at least some of the curvature in reference-dependent utility that we observe behaviorally. The iterative Bush and Mosteller-style calculation of average subjective value also induces systematic errors in our estimates of probability that can be well explained by the learning rate a subject employs. We know less about linguistically communicated probabilities, systematic distortions of those probabilities, and how these subjective probabilities combine with learned subjective values. We know that these are systematically misrepresented at some point in the nervous system. We do not yet know where, but we know that the products of these probabilities and subjective values are computed and represented in the final common areas for valuation that feed the choice networks.

In this chapter, I attempt to encapsulate these interdisciplinary constraints in a more mathematical form. Let me be clear that the pages that follow are not a complete model; rather, the contents encapsulate the set of existing constraints any future model must respect. For economists and more mathematically trained psychologists and neurobiologists, the pages that follow provide a compact précis of the second and third sections of this book. They also provide a common nomenclature for (and a formal definition of) the linked objects that I believe form the core of neuroeconomic theory today. For neoclassically trained economists in particular, the pages that follow should make my goals and intentions more clear. For some scholars, however, the pages that follow may provide more mathematical detail than is desirable. My suggestion for these scholars would be to skip over the sections that follow and proceed immediately to the concluding chapter of this book.

Subjective Value-Related Signals

The core set of ideas around which initial neuroeconomic theories will be built are the linkages between measurable neural activity and utility-like concepts derived from economics. The key insight provided by this approach is that existing notions of utility provide a starting point as we search for the neural mechanisms of choice. As neural correlates for utility come to be identified, we can use the observed structure of that neural representation to refine economic-level theories that constrain and define our understanding of utility-like objects. This is the iterative interaction that forms the core of the neuroeconomic approach. The very first step in this process is thus a definition of the observable neurobiological object that we hope to relate to the economic object we call utility, an object with properties we hope to refine. We refer to this object, or more precisely this set of objects, as *subjective values* (SVs) to distinguish their specific properties from the properties of the behaviorally revealed utility to which they are conceptually linked.

Subjective Values

SVs are real numbers ranging from 0 to 1,000. They take action potentials per second as their natural units. SVs have the following properties:

1. Mean SVs predict choice stochastically.[1] Average choice identifies the option having the highest mean SV. Instantaneous SVs are the sum (see below) of mean SV and a single noise term (see below). Instantaneous SVs predict trial-by-trial choice with greater accuracy than do mean SVs. Choice identifies the option with the highest instantaneous SV. This means that SV theory will be most closely allied with random utility-type models from economics. (In other words, the random utilities of McFadden [2000] are homomorphic, at least in a limited way, to instantaneous SVs. More traditional utilities such as those of Samuelson [1938] are similarly homomorphic to mean SVs.)
2. Mean SVs are defined as the mean firing rates of specific populations of neurons, the identification of which follows. For this reason, SVs

---

1. This relationship to choice is critical because it means that the theory of utility and the theory of subjective value share a common object, which allows for formal linkage of the two sets of theoretical constructs, a point taken up in the first section of this book.

are linearly proportional to the BOLD signal[2] from fMRI as measured in these same populations.

3. When choice behavior obeys GARP, the SVs obey all of the ordinal constraints on utility imposed by GARP. (This is the *central linking hypothesis of neuroeconomics*.)

4. SVs are *always* consistent with choice, though stochastically, even when choice is not consistent with standard economic theories such as GARP or EU. Thus, changes in theoretical notions of utility aimed at strengthening the central linking hypothesis of neuroeconomics necessarily strengthen the predictive power of the modified theory.

5. SVs have a unique anchor point called the *baseline firing rate*. They inherit this property from neuronal spike rates, which always have an anchoring point called the baseline firing rate. All SVs are encoded cardinally in firing rates relative to this baseline. This means that mean SVs are fully cardinal and unique representations. (This is a property that SVs do not share with post-Pareto notions of utility.)

I want to be extremely clear about what these properties mean. SVs are in many ways like utilities. These two objects are linearly correlated with one another, a correlation that I refer to as the *central linking hypothesis of neuroeconomics*.[3] Their utility-like properties, specified by this linking hypothesis, are of course the very features that allowed us to begin the search for SVs in the nervous system. And like utilities, SVs are inextricably linked to choice. When a subject obeys the axioms of GARP, a neoclassical Soft-theory, we say that he or she chooses as if the choices reflected an underlying monotonic utility function. If GARP were a Hard-theory, we would say that he or she chooses because the choices reflect the presence, in his or her brain, of a group of neurons whose firing rate is a

---

2. I assume here that mean neural activity and the BOLD signal are linearly correlated. I recognize that this is a strong (although widely held) assumption that will eventually have to be relaxed as we learn more about BOLD. See Niv et al. (2008) and Logothetis and Wandell (2004) for more on this point.

3. Many scholars, particularly economists, may find the assertion of a linear relationship here unnecessarily restrictive. Let me respond that all of our available empirical data argue for this linear relationship (e.g., Louie and Glimcher, 2010). If those empirical data are correct, this has profound implications for the cardinality of utility-like objects. It should not escape the attention of a political economist that this may be of tremendous significance.

monotonic function of quantity that guides choice through an argmax-like operation. Unfortunately GARP is only sometimes true. Sometimes choosers violate GARP.

The empirical data we have today strongly suggest that the firing rates of a particular group of neurons guide choice through an argmax-like (or winner-take-all–like) operation. The empirical data we have tie the firing rates of these neurons to choice *at all times*. *When behavior obeys GARP, these firing rates must have the properties of utilities, as specified by GARP.* This simple fact communicates much of the power and beauty of the economic approach. If GARP tells us that under specific behavioral conditions

$$U(a) \geq U(b) \geq U(c)$$

then

$$SV(a) \geq SV(b) \geq SV(c)$$

It is equally important, however, to realize that when GARP fails to predict choice, when choosers violate the axioms of that theory, then that theory no longer constrains SVs. Once behavior lies outside the predictive range of that particular theory, so does SV.

This should reveal why GARP and for that matter such other theories as expected utility are critical to empirical neuroeconomics. It is not that GARP (or EU) is a globally correct theory, but rather that GARP and EU are important tools because they tell us what SVs (or expected SVs) *must* look like under many conditions. In fact, it is this very feature that has already allowed us to identify SVs in the nervous system.

Subjective Values and Probabilistic Events

SVs and traditional utilities, however, differ from one another in another very important respect that I need to emphasize. We know, at a mechanistic level, that probabilistic rewards can influence choice behavior in two very distinct ways.

Consider pushing a button that yields $10 with a probability of 5%. Imagine that I place you alone in a room with that button and you begin to press it repeatedly. We know how you learn the value of this button; that algorithm was the topic of Chapter 13. On each trial you press the button. The outcome, winning $10 or $0, gives rise to a reward prediction error (RPE). From Chapter 12:

RPE = reward expected − reward obtained

That RPE is multiplied by a learning rate and used to update your estimate of the value of that action, a point taken up below. What I want to point out here is that when you learn the value of an action in this way, the probability is bundled directly into your estimate of the value of that action. Your estimate of the value of that action includes the probability, but you cannot extract that probability from this estimate. If I told you verbally that I had changed the probability, this is not information that you could use accurately to guide choice through *this* reinforcement learning-based mechanism for computing SV. To put this more formally, the reinforcement learning mechanism incorporates probability into your estimate of what pushing that button is worth, but in a *non-invertible* way.

The critical idea is that what you have learned through experience about the value of pushing that button is behaving more like a utility than like an expected utility, even though the underlying event is probabilistic. Let me say this another way. When Samuelson developed WARP and Houthakker developed GARP, there was no barrier to the inclusion of probabilistic events as prizes in their axioms. In those theories, we could easily ask a subject whether she preferred a 50% chance of winning one apple to a 25% chance of winning two apples. What we could not do with those theories, however, was to use these probabilities to infer things about the curvature of the utility function for apples *cum* apples. Probabilistic events could be included in prizes, but the theory had nothing to say about these probabilities *cum* probabilities. Exactly the same thing is true about the SVs of probabilistic events learned by experience.

Von Neumann and Morgenstern, when they added the independence axiom to the toolkit of neoclassical economics developed a method for treating probabilities *as* probabilities. They developed a representational theory of probabilities that could be used to tell us about the curvature of the utility function for apples *cum* apples. At a theoretical level, the independence axiom turned probabilities into a ruler for measuring utilities. At an empirical level, von Neumann and Morgenstern showed us how to measure curvature by presenting people with symbolically communicated lotteries. They used symbolic probabilities to specify utility function curvature through the tool of expected utilities. (This is a point developed in more detail in Chapter 3.)

To preserve this set of features, I adopt here the convention that when the values of probabilistic events are non-invertibly encoded, we must treat them, using tools related to GARP, as SVs. Only when probabilities are invertibly encoded, only when we can separate probability and SV (as indicated by behavioral or neural measurements), do we refer to the object specified by these properties as an *expected SV*. Fortunately, these two encoding systems turn out to be easy to identify even at the behavioral level. In general, Bush and Mosteller-like learning systems that embed probabilities in SVs show an underweighting of low probabilities and an overweighting of high probabilities (a point developed in Chapter 13). In contrast, symbolically communicated probabilities typically produce choices that can be characterized as an overweighting of low probabilities and an underweighting of high probabilities (a point developed in Chapter 5). In practice, this is probably the best tool for discriminating these two processes embedded in any standard neuroeconomic model.

In any case, I define here the concept of SV (both instantaneous and mean). SVs are both firing rates and, via a few transformations, choice. They thus inherit properties from both neurons and from choice. The properties they inherit from choice, properties *necessarily* specified by economic theories of choice, are described above. From neurons they inherit the fact that they are real numbers ranging from 0 to 1,000, have fixed variance, and are unique and fully cardinal.

The fact that SVs have significant variance also has a number of important implications for how these objects relate to economic theory and choice. These implications are discussed below where stochasticity is covered.

To summarize, SV is encoded directly as firing rate in the valuation mechanisms of the human brain. Each object in a choice set has an SV, SV_j.

Choice is the process of selecting the object with the highest SV from the choice set.

Variability in SV, the physical instantiation of our preferences, reflects variations in our preferences. This is not the only source of variance in our choices. (Independent variance in the fronto-parietal networks, which is described below, can induce stochasticity unrelated to random utilities/random SVs.) Further, let me be clear that whenever a subject learns the value of a probabilistic choice object by experience, the average of that probabilistic value (as computed by an iterative Bush and Mosteller-like computation) is fully captured in SV. SVs capture some kinds of probabilistic goods, those valued through repeated sampling. *The concept of an expected SV is reserved for symbolically communicated probabilities.*

The location in the nervous system at which SV (as distinct from *expected* SV) is represented is not known with certainty. Current evidence suggests that neurons in the dorsal striatum almost certainly encode the SVs of actions, although some doubt remains over whether these are actually expected SVs. Several frontal areas are also candidates for encoding SV, but because not all experiments allow us to distinguish expected SV from SV, uncertainties remain about the neural instantiation of this object.

Expected SV

Expected SV (ESV) is the product of linguistically or symbolically communicated probabilities and SV. It is also a cardinal measure, similar in all respects to SV, whose properties it inherits. It is ESV that is known to be represented in areas like the medial prefrontal cortex. It is this stochastically varying object that is passed to the fronto-parietal networks for choice. One central goal of neuroeconomics will be to develop a complete theory of ESV. It has been my core argument that if we had a complete theory of ESV and a complete form of the central linking hypothesis of neuroeconomics, we would necessarily be able to complete (in the positive sense) a full economic-level theory of choice.

For all of the reasons described above, when choice behavior obeys the axioms of expected utility theory (EU), ESVs are *linearly proportional* to the expected utilities embedded in that theory. Under these conditions, if (for example) a lottery yielding prize a with probability p is considered,

$Eu(a, p) = p \times a^{0.6}$, then $ESV(a, p) = p \times (k_1 + k_2 a^{0.6})$ *See note*[4]

Let me repeat that p's appear in this representation only when they are communicated to subjects symbolically and when they can, in a mechanistic sense, be invertibly removed from ESVs to yield SVs. In this way we reserve ESVs for the class of probability-related objects that originally interested von Neumann and Morgenstern (1944).

We know that the medial prefrontal cortex encodes an ESV signal encoded in spike rates. While there is debate about whether the ventral striatum encodes an RPE *and* either ESV or SV, current evidence leans strongly to SV.

Relative Expected Subjective Value

We define the (mean) relative ESV of a single option j as:

$$\overline{RSV_j} = \frac{ESV_j + \beta}{\sum_{k=1}^{K} ESV_k + \sigma^2}$$

where RSV is relative expected subjective value, K is the set of all options in a choice set (including j), σ is an empirically measured saturation constant of the type first described in the cerebral cortex by David Heeger (1992a, 1992b), and β is an empirically measured additive baseline term also of the kind first defined in cortex (Louie and Glimcher, 2010; Reynolds and Heeger, 2009). Our current evidence suggests that choices are actually made between options by comparing mean RSV_j's after corruption by noise. This is the second source of noise in the architecture, and it is conceptually distinct from random utility-like fluctuations. This noise induces stochasticity in choice that is independent of the stochastic fluctuations of ESV.

RSV has been clearly documented in the posterior parietal segments of the choice network (Dorris and Glimcher, 2004; Louie and Glimcher, 2010; Platt and Glimcher, 1999). There is evidence that this term is also encoded in other elements of the choice network (Basso and Wurtz,

---

4. When choice is not a linear function of probability, when the equation on the left does not hold, ESV is also not a linear function of probability.

1997; McCoy and Platt, 2005). It seems likely that all elements of the fronto-parietal network employ RSV.

The RSV equation described above has been linked to normative models of information encoding by Schwartz and Simoncelli, a point taken up in Chapter 10. They have pointed out that a more general formulation of this equation can be used to define an encoding scheme that maximizes joint information (in this case about ESVs) across any neuronal population.

Stochastic Terms

The existing neural data suggest two classes of noise that influence choice: one at the level of the valuation system and one at the level of the choice system. In economic terms, the first can be viewed as roughly corresponding to random utility distributions (McFadden, 1974) and to stochasticity in the representation of probability that gives rise to a random expected utility-like representation that can be roughly related to the axioms of Gul and Pesendorfer (2006). The second class can be seen as corresponding to the trembling hand (Selten, 1975) notion of stochastic behavior from economics. There is compelling evidence for both classes of stochasticity.

SV *noise* (from class 1) is a random term, ε_1, drawn from a distribution (independently at each time point t) assumed to be Poisson and added to mean SV to yield the instantaneous SV of object j at time t. It is always present. Thus the SV at time t is

$$SV_{jt} = \overline{SV_j} + [\eta_{1t} \times (\varepsilon_{1t} - \overline{SV_j})]$$

where ε_1 is drawn (at each time t) from a Poisson distribution with a mean of $\overline{SV}$ and η_1 is a noise scaling constant ranging from 1.15 to 0. ε_1 is Poisson distributed with a mean of $\overline{SV}$ because this is a fundamental property of the neurons that carry SV. η_1 allows for changes in the degree of variance. It has a maximal possible value of 1.15 based upon empirical data about the limits of neuronal stochasticity. These were points taken up in Chapters 9 and 10.

It is important to note that we are hypothesizing that SV_{jt} is preference for object i at time t. That means that if, at a particular moment, ε_{1t} is high, then at that particular moment our preference for j is high.

This means that SV_{jt} has all of the properties of a random utility with the underlying distribution defined as a scaled Poisson variance.

Expectation noise (from class 1) is a random term drawn from a distribution assumed to be Poisson and added to subjectively transformed probabilities. We know little today about where subjective probabilities are represented, but we do know that they must be represented by neuronal firing rates. This means that we can define the instantaneous expectation π at time t for probability j as

$$\pi(P_{jt}) = \overline{P}_j + [\eta_{2t} \times (\varepsilon_{2t} - \overline{P}_j)]$$

where ε_2 is again drawn from a Poisson distribution with a mean of $\overline{P}$ and η_2 is a noise scaling constant ranging from 1.15 to 0. ε_2 is Poisson-distributed with a mean of $\overline{P}$ because this is a fundamental property of the neurons that carry ESV. η_2 allows for changes in the degree of variance. It has a maximal possible value of 1.15 based upon empirical data about the limits of neuronal stochasticity.

One final note bears on the combination of P_j and SV_j when ESVs are produced. Our behavioral evidence suggests that mean ESVs are the product of mean expectations and mean SVs. Neuronal data suggest, oddly enough, that the variances of these two terms do not necessarily multiply. Cortical neurons receive thousands of Poisson varying inputs and maintain a Poisson varying output. Although the algorithmic process by which this is accomplished is not well understood, we know that it occurs. Thus, when P_{jt} and SV_{jt} are combined to yield an instantaneous ESV, variation in that quantity is best described as having an intrinsically scaled variance that cannot necessarily be inferred from the variances of P_j and SV_j. In any case, the stochastically varying product, ESV_{jt}, would behave largely like a random expected utility (Gul and Pesendorfer, 2006) with scaled Poisson variance.

Cortical noise before choice (from class 2) is a final noise source added (as a stochastic time series) to RSV_j before choice occurs. The source of this term is noise intrinsic to cortical neurons in the fronto-parietal network, which requires that it also be Poisson in distribution at the mechanistic point of addition.

$$RSV_{jt} = \overline{RSV}_j + [\eta_{3t} \times (\varepsilon_{3t} - \overline{RSV}_j)]$$

Neuronal pooling that occurs during the choice process and adjustability of the inter-neuronal correlation term may be used to reduce this variance and thus are reflected in the magnitude of the term η_3 (Krug and Parker, 2004). For more on the theoretical implications of this, see Glimcher (2005).

From a logical point of view, ε_3 can be seen as giving rise to errors in the choice process, with η_3 scaling the magnitude of those errors. We can thus think of η_3 as setting the slope of the stochastic choice function, typically represented as a logit, relating the relative values of two options under consideration to choice probabilities.

Learning-Related Signals

Experienced SV

Experienced SV (ExperSV) is a pattern of neuronal firing, much like SV, that encodes the SV of current states of the world. The neural location of ExperSV is not known, though the activity of dopamine neurons provides overwhelming evidence that it is present as one of the inputs to those midbrain neurons. For reasons that will be described below, ExperSV actually serves as one source of the utility-like properties of SV. ExperSV is related to true states of the outside world by two transformations. First, a non-recoverable reference point is subtracted from the true state of the world. The remainder is then monotonically transformed to ExperSV. Thus, for a good j provided in quantity x,

$$ExperSV_{jt} = f_j(x_j) - \beta_{jt}$$

where f_j is a monotonic transform of magnitude (typically but not always concave; e.g., Stevens, 1961) specific to the neural system encoding good j, x_j is the quantity of good j encountered, and β_{jt} is the current value of the non-recoverable baseline for good j, typically defined independently for each of the neural transduction systems.

At least one anatomical source of the transformation set f_i is the sensory transduction systems of the nervous system. Fairly direct inputs to the dopamine neurons from these transduction systems likely carry ExperSV for many consumable rewards. There is some evidence that many of these signals originate in the nucleus of the solitary tract, a point taken up in Chapter 4. The location of monetary ExperSV signals is not completely known, although dopamine firing rates, again, point at their existence. Some single-neuron evidence (Nakamura et al., 2008) suggests that the serotonergic neurons of the midbrain raphe also encode ExperSV for primary rewards.

Forecast Expected Subjective Value

Forecast expected subjective value ($ESV_{forecast}$) is a discounted rational expectation of all future rewards. At the level of theory, $ESV_{forecast}$ is similar to the rational expectation, or reference point, of Kőszeki and Rabin. Thus, it is also identical to the reward prediction term employed in learning models such as those of Sutton and Barto. Both of these theories would define $ESV_{forecast}$ (although one would define it for use in learning and the other for use in choice) as

$$ESV_{forecast} = SV_t + \gamma^1 ESV_{t+1} + \gamma^2 ESV_{t+2} + \gamma^3 ESV_{t+3} + \gamma^4 ESV_{t+4} \cdots$$

where γ, the discount parameter, captures the decline in value of the stream of all future rewards as a function of time.

$ESV_{forecast}$ is a critical term for the theory because it serves as the reference point against which all "utilities" (or more accurately, SVs) are represented and learned. Mechanistically this arises because the values of goods or actions are learned as errors, in the units of ExperSV, from $ESV_{forecast}$. When we encounter a new good, we have to learn its SV. We do that by taking the reference-dependent sensory inputs of ExperSV and subtracting from them $ESV_{forecast}$.

Clear evidence about the location of $ESV_{forecast}$ is not now available. We do know that the activity of midbrain dopamine neurons also reflects the input of this signal. That leads to the suggestion that the output of the striatum directed towards the midbrain dopamine neurons must contain $ESV_{forecast}$. Some single-neuron studies in the output areas of the basal ganglia provide evidence for this signal (Handel and Glimcher, 1999, 2000). Single neurons in the striatum (Lau and Glimcher, 2007; Samejima et al., 2005) have been shown to carry a signal that may also reflect $ESV_{forecast}$.

Reward Prediction Error

Reward Prediction Error (RPE) is defined here as it is in learning studies, and as summarized in Chapter 12. Put extremely (perhaps too) briefly, it is

$$RPE = (ExperSV - ESV_{forecast})$$

Our current evidence indicates that RPE is encoded in the activity of the midbrain dopamine neurons and in the neurons of the habenula (Matsumoto and Hikosaka, 2007, 2008b). RPE is positively correlated with activity in the dopamine neurons and negatively correlated with activity in the habenula. It has been hypothesized that other signals encoding very negative RPEs may yet be identified (Balleine et al., 2008; Bayer and Glimcher, 2005; Daw et al., 2002; Glimcher, 2008). It is not known whether the learning rate constant, α (see Chapter 12), which modulates the RPE term and is used to update SVs

$$SV_{j(t+1)} = SV_{jt} + \alpha RPE_t$$

is encoded in dopamine firing rates as well, or whether this term is multiplied with the dopaminergic signal in dopamine target areas.

Structure of the Learned Subjective Value Function

Given that ExperSV is the product of a non-stationary sensory system, we can therefore conclude that ExperSV is influenced by the metabolic current state of the animal. For example, if blood glucose levels are high, then the ExperSV of a dried apricot is lower than it would be in a low-blood-glucose state. In principle this should induce significant violations of rationality in the form of intransitivities, if we measure over a long enough time period. We can overcome many (but not all) of these intransitivities in behavior if SVs are, unlike traditional utilities, a function of both the value of a good and the state of the chooser.

Thus it is tempting to hypothesize that ESVs, *with regard to behavior,* are a function of both state and value, a representation of the "utility function" that has the effect of minimizing intransitivities in a reference-dependent system

$$ESV = g[(ExperSV - SV_{forecast}), (State)]$$

where *state* is an observable internal state variable, such as blood glucose level.

Relationship Between Theoretical Variables and Neural Activity

Formally (and of course too simplistically), ESV (and most of the terms described above) can be seen as a neuronal sum of the form

$$ESV_j = \frac{\sum_i \omega_{ij} x_{ij}}{\sum_i \omega_{ij}}$$

where the term i indexes each of the neurons in the brain, x_{ij} is the firing rate of the ith neuron to good j, and ω_{ij} is a weight ranging from 0 to 1 describing the additive contribution of that neuron to the ESV of object or action j. This object places into the language of economics the standard neurobiological insight that a weighted sum of neurons, often arranged in topographic maps, encodes behaviorally relevant variables. The ESV of a particular object j in the external world is thus simply represented as the average weighted firing rate of a subpopulation of neurons that encode the SV of that object. In a topographically mapped action–encoding region such as the superior colliculus, this is equivalent to saying that activity in a restricted region of the map encodes value for a particular action (but note that in the superior colliculus it is RSV that is encoded). However, this definition specifically excludes distributed nonlinear encoding schemes.

For an empirical neurophysiologist or functional magnetic resonance imager looking for any of these variables in the brain, two questions then become paramount:

1. Is there a firing rate pattern (or a BOLD activation, in the case of fMRI) we can identify in the brain that is linearly correlated with one of these theoretical objects?
2. What is the most compact population of neurons (both in number of neurons and in anatomical extent of the population) that can maintain this linear correlation with that object (i.e., the smallest population of neurons for which ω_{ij} is not equal to zero)?

Normative Neuroeconomics

Most economists discriminate between two classes of economic theory: the *positive* and the *normative*. Positive economics is about prediction. Asking whether a theory can be used to accurately describe human behavior is a positive question. Normative theory is about optimality, well-being, and efficiency.

All of the modern neoclassical theories begin with a clear statement of axioms. So far, I have focused exclusively on the positive features of these theories, but most of these axiom sets have normative implications that we have not discussed. Consider something as simple as an axiom on transitivity, such as the one around which GARP is organized. I begin by asserting that if I see apples chosen over oranges and oranges over pears, I am therefore prevented from drawing the conclusion that my subject strictly prefers pears to apples. If apples ≻ oranges ≻ pears, then a chooser cannot show pears ≻ apples.

In a positive sense, I test my theory to see if it is predictive. If a subject actually did choose apples over oranges and oranges over pears, but strictly preferred pears to apples, then my theory would have no predictive power. It would be false in the positive sense. But I still might quite reasonably believe that my theory was normatively valuable. After all, a subject who actually showed these preferences could be induced to buy a pear from me, sell me back that pear at a loss for an orange, then sell me back the orange at an additional loss for an apple, then to sell me back the apple at a loss for the original pear. At the end of that process he would be poorer, would still own the original pear, and would be convinced that each of his decisions was reasonable. He would have lost money and gained nothing, but he would still tell you that he wanted to repeat this set of decisions. While transitivity has no positive (predictive) power when it comes to this individual, everyone would probably agree that this subject's preferences were compromising his welfare (because they violated transitivity). We might even argue that if we observed a subject robustly violating such an axiom we would do him a favor by restricting the ability of others to pump money out of his pockets.

Normative issues have figured in neuroeconomic discourse since its inception, and the role of neuroeconomics in normative theory has come under particularly intense scrutiny in recent years. Princeton's Daniel Kahneman (e.g., Kahneman, 2008), who has argued strongly against neoclassical notions of how to maximize welfare, has expressed a strong interest in neuroeconomic measurement. Stanford University's Doug Bernheim (2008), to take another example, has begun to ask hard questions about neuroeconomics and welfare in a more neoclassical vein. These scholars, and others like them, press neuroeconomists to answer such questions as, can we use brain scanners to tell us what is best for people? Can we use neural data to overrule the choices people make and leave them better off by doing so?

These are key problems in neuroeconomics, and all of them rest squarely on the relationship between brain activations, welfare, and utility. Can brain activations provide better information about what makes people well off than does choice? If you believe, as Kahneman does, that the utility that guides choices is distinct from the brain mechanisms with which we experience well-being, then brain scans might be a better tool for maximizing welfare than choice. If you believe that utility can be more accurately measured with a brain scanner than with choice (an idea that many reasonably find an oxymoron), then brain scans again might be a better tool for maximizing welfare than choice. If we can identify neural signals that obey the axioms of choice more precisely than does behavioral choice, then once again, brain scans might be a better tool for maximizing welfare than choice.

For all of these reasons, it may be tempting to use some of the insights from positive neuroeconomics presented here to draw normative conclusions about welfare. Let me, however, sound a note of caution. First, the theory and data presented here are explicitly positive in nature. We do not yet have a neural theory of welfare. There is no conceptual bar to the generation of such a theory, but that theory does not yet exist, and for that reason alone one should go cautiously. A second reason to go cautiously arises from the nature of the neural representation of SV. We know that activity in the fronto-parietal choice network represents RSV. Critically, RSV cannot be cardinally transformed to a notion of welfare, specifically because it is SV *relative* to the choice set under consideration. But that may also be true of *every* neural representation of SV. The Schwartz-Simoncelli equation discussed in Chapter 10 implies that all neural representations of SV encode that quantity relative to the set of all previously encountered rewards. If that is true, it implies a strongly ordinal property for inter-individual comparisons of SV that has yet to be fully explored.

For these reasons, my normative counsel, for what it is worth, is to *go slowly*. The tools for measuring individual human brain activations are primitive at best, and our theoretical tools are limited. The neuro-economics of welfare will simply have to wait unless we choose to be terribly incautious, because the risks of an overzealous application of neuroeconomics in the normative domain are significant.

Conclusions

My goals in presenting the basic features of the standard neuroeconomic model in this way are twofold. First, I hope to provide a fairly unified notation, a single common language for the basic objects already known to be required by neuroeconomic discourse. Second, I hope to summarize, in a general way, the main features of the human decision-making system. This presentation is both incomplete and too general. The presentation is incomplete because there are many features of the human choice architecture that have been discussed in the preceding pages that are not captured in this brief summary. There are also elements of the human system (for example, how we learn discounted values) that we understand but that are not discussed in this book. The presentation is too general because I do not provide a complete mathematical model of the choice process. Instead, I outline key features that all complete theories must include. I avoid a complete specification of one exemplar from this class of complete theories because it would be quickly shown to be wrong in the specific details not constrained by the observations we already have in hand, and because it would show terrible hubris to specify a complete model of the human choice system at a neuroeconomic level while we are still at this early state of neuroeconomic research. Even I realize that such a model would be premature at this point.

My hope is that the presentation does, however, make it clear that what we already know places significant constraints on the class of Hard-economic theories. Complete theories of decision making based exclusively on choice probabilities, for example, cannot coexist with economic theory and data (because they do not incorporate transitivity as a primitive). Traditional economic theories rooted in marginal utilities are incompatible with the human choice architecture (because they do not include the reference point as a primitive). These are constraints that anyone working on a "because" theory of choice must respect. If the past decade is any indication, there can be no real doubt that additional constraints will emerge at a breakneck pace in the years to come. I hope that the preceding pages have offered a foundation on which these future neuroeconomic analyses can be built.

17

Conclusions

Summary

This book has presented, in three main parts, a framework for understanding the relationship between the brain, the mind, and choice. In the first section I argued that the history of science, at least for the last 100 years, has been one of interdisciplinary reduction. To be more precise, I argued that this history has been one of *partial* reduction, a process that the great biologist E. O. Wilson (1998) has called *consilience*. In the 1950s and 1960s, to take one particularly striking example of this kind of consilience, chemistry and biology came to be reductively linked by the insights of biochemistry. Both of those parent disciplines survived this linkage, but in altered forms: the development of biochemistry changed and strengthened both of its parent disciplines. The central premise of this book is that the same process is now at work bridging the social and natural sciences by linking and modifying the disciplines of neuroscience, psychology, and economics.

If we accept that the interdisciplinary linkages that have characterized the natural sciences will spread across the cultural divide that separates them from the social sciences, then we can use what we know about the past to make a few predictions about what neuroeconomics will look like in a decade or two. On historical grounds alone it seems obvious that neuroscience and psychology must strive to explain the great empirical regularities described (albeit imperfectly) by contemporary economics.

The fundamental representational theories of economics (Samuelson, 1938; von Neumann and Morgenstern, 1944) tell us that choosers, who show the common regularity of "consistency," behave *as if* they had a single internal representation of the idiosyncratic values of their options. These theories suggest that choosers behave as if they somehow select from those representations the single option having the highest idiosyncratic value. But choosers do not always show consistency, just as biologists working before biochemistry knew that the Mendelian laws of inheritance were often violated. Organisms as simple as corn plants had been shown, before the dawn of biochemistry, to possess law-violating "jumping genes" (McClintock, 1983), which a few scientists felt would ultimately falsify our biological understanding of heredity. But the complete abandonment of biological theory never occurred; instead, biochemistry expanded the reach of the laws of heredity. What I have endeavored to point out in these pages is that it has always been the great, though imperfectly described, regularities of "higher" disciplines around which interdisciplinary synthesis can be meaningfully built even when the detailed predictions of those "laws" have been greatly limited in their applicability or accuracy.

Accordingly, I have argued that any search for neuroeconomics must begin with a search for two objects. First, we must seek to describe the neural and psychological correlates of utility, obviously under conditions in which choosers behave consistently. Second, we must look for the mechanism that transforms this correlate of utility into choice. Only after that initial search begins to bear clear fruit can the discipline realize its true potential by modifying the way economics defines and identifies the great empirical regularities of human choice behavior.

The model of the primate choice architecture presented here is thus a two-stage mechanism. I have presented a large quantity of evidence suggesting that circuits of the frontal cortex and the basal ganglia construct a utility-like representation of the values of our options and that these utility-like signals are passed to a fronto-parietal network of areas that selects from among the currently available options the single option having the highest subjective value. The degree to which these two stages are truly separable will be resolved only by future inquiry. Economics has struggled for centuries with the issue of whether choice and utility can be truly separated, and it will be one job of neuroeconomics to provide the *because*-level theories that test that division.

Our examinations have also revealed, however, a number of mechanisms that violate the great regularity of consistent choice around which much of contemporary economics is organized. These are the insights that will reshape economics just as the discovery of "transposons"—mobile chemical objects, pieces of DNA—reshaped the biological laws of heredity.

Although I have presented many examples of these neuroeconomic findings that call for revisions to standard neoclassical economic theory, in my opinion four observations stand out as critical for the first revision of economics by neuroeconomics:

1. <u>Reference dependence</u>, dealt with primarily in Chapters 4, 12, and 13. Everything we know about the brain tells us that the values of options are encoded in a reference-dependent way. In fact, one can even see reference dependence as a biological solution to an environmental challenge, a kind of optimization under constraint. Any future science of choice must respect the fact that whatever empirical regularities characterize the decisions we make, these regularities are the product of a mechanism that inescapably employs a reference point.

2. <u>Cortical areas do not represent the absolute values of anything</u>, as seen in the study of efficient neural coding in Chapter 10. The cortical representation of anything, whether the brightness of a light or the value of a jar of jelly, is efficient, compact and as a result heavily normalized. Again, one can see this as an optimization under constraint. Neurons are costly to maintain, and evolution appears to push us to efficiently use what neurons we have. This constraint on how our brains represent subjective value has profound implications for everything from welfare economics to the influence of irrelevant alternatives on consumer choice. Although closely related to reference dependence, it also imposes a set of regularities on how we store value and choose. Any future reduced-form economic-style model must account for this.

3. <u>Stochasticity in choice</u>, a point developed principally in Chapter 9. Since McFadden's (1974) groundbreaking work in economics, we have had powerful tools for thinking about randomness in choice. At least since the first studies of synaptic release, we have thought of neurons as including a random component (Mainen and Sejnowski, 1995; Stevens, 2003). Although psychologists have been slower to acknowledge this point, we have also known for some time that

humans and animals can appear truly random in their behavior (Neuringer, 2002). The information we have today clearly links these three traditions and identifies stochasticity, constrained by the distributional structure of neural variance, as a core feature of any future approach to choice.

4. The impact of learning on choice, detailed in Chapters 12 and 13. Psychologists since Pavlov have studied learning, but they have only recently begun to think of its impact on choice. Neurobiologists have now specified much of the algorithmic structure of the machines in our skulls that learn. Oddly, though, economics has almost entirely overlooked learning in its search for the sources of utility. We know so much today about how we learn the values of our actions, and sometimes the details of that mechanism explain ways in which we violate consistency in our choices. Many features of those mechanisms are even normative (Sutton and Barto, 1998). In the years to come, the mechanism for learning value will without a doubt figure in any explanation of choice.

Of course there are many other detailed features of any standard neuroeconomic model of choice that will be important. In fact, there are many important findings that I have not discussed in these pages. For example, we know much more about inter-temporal choice than these pages have revealed. We already have first hints about how we learn the values of goods that we choose today but receive tomorrow (Kobayashi and Schultz, 2008; Schultz, 2007). We know that an odd kind of temporal reference dependence seems to influence our inter-temporal choices, and we even have hints about how inconsistencies in inter-temporal choice may arise from constraints on mechanism (Kable and Glimcher, 2007, 2009, 2010). Inter-temporal choice is just one such example; the list of mechanisms and constraints about which we have important information grows almost daily. Neuroeconomics has forged the rudiments of a new theory of choice in only a decade; it is hard to imagine what we will understand a decade hence.

Unanswered Questions

Although it may be hard to imagine what we will know in a decade, we can identify the key gaps in our understanding of choice today. These are gaps in understanding that hold us back and that we must endeavor to fill. In 1900 the German mathematician Daniel Hilbert identified 24 unanswered problems in mathematics that he felt were critical to the future of mathematics. A century later, only half of those problems have been solved, but our progress in mathematics has been shaped by those questions that have been answered. In that spirit, I want to identify six huge unsolved problems in neuroeconomics. It is my belief that our understanding of these issues will strongly shape the future of neuroeconomics.

1. Where Is Subjective Value Stored and How Does It Get to Choice?

We know that the fronto-parietal choice networks encode the normalized expected subjective values of options in a choice set. These areas appear to receive expected subjective value signals from final common valuation areas like the medial prefrontal cortex and the striatum. We even have good reason to believe that the activity of medium spiny neurons in the striatum encodes the learned subjective values of actions. But it is also true that we humans can associate values with literally thousands of choice objects. We can place values on everything from artworks to cold cereals. An art dealer might be able to consistently place values on 10,000 paintings. A child might be able to place consistent values on 50 kinds of cold cereal. Where in the brain are these valuations stored? How does that storage mechanism relate to the systems for episodic memory known to exist in the medial temporal lobe? By what route do signals representing these stored values propagate to the choice mechanism? This is a huge and almost entirely unexplored set of questions that are critical for understanding choice.

2. Who Says When It Is Time to Choose?

We know that the fronto-parietal choice networks can perform a winner-take-all computation, a computation that I have argued is the physical instantiation of most choice. We know that a group of reciprocally interconnected networks that range in location from the orbitofrontal cortex to the brainstem encode the expected subjective values of the options in a choice set. Overwhelming evidence now suggests that changes in the inhibitory and excitatory tone of one or more of these networks can force these systems to converge—to choose. What causes the global state of one or more of those networks to change? What mechanism says that it is "time to choose"? Is it more than one mechanism? In a similar way, what presets the state of these networks when choosers perform reservation-based choice as in the reaction-time studies of Shadlen and his colleagues (e.g., Gold and Shadlen, 2007)? Although almost never mentioned, we are almost completely ignorant about the location and structure of the mechanism that chooses to choose.

3. What Is the Neural Mechanism of Complementarity?

Perhaps the most subtle of these six questions is the question of how the economic phenomenon we call "substitution"—or more precisely "complementarity"—arises. Consider an indifference curve in a two-good budget space, a choice between rising quantities of apples and oranges, of the kind presented in Chapter 3. If we thought of the subjective value of apples as represented by a compressive utility curve and orange values as having a similar utility curve, we could construct curvilinear "indifference curves" in our budget space that showed all of the combinations of apples and oranges that yielded equivalent utility, as shown in Figure 17.1a.

We could even transform the two axes into units of utility, and if we constrain ourselves to think about the problem this way, our indifference curves can be thought of as straight lines, as in Figure 17.1b.

If indifference curves in budget spaces always behaved in this way— if the subjective values of apples and oranges were always completely independent processes—then these indifference curves could (in units of utility) always be thought of as the straight lines in Figure 17.1b. A given fraction of oranges could always be replaced with a given fraction of apples. Apples and oranges could be thought of as perfect substitutes, at least in units of utility.

Unfortunately, real goods do not always behave this way when people choose among them. That should be obvious. The value of a beer may actually increase if we consume it with potato chips. The value of a left shoe, to take a more classical economic example, depends almost entirely on our possession of a right shoe. The utility functions for goods

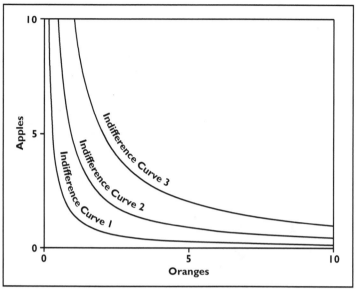

A

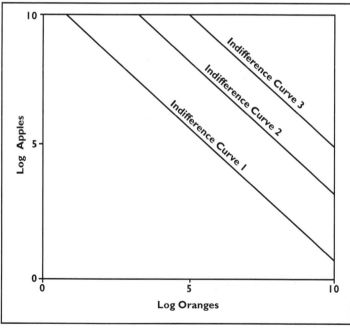

B

Figure 17.1

interact, a property that economists refer to as complementarity, and this imposes curvature in the indifference curves even when those indifference curves are plotted in units of utility.

The algorithmic model of valuation I have presented so far in this book is entirely unable to produce this kind of curvature. In the language of neuroscience, it is an entirely feed-forward model. What is important here is that feed-forward models of valuation cannot produce curved indifference functions in utility spaces. They cannot produce indifference curves in which the "elasticity of substitution" varies. This class of model can account only for indifference curves that show perfect substitutability (in units of utility), and economists have known for centuries that many indifference curves do not have this property. What that means, of necessity, is that subjective values are a good deal more complex than I have made them look so far. A complete theory of subjective value will have to respect this fact. To put that in more standard neurobiological terms, the theory of subjective value will have to include both "feed-forward" and "feed-back" influences, and a core feature of the model I have presented here is that it lacks this property.

This means that future theories of the neurobiological basis of choice will have to be much more complex. This is a kind of complexity that is being explored today in the primate visual system, where the interactions of "bottom-up" and "top-down" mechanisms are under active investigation. It is unclear at this time just what such a theory would look like for choice, but we must bear in mind that the feed-forward models of choice popular today bear within them this critical flaw.

4. How Does Symbolic Probability Work?

In Section 3 of this book I pointed out that two distinct mechanisms seem to operate when we represent the *expected* subjective values of probabilistic events. The first of these mechanisms is a device for iterative subjective value estimation that "learns" the long-run average value of an action or an object from repeated sampling. This is the mechanism we associate with the neurotransmitter dopamine and with reinforcement learning. One interesting feature of this mechanism is that it does not represent probabilities explicitly; instead, it inextricably bundles probability and value together. But we also know that humans (and perhaps other primates as well) can explicitly encode probability and use that information to guide choice. We even know that these explicitly encoded probabilities influence choice in inconsistent ways (Allais, 1953; Kahneman and Tversky, 1979). How does that work? Where are explicit probabilities, separable from utilities or subjective values, encoded in the brain? How do these symbolic probabilities influence choice? Although we have growing information about the neural representation of symbolic numbers (Hubbard et al., 2005), and at least some of these neural mechanisms reside in or near the fronto-parietal choice networks, we know next to nothing about the neurobiology of probability. Understanding those mechanisms will be the key to understanding expected subjective value.

5. How Do State and the Utility Function Interact?

We all agree that utility functions are state dependent. How much we value food depends on how hungry we are. But how important is this to choice? Economists have tended to trivialize this problem when they argue that utility functions are state dependent and then go no farther. But what form does this state dependence take? We simply do not know. What are the specific functions that relate state to subjective value? How does this influence learning? Does state-dependent utility during learning influence choices made later when behavioral state has changed? Is this a major source of inconsistency in our choice behavior, or are there compensatory mechanisms that limit the influence of state on what we learn about the values of goods and actions? Do the mechanisms for valuation separate state-dependent values experienced during learning from state-dependent values at the time of choice?

6. What Is the Neural Organ for Representing Money?

Money is one of the most puzzling of human inventions. All animals place values on sources of food, water, and reproduction, and humans seem to be no exception to this rule. Money is different. In our distant social past, societies did not have money. Economies functioned on the direct trade of (consumable) goods that had real values. The economic theory of money tells us that currencies arose to facilitate these trades.

But what is striking to a biologist is the speed with which these currencies have penetrated nearly all human societies. Money has arisen at a speed that defies evolution; it could not be the case that the rise of currencies reflects the evolution of a neural circuit specifically for monetary valuation. Instead, our ability to value money must reflect the conscription of a pre-existing neural mechanism, but what mechanism is that?

We already have some evidence suggesting that neural circuits for the valuation of food rewards, water rewards, and monetary rewards are partially distinct, but then what is the evolutionary origin of the mechanism that values money? Understanding the natural object that our monetary systems evolved to value might well explain some of the inconsistencies we observe when humans place subjective values on money.

One serious possibility is that money attaches itself to the neural mechanisms that evolved for placing values on social interactions. Primates are, as a general rule, highly social species. Many primates build social alliances and trade support in conflicts with one another. It may be that the evolved ability of our distant ancestors to make and trade social treaties lies at the root of our ability to place values on fiat currencies. Currently that is pure speculation. What is certain is that if we want to understand the behavioral inconsistencies that plague monetary interactions, we will have to understand the neural organ that allows us to value money. The algorithmic structure, let alone the identity, of that organ remains one of the greatest mysteries in neuroeconomics today.

Normative Issues

While these six problems reflect some of the most glaring limitations of our current knowledge, before closing I want to return to the normative issues that I believe place an even more important set of limitations on neuroeconomics today. Unlike traditional economic theories of utility, the neuroeconomic theory of expected subjective value is by construction a logically reducible theory. If we refer to expected subjective value (ESV) as an economic object, we include in that reference (at least in principle) a description at the level of psychology, at the level of neuro-biology, and even at levels of reduction beneath those. So inasmuch as

ESV is a reducible concept and unique (in the mathematical/economic sense), ESV can be directly compared across individuals.[1]

It may turn out that, as neuroeconomics matures, new constraints emerge on ESV and objects like it, but it seems almost inescapable that our growing ability to measure objective brain states will grant us the ability to objectively compare mental state between individuals. We already know that saying Oskar impulsively prefers immediate rewards is the same as saying that Oskar's medial prefrontal cortex shows a steeply hyperbolic discount function. We already know that orbitofrontal firing rates 10 Hz above baseline correspond to a specific level of preference for an apple juice reward. We even know that the brain of a monkey whose area LIP fires 50 spikes in response to a photograph of his paramour will pay more to look at a picture of her than will a monkey whose brain fires only 10 spikes in response to that same photograph. It is hard to believe that these cardinal observations will not lead to direct inter-individual comparisons of welfare at some point.

So what do current models of the architecture for human choice tell us normatively? Do these new measurements and theories give us new tools to maximize individual welfare? Do these new measurements and theories challenge Pareto's century-old conclusion that scientists cannot mathematically compute the welfare of a society from the welfare of its individuals? The ability to measure ESV uniquely in the human brain could have profound implications for normative theory, whether we like it or not.

To me, trying to use neural measurements to assess welfare today seems reckless and unwarranted for at least three reasons. First, it seems reckless because we would undoubtedly make errors at this early stage, and the choosers would pay the price associated with those errors.

---

1. I am aware that the full reduction of ESV (or alternatively, the reduction of SV, which would be as effective) may fail, in the philosophical sense. This is a point engaged in Chapter 2, where I was quick to point out that the vast bulk of neuroeconomics will require only partial reducibility. I want to be clear that the social welfare issue raised here requires that at least one concept from the discipline (for example, ESV or SV) be fully reducible. If that is not the case, then the relevance of this issue to *social* welfare will be more circumscribed. I take the time to describe the strong form of the theory, though, because it is important and because it places a bound on what we can and cannot say about the future.

Second, we know that ESV violates much of the normative theory that we have in hand, notably the independence axiom, so being able to uniquely measure ESV still leaves us with a host of traditional, and unsolved, problems from economics and political economy. The third, and most important, reason not to consider maximizing ESV as a social goal is that we do not know that ESV is the quantity that should be maximized. Until we have an actual neurobiological-level theory of welfare, a theory of where and how brain activations relate to well-being, using brain activations to make guesses about how to maximize welfare will be a mistake. For these reasons and a host of others that are beginning to be discussed in the neuroeconomic literature, it seems clear that the normative use of objects such as ESV should be proscribed until we know far more than we do now.

Pareto and the neoclassicists who followed him argued against classic utilitarianism on two grounds: because they knew that it was mathematically impossible to compare utilities across individuals, and because they were convinced it was wrong to impose any social welfare function on a society from above. Neuroeconomics may eliminate the first of Pareto's barriers to this kind of social engineering by replacing utility with subjective value, but just because you can doesn't mean you should. That is a point that any responsible scientist must bear in mind as neuroeconomics matures.

Finis

Over the past decade, a lively and beneficial debate has accompanied the birth of neuroeconomics. Some economists have asked whether the mechanism by which we choose should be of interest to their discipline. Others have wondered whether what we know today about the brain could really tell us anything interesting about choice. On the other side, neurobiologists and psychologists have wondered, given the explanatory limits of contemporary economics, whether that science will be of any use in understanding how humans and animals choose. The history of science and the work of scholars in all three disciplines during this first decade of neuroeconomics have now provided us with clear answers to those questions. What we know about the brain can tell us much about the structure of choice, as long as we let the great empirical and theoretical regularities of the social sciences guide us. Economics is, in the words of the 19th-century economist Thorstein Veblen, finally becoming an "evolutionary science," and that science has already shown itself to be a powerful tool for understanding human behavior. While we cannot know what economics, the psychology of judgment and decision, and the neurobiology of choice will look like in the future, there can be little doubt that their consilience is upon us.

References

Adelson, E. H. (1995). Checker Shadow Illusion. Retrieved October 15, 2009, from Edward H. Adelson's Web site: http: //web.mit.edu/persci/people/ adelson/checkershadow_illusion.html

Aharon, I., Etcoff, N., Ariely, D., Chabris, C., O'Connor, E., and Breiter, H. (2001). Beautiful faces have variable reward value: fMRI and behavioral evidence. *Neuron*, 32(3): 537-551.

Allais, M. (1953). Le comportement de l'homme rationel devant le risque. Critique des postulats et axiomes de l'ecole américaine [Rational behavior under risk: criticism of the postulates and axioms of the American school]. *Econometrica*, 21(4): 503-546.

Andersen, R. A. (1989). Visual and eye movement functions of the posterior parietal cortex. *Annual Review of Neuroscience*, 12: 377-403.

Anderson, A. K., and Phelps, E. A. (2002). Is the human amygdala critical for the subjective experience of emotion? Evidence of intact dispositional affect in patients with amygdala lesions. *Journal of Cognitive Neuroscience*, 14(5): 709-720.

Arnauld, A., and Nicole, P. (1662; 1996). *La Logique, ou l'art de penser (Logic or the Art of Thinking)*, J. V. Buroker (trans. and ed.) Cambridge: Cambridge University Press, 1996.

Atick, J. J., and Redlich, A. N. (1990). Towards a theory of early visual processing. *Neural Computation*, 2(3): 308-320.

Atick, J. J., and Redlich, A. N. (1992). What does the retina know about natural scenes? *Neural Computation*, 4 (2): 196-210.

Attneave, F. (1954). Some informational aspects of visual perception. *Psychological Review*, 61: 183-193.

Augustine, J. R. (1996). Circuitry and functional aspects of the insular lobe in primates including humans. *Brain Research Reviews*, 22(3): 229-244.

Baccus, S. A. (2006). From a whisper to a roar: Adaptation to the mean and variance of naturalistic sounds. *Neuron*, 51: 682-684.

Bailey, P., and von Bonin, G. (1951). *The Isocortex of Man*. Urbana: University of Illinois Press.

Balleine, B. W., Daw, N. D., and O'Doherty, J. P. (2008). Multiple forms of value learning and the function of dopamine. In: P. W. Glimcher, C. F. Camerer, E. Fehr, and R. A. Poldrack (eds.), *Neuroeconomics: Decision Making and the Brain*. London: Academic Press, pp. 367-386.

Barlow, H. B. (1961a). The coding of sensory messages. In: Thorpe and Zangwill (eds.), *Current Problems in Animal Behaviour*. New York: Cambridge University Press, pp. 330-360.

Barlow, H. B. (1961b). Possible principles underlying the transformation of sensory messages. In: W. A. Rosenblith (ed.), *Sensory Communication*. Cambridge, MA: MIT Press, pp. 217-234.

Basso, M. A., and Wurtz, R. H. (1997). Modulation of neuronal activity by target uncertainty. *Nature*, 389: 66-69.

Basso, M. A., and Wurtz, R. H. (1998). Modulation of neuronal activity in superior colliculus by changes in target probability. *Journal of Neuroscience*, 18: 7519-7534.

Bayer, H. M., Lau, B., and Glimcher, P. W. (2007). Statistics of midbrain dopamine neuron spike trains in the awake primate. *Journal of Neurophysiology*, 98(3): 1428-1439.

Bayer, H. M., and Glimcher, P. W. (2005). Midbrain dopamine neurons encode a quantitative reward prediction error signal. *Neuron*, 47: 129-141.

Baylor, D. A., Nunn, B. J., and Scnapft, J. L. (1987). Spectral sensitivity of cones of the monkey *Macaca fascicularis*. *Journal of Physiology*, 390: 145-160.

Bechara, A., Tranel, D., Damasio, H., Adolphs, R., Rockland, C., and Damasio, A. R. (1995). Double dissociation of conditioning and declarative knowledge relative to the amygdale and hippocampus in humans. *Science*, 269(5227): 1115-1118.

Beck, J. M., Ma, W. J., Kiani, R., Hanks, T., Churchland, A. K., Roitman, J., Shadlen, M. N., Latham, P. E., and Pouget, A. (2008). Probabilistic population codes for Bayesian decision making. *Neuron*, 60(6): 1142-1152.

Becker, G. M., DeGroot, M. H., and Marshack. (1964). Measuring utility by a single-response sequential method. *Behavioral Science*, 9: 226-232.

Belova, M. A., Paton, J. J., and Salzman, C. D. (2008). Moment-to-moment tracking of state value in the amygdala. *Journal of Neuroscience*, 28(40): 10023-10030.

Belovsky, G. E. (1984). Herbivore optimal foraging: a comparative test of three models. *American Naturalist*, 124: 97-115.

Bernheim, D. (2008). The psychology and neurobiology of judgment and decision making: what's in it for economists? In: P. W. Glimcher, C. F. Camerer, E. Fehr, and R. A. Poldrack (eds.), *Neuroeconomics: Decision Making and the Brain*. London: Academic Press, pp. 115-125.

Bernoulli, D. (1738; 1954). Exposition of a new theory on the measurement of risk. *Econometrica*, 22: 23-36.

Bernstein, N. (1961; 1984). Trends and problems in the study of physiology of activity. *Questions of Philosophy* 6. Reprinted in: H. T. A. Whiting (ed.), *Human Motor Actions: Bernstein Reassessed*. Amsterdam: North-Holland.

Berridge, K. C., Robinson, T. E., and Aldridge, J. W. (2009). Dissecting components of reward: 'liking', 'wanting', and learning. *Current Opinion in Pharmacology*, 9: 65-73.

Bertino, M., Beauchamp, G. K., and Engelman, K. (1982). Long-term reduction in dietary sodium alters the taste of salt. *American Journal of Clinical Nutrition*, 36: 1134-1144.

Bertino, M., Beauchamp, G. K., and Engelman, K. (1986). Increasing dietary salt alters salt taste preference. *Physiology & Behavior*, 38: 203-213.

Bliss, T. V., and Lomo, T. (1973). Long-lasting potentiation of synaptic transmission in the dentate area of the anaesthetized rabbit following stimulation of the perforant path. *Journal of Physiology*, 232(2): 331-356.

Borg, G., Diamant, H., Strom, L., and Zotterman, Y. (1967). The relation between neural and perceptual intensity: A comparative study on the neural and psychophysical response to taste stimuli. *Journal of Physiology*, 192(13): 13-20.

Born, R. T., and Bradley, D. C. (2005). Structure and function of visual area MT. *Annual Review of Neuroscience*, 28: 157-189.

Brafman, R. I., and Tennenholtz, M. (2003). R-MAX—A general polynomial time algorithm for near-optimal reinforment learning. *Journal of Machine Learning Research*, 3: 213-231.

Breedlove, S. M., Rosenzweig, M., Watson, N., and Fraser, S. (2007). *Biological Psychology: An Introduction to Behavioral, Cognitive, and Clinical Neuroscience*, 5th ed. Sunderland, MA: Sinauer Associate Publishers.

Breiter, H. C., Aharon, I., Kahneman, D., Dale, A., and Shizgal, P. (2001). Functional imaging of neural responses to expectancy and experience of monetary gains and losses. *Neuron*, 30(2): 619-639.

Bres, M. (2006). The effects of prey relative abundance and chemical cues on prey selection in rainbow trout. *Journal of Fish Biology*, 35(3): 439-445.

Britten, K. H., and Heuer, H. W. (1999). Spatial summation in the receptive fields of MT neurons. *Journal of Neuroscience*, 19(12): 5074-5084.

Britten, K. H., Shadlen, M. N., Newsome, W. T., and Movshon, J. A. (1993). Responses of neurons in macaque MT to stochastic motion signals. *Visual Neuroscience*, 10: 1157-1169.

Broad, C. D. (1925). *The Mind and its Place in Nature*. New York: Harcourt, Brace & Company, Inc.

Brodmann, K. (1909; 1999). *Vergleichende Lokalisationslehre der Grosshirnrinde (Brodmann's Localisation in the Cerebral Cortex: The Principles of Comparative Localisation in the Cerebral Cortex based on the Cytoarchitectonics)*, translated and edited by L. Garey. London: Imperial College Press.

Brown, J. W., and Braver, T. S. (2005). Learned predictions of error likelihood in the anterior cingulate cortex. *Science*, 307(5712): 1118-1121.

Bruce, C. J., and Goldberg, M. E. (1985). Primate frontal eye fields: I. Single neurons discharging before saccades. *Journal of Neurophysiology*, 53(3): 603-635.

Burns, M. E., and Baylor, D. A. (2001). Activation, deactivation, and adaptation in vertebrate photoreceptor cells. *Annual Review of Neuroscience*, 24: 779-805.

Bush, R. R., and Mosteller, F. (1951a). A mathematical model for simple learning. *Psychological Review*, 58: 313-323.

Bush, R. R., and Mosteller, F. (1951b). A model for stimulus generalization and discrimination. *Psychological Review*, 58: 413-423.

Cajal, S. R. Y. (1909; 1995). *Histologie du système nerveux de l'homme et des vertébrés (Histology of the Nervous System of Man and Vertebrates)*, translated by N. Swanson and L. Swanson. New York: Oxford University Press.

Camerer, C., Loewenstein, G., and Prelec, D. (2005). Neuroeconomics: How neuroscience can inform economics. *Journal of Economic Literature*, XLIII: 9-64.

Caplin, A., and Dean, M. (2007). The neuroeconomic theory of learning. *American Economic Review*, 97(2): 148-152.

Caplin, A., and Dean, M. (2008). Axiomatic neuroeconomics. In: P. W. Glimcher, C. F. Camerer, E. Fehr, and R. A. Poldrack (eds.), *Neuroeconomics: Decision Making and the Brain*. London: Academic Press, pp. 21-31.

Caplin, A., Dean, M., Glimcher P. W., and Rutledge, R. (2010). Measuring beliefs and rewards: a neuroeconomic approach. *Quarterly Journal of Economics*, 125:3.

Caplin, A., and Leahy, J. (2001). Psychological expected utility theory and anticipatory feelings. *Quarterly Journal of Economics*, 116(1): 55-79.

Carandini, M., and Heeger, D. J. (1994). Summation and division by neurons in visual cortex. *Science*, 264: 1333-1336.

Carandini, M., Heeger, D. J., and Movshon, J.A. (1997). Linearity and normalization in simple cells of the macaque primary visual cortex. *Journal of Neuroscience*, 17: 8621-8644.

Carlsson, A. (2000). A half-century of neurotransmitter research: impact on neurology and psychiatry. Nobel Prize Lecture presented at Karolinska Institutet, Stockholm. Full text of speech retrieved November 2008 from http://nobelprize.org/nobel_prizes/medicine/laureates/2000/carlsson-lecture.html.

Carnap, R., Hahn, H., and Neurath, O. (1929; 1996). *Wissenschaftliche Weltauffassung. Der Wiener Kreis. (The Scientific Conception of the World. The Vienna Circle)*. Reprinted and translated in S. Sarkar (ed.), *The Emergence of Logical Empiricism: From 1900 to the Vienna Circle*. New York: Garland Publishing, pp. 321-340.

Chen, M. K., Lakshminarayanan, V., and Santos, L. R. (2006). How basic are behavioral biases? Evidence from capuchin monkey trading behavior. *Journal of Political Economy*, 114(3): 517-537.

Chib, V. S., Rangel, A., Shimojo, S., and O'Doherty, J. P. (2009). Evidence for a common representation of decision values for dissimilar goods in human ventromedial prefrontal cortex. *Journal of Neuroscience*, 29(39): 12315-12320.

Cisek, P., and Kalaska, J. F. (2002). Simultaneous encoding of multiple potential reach directions in dorsal premotor cortex. *Journal of Neurophysiology*, 87(2): 1149-1154.

Colby, C., and Goldberg, M. (1999). Space and attention in parietal cortex. *Annual Review of Neuroscience*, 22: 319-349.

Contreras, R. J., and Frank, M. (1979). Sodium deprivation alters neural responses to gustatory stimuli. *Journal of General Physiology*, 73: 569-594.

Cooper, F. E., Bloom, R. H., and Roth, J. R. (2003). *The Biochemical Basis of Neuropharmacology*. New York: Oxford University Press.

Curtis, C. E., and Connolly, J. D. (2008). Saccade preparation signals in the human frontal and parietal cortices. *Journal of Neurophysiology*, 99(1): 133-145.

Dan, Y., Atick, J. J., and Reid, C. R. (1996). Efficient coding of natural scenes in the lateral geniculate nucleus: Experimental test of a computational theory. *Journal of Neuroscience*, 16(10): 3351-3362.

Das, A., and Gilbert, C. D. (1999). Topography of contextual modulations mediated by short-range interactions in primary visual cortex. *Nature*, 399: 665-661.

Daugman, J. G. (1985). Uncertainty relation for resolution in space, spatial frequency, and orientation optimized by two-dimensional visual cortical filters. *Journal of the Optical Society of America A*, 2: 1160-1169.

Daw, N. D., Kakade, S., and Dayan, P. (2002). Opponent interactions between serotonin and dopamine. *Neural Networks*, 15: 603-616.

Daw, N. D., Niv, Y., and Dayan, P. (2005). Uncertainty-based competition between prefrontal and dorsolateral striatal systems for behavioral control. *Nature Neuroscience*, 8: 1704-1711.

Daw, N. D., O'Doherty, J. P., Dayan, P., Seymour, B., and Dolan, R. J. (2006). Cortical substrates for exploratory decisions in humans. *Nature*, 441: 876-879.

Daw, N. D., and Shohamy, D. (2008). The cognitive neuroscience of motivation and learning. *Social Cognition*, 26: 593-620.

Dayan, P. (2008). The role of value systems in decision making. In: C. Engel and W. Singer (eds.), *Better than Conscious? Decision Making, the Human Mind, and Implications for Institutions*. Frankfurt, Germany: MIT Press, pp. 51-70.

Dayan, P., and Daw, N. D. (2008). Decision theory, reinforcement learning, and the brain. *Cognitive, Affective, and Behavioral Neuroscience*, 8(4): 429-453.

Dean, A. F. (1983). Adaptation-induced alteration of the relation between response amplitude and contrast in cat striate cortical neurones. *Vision Research*, 23(3): 249-256.

Deaner, R. O., Khera, A. V., and Platt, M. L. (2005). Monkeys pay per view: Adaptive valuation of social images by rhesus macaques. *Current Biology*, 15: 543-548.

Delgado, M. R., Nystrom, L. E., Fissell, C., Noll, D. C., and Fiez, J. A. (2000). Tracking the hemodynamic responses to reward and punishment in the striatum. *Journal of Neurophysiology*, 84(6): 3072-3077.

DeShazo, J. R., and Fermo, G. (2002). Designing choice sets for stated preference methods: the effects of complexity on choice consistency. *Journal of Environmental Economics and Management*, 44: 123-143.

De Valois, K. K., De Valois, R. L., and Yund, E. W. (1979). Responses of striate cortex cells to grating and checkerboard patterns. *Journal of Physiology*, 291: 483-505.

Dodd, J. V., Krug, K., Cumming, B. G., and Parker, A. J. (2001). Perceptually bistable three-dimensional figures evoke high choice probabilities in cortical area MT. *Journal of Neuroscience*, 21(13): 4809-4821.

Dorris, M. C., and Glimcher, P. W. (2004). Activity in posterior parietal cortex is correlated with the subjective desireability of an action. *Neuron*, 44: 365-378.

Dorris, M. C., Klein, R. M., Everling, S., and Munoz, D. P. (2002). Contribution of the primate superior colliculus to inhibition of return. *Journal of Cognitive Neuroscience*, 14: 1256-1263.

Dorris, M. C., and Munoz, D. P. (1995). A neural correlate for the gap effect on saccadic reaction times in monkey. *Journal of Neurophysiology*, 73(85): 2558-2562.

Dorris, M. C., and Munoz, D. P. (1998). Saccadic probability influences motor preparation signals and time to saccadic initiation. *Journal of Neuroscience*, 18: 7015-7026.

Edelman, J. A., and Keller, E. L. (1996). Activity of visuomotor burst neurons in the superior colliculus accompanying express saccades. *Journal of Neurophysiology*, 76(2): 908-926.

Elliot, R., Friston, K. J., and Dolan, R. J. (2000). Dissociable neural responses in human reward systems. *Journal of Neuroscience*, 20(16): 6159-6165.

Elliot, R., Newman, J. L., Longe, O. A., and Deakin, J. F. (2003). Differential response patterns in the striatum and orbitofrontal cortex to financial reward in humans: a parametric functional magnetic resonance imaging study. *Journal of Neuroscience*, 23(1): 303-307.

Ellsberg, D. (1961). Risk, ambiguity, and the savage axioms. *Quarterly Journal of Economics*, 75: 643-669.

Etcoff, N. (1999). *Survival of the Prettiest*. New York: Doubleday.

Evarts, E. V., and Tanji, J. (1974). Gating of motor cortex reflexes by prior instruction. *Brain Research*, 71: 479-494.

Evarts, E. V., and Tanji, J. (1976). Reflex and intended responses in motor cortex pyramidal tract neurons of monkey. *Journal of Neurophysiology*, 39: 1069.

Falkenstein, M., Hohnsbein, J., Hoorman, J., and Blanke, L. (1990). Effects of errors in choice reaction tasks on the ERP under focused and divided attention. In: C. H. M. Brunia, A. W. K. Gaillard, and A. Kok (eds.), *Psychophysiological Brain Research*, Volume 1. Tilburg, the Netherlands: Tilburg University Press, pp. 192-195.

Falkenstein, M., Hohnsbein, J., Hoorman, J., and Blanke, L. (1991). Effects of crossmodal divided attention on late ERP components. II. Error processing in choice reaction tasks. *Electroencephalography and Clinical Neurophysiology*, 78(6): 447-455.

Falmagne, J. (1985). *Elements of Psychophysical Theory.* New York: Oxford University Press.

Fechner, G. T. (1860; 1966). *Elements of Psychophysics,* H. E. Adler (trans.). New York: Holt, Rinehart and Winston.

Fibiger, H. C., and Phillips, A. G. (1986). Reward, motivation, cognition: psychobiology of mesotelencephalic dopamine systems. In: F. E. Bloom and S. D. Geiger (eds.), *Handbook of Physiology: The Nervous System IV.* Bethesda, MD: American Physiology Society, pp. 647-675.

Fiorillo, C. D., Tobler, P. N., and Schultz, W. (2003). Discrete coding of reward probability and uncertainty by dopamine neurons. *Science,* 299: 1898-1902.

Fishburn, P. C., and Rubinstein, A. (1982). Time preference. *International Economics Review,* 23: 677-694.

Fodor, J. (1974). Special sciences and the disunity of science as a working hypothesis. *Synthese,* 28: 77-115.

Fox, C., and Poldrack, R. A. (2009). Prospect theory and the brain. In: P. W. Glimcher, C. F. Camerer, E. Fehr, and R. A. Poldrack (eds.), *Neuroeconomics: Decision Making and the Brain.* London: Academic Press, pp. 145-173.

Friedman, M. (1953). *Essays in Positive Economics.* Chicago: University of Chicago Press.

Friedman, M., and Savage, L. J. (1948). The utility analysis of choices involving risk. *Journal of Political Economy,* 56(4): 279-304.

Friedman, M., and Savage, L. J. (1952). The expected-utility hypothesis and the measurability of utility. *Journal of Political Economy,* 60(6): 463-474.

Freud, S. (1923; 1961). *Das Ich und das Es* (The Ego and the Id). Translated in: J. Strachey (ed.), *The Standard Edition of the Complete Psychological Works of Sigmund Freud.* New York: W. W. Norton and Company.

Fromm, C., and Evarts, E. V. (1982). Pyramidal tract neurons in somatosensory cortex: Central and peripheral inputs during voluntary movement. *Brain Research,* 238(1): 186-191.

Fudenberg, D., and Tirole, J. (1991). *Game Theory.* Massachusetts: MIT Press.

Futuyma, D. (1998). *Evolutionary Biology,* 3rd ed. Sunderland, MA: Sinauer Associates.

Gabor, D. (1946). Theory of communication. *Journal of IEE, London,* 93: 429-457.

Gabor, D. (1971). *Holography.* Nobel Prize Lecture presented at Imperial Colleges of Science and Technology, London. Full text of speech retrieved November 2008 from: http://www.huwu.org/nobel_prizes/physics/laureates/1971/gabor-lecture.html

Gehring, W. J., Goss, B., Coles, M. G. H., Meyer, D. E., and Donchin, E. (1993). A neural system for error-detection and compensation. *Psychological Science,* 4: 385-390.

Gigerenzer, G., Todd, P. M., and ABC Research Group. (1999). *Simple Heuristics That Make Us Smart*. New York: Oxford University Press.

Gilovich, T., Vallone, R., and Tversky, A. (1985). The hot hand in basketball: On the misperception of random sequences. *Cognitive Psychology*, 17: 295-314.

Gläscher, J., Hampton, A. N., and O'Doherty, J. P. (2009). Determining a role for ventromedial prefrontal cortex in encoding action-based value signals during reward-related decision making. *Cerebral Cortex*, 19(2): 483-495.

Glascher, J., Daw, N. D., Dayan, P., and O'Doherty, J. (2009a). The human brain computes two different prediction errors. *Frontiers in Systems Neuroscience. Conference Abstract: Computational and systems neuroscience*. doi: 10.3389/conf. neuro.06.2009.03.270

Glimcher, P. W. (2003a). *Decisions, Uncertainty, and the Brain: The Science of Neuroeconomics*. Cambridge, MA: MIT Press.

Glimcher, P. W. (2003b). The neurobiology of visual-saccadic decision making. *Annual Review of Neuroscience*, 26: 133-179.

Glimcher, P. W. (2005). Indeterminacy in brain and behavior. *Annual Review of Psychology*, 56: 25-56.

Glimcher, P. W. (2008). Choice: towards a standard back-pocket model . In: P. W. Glimcher, C. F. Camerer, E. Fehr, and R. A. Poldrack (eds.), *Neuroeconomics: Decision Making and the Brain*. London: Academic Press, pp. 503-521.

Glimcher, P. W., and Rustichini, A. (2004). Neuroeconomics: The consilience of brain and decision. *Science*, 306: 447-452.

Glimcher, P. W., and Sparks, D. L. (1992). Movement selection in advance of action in the superior colliculus. *Nature*, 355: 542-545.

Gold, J. I., and Shadlen, M. N. (2003). The influence of behavioral context on the representation of a perceptual decision in developing oculomotor commands. *Journal of Neuroscience*, 23: 632-651.

Gold, J. I., and Shadlen, M. N. (2007). The neural basis of decision making. *Annual Review of Neuroscience*, 30: 374-535.

Grace, A. A., and Bunney, B. S. (1983). Intracellular and extracellular electrophysiology of nigral dopaminergic neurons—1. Identification and characterization. *Neuroscience*, 10(2): 301-315.

Graybiel, A. M. (2002). Guide to the anatomy of the brain: the basal ganglia. In: J. H. Byrne, (ed.), *Encyclopedia of Learning and Memory*, 2nd ed. New York: MacMillan.

Green, D. M., and Swets, J. A. (1966; 1988). *Signal Detection Theory and Psychophysics*. New York: Wiley. Reprinted: Los Altos, CA: Peninsula Publishing.

Gul, F., and Pesendorfer, W. (2001). Temptation and self-control. *Econometrica*, 69: 1403-1435.

Gul, F., and Pesendorfer, W. (2006). Random expected utility. *Econometrica*, 74: 121-146.

Gul, F., and Pesendorfer, W. (2008). The case for mindless economics. In: A. Caplin and A. Schotter (eds.), *The Foundations of Positive and Normative Economics*. New York: Oxford University Press, pp. 3-41.

Güth, W., Schmittberger, R., and Schwarze, B. (1982). An experimental analysis of ultimatum bargaining. *Journal of Economic Behavior and Organization*, 3: 367-388.

Haber, S. N., Fudge, J. L., and McFarland, N. R. (2000). Striatonigrostriatal pathways in primates form an ascending spiral from the shell to the dorsolateral striatum. *Journal of Neuroscience*, 20(6): 2369-2382.

Hall, W. C., and Moschovakis, A. (eds.) (2003). *The Superior Colliculus: New Approaches for Studying Sensorimotor Integration*. New York: CRC Press.

Handel, A., and Glimcher, P. W. (1999). Quantitative analysis of substantia nigra pars reticulata activity during a visually guided saccade task. *Journal of Neurophysiology*, 82(6): 3458-3475.

Handel, A., and Glimcher, P. W. (2000). Contextual modulation of substantia nigra pars reticulata neurons. *Journal of Neurophysiology*, 83(5): 3042-3048.

Harbaugh, W. T., Krause, K., and Berry, T. (2001). On the development of rational choice behavior. *American Economic Review*, 91(5): 1539-1545.

Hare, T. A., Camerer, C. F., and Rangel, A. (2009). Self-control in decision-making involves modulation of the vmPFC valuation system. *Science*, 324(5927): 646-648.

Hare, T. A., O'Doherty, J., Camerer, C. F., Schultz, W., and Rangel, A. (2008). Dissociating the role of the orbitofrontal cortex and the striatum in the computation of goal values and prediction errors. *Journal of Neuroscience*, 28(22): 5623-5630.

Hebb, D. O. (1949). *The Organization of Behavior: A Neuropsychological Theory*. New York: Wiley.

Heeger, D. J. (1992a). Half-squaring in responses of cat striate cells. *Visual Neuroscience*, 9: 427-443.

Heeger, D. J. (1992b). Normalization of cell responses in cat striate cortex. *Visual Neuroscience*, 9: 181-197.

Heeger, D. J. (1993). Modeling simple-cell direction selectivity with normalized, half-squared, linear operators. *Journal of Neurophysiology*, 70(5): 1885-1898.

Heeger, D. J., Simoncelli, E. P., and Movshon, J. A. (1996). Computational models of cortical visual processing. *Proceedings of the National Academy of Sciences USA*, 93: 623-627.

Helm, M. C., Özen, G. and Hall, W. C. (2004). Organization of the Intermediate Gray Layer of the Superior Colliculus. I. Intrinsic Vertical Connections. *Journal of Neurophysiology*, 91: 1706-1715.

Herrnstein, R. J. (1961). Relative and absolute strength of response as a function of frequency of reinforcement. *Journal of the Experimental Analysis of Behavior*, 4: 267-272.

Herrnstein, R. (1997). *The Matching Law*. Cambridge, MA: Harvard University Press. (A posthumous collection of the papers edited by H. Rachlin and D. I. Laibson).

Hertwig, R., Barron, G., Weber, E. U., and Erev, I. (2004). Decisions from experience and the effect of rare events in risky choice. *American Psychological Society*, 15(8): 534-539.

Hertz, J., Krogh, A., and Palmer, R. G. (1991). *Introduction to the Theory of Neural Computation*. Reading, MA: Addison-Wesley.

Hikosaka, O., Takikawa, Y., and Kawagoe, R. (2000). Role of the basal ganglia in the control of purposive saccadic eye movements. *Physiological Reviews*, 80: 953-978.

Holt, D. J., Graybiel, A. M., and Saper, C. B. (1997). Neurochemical architecture of the human striatum. *Journal of Comparative Neurology*, 384: 1-25.

Horvitz, J. C. (2000). Mesolimbocortical and nigrostriatal dopamine responses to salient non-reward events. *Neuroscience*, 96: 651-656.

Horvitz, J. C. (2009). Stimulus-response and response-outcome learning mechanisms in the striatum. *Behavioural Brain Research*, 199(1): 129-140.

Horwitz, G. D., Batista, A. P., and Newsome, W. T. (2004). Representation of an abstract perceptual decision in macaque superior colliculus. *Journal of Neurophysiology*, 91: 2281-2296.

Horwitz, G. D., and Newsome, W. T. (2001a). Target selection for saccadic eye movements: direction selective visual responses in the superior colliculus induced by behavioral training. *Journal of Neurophysiology*, 86: 2527-2542.

Horwitz, G. D., and Newsome, W. T. (2001b). Target selection for saccadic eye movements: prelude activity in the superior colliculus during a direction discrimination task. *Journal of Neurophysiology*, 86: 2543-2558.

Houthakker, H. S. (1950). Revealed preference and the utility function. *Economica*, 17: 159-174.

Hsu, M., Bhatt, M., Adolphs, R., Tranel, D., and Camerer, C. F. (2005). Neural systems responding to degrees of uncertainty in human decision making. *Science*, 310(5754): 1680-1683.

Hubbard, E. M., Piazza, M., Pinel, P., and Dehaene, S. (2005). Interactions between number and space in parietal cortex. *Nature Reviews Neuroscience*, 6: 435-448.

Hubel, D. H. (1988). *Eye, Brain, and Vision*. New York: Scientific American Library.

Hubel, D. H., and Wiesel, T. N. (1977). Ferrier lecture. Functional architecture of macaque monkey visual cortex. *Proceedings of the Royal Society of London: Biological Sciences*, 198: 1-59.

Isa, T., Kobayashi, Y., and Saito, Y. (2003). Dynamic modulation of signal transmission in the local circuit of mammalian superior colliculus.

In: W. C. Hall and A. K. Moschovakis (eds.), *The Superior Colliculus: New Approaches for Studying Sensorimotor Integration.* Boca Raton, FL: CRC Press, pp. 159-171.

Iyengar, S. S., and Lepper, M. R. (2000). When choice is demotivating: Can one desire too much of a good thing? *Journal of Personality and Social Psychology,* 79(6): 995-1006.

Johnson, D. H. (1996). Point process models of single-neuron discharges. *Journal of Computational Neuroscience,* 3: 275-299.

Jones, J. P., and Palmer, L. A. (1987). An evaluation of the two-dimensional Gabor filter model of simple receptive fields in cat striate cortex. *Journal of Neurophysiology,* 58(6): 1233-1258.

Jones, J. P., Stepnoski, A., and Palmer, L. A. (1987). The two-dimensional spectral structure of simple receptive fields in cat striate cortex. *Journal of Neurophysiology,* 58: 1212-1232.

Kaas, J. H. (1987). The organization and neocortex in mammals: Implications for theories of brain function. *Annual Review of Psychology,* 38: 124-151.

Kable, J. W., and Glimcher, P. W. (2007). The neural correlates of subjective value during intertemporal choice. *Nature Neuroscience,* 10(12): 1625-1633.

Kable, J. W., and Glimcher, P. W. (2009). The neurobiology of decision: Consensus and controversy. *Neuron,* 63(6): 733-745.

Kahnemen, D. (2008). Remarks on neuroeconomics. In: P. W. Glimcher, C. F. Camerer, E. Fehr, and R. A. Poldrack (eds.), *Neuroeconomics: Decision Making and the Brain.* London: Academic Press, pp. 523-526.

Kahneman, D., Knetsch, J. L., and Thaler, R. H. (1990). Experimental tests of the endowment effect and the Coase theorem. *Journal of Political Economy,* 98: 1325-1348.

Kahneman, D., Slovic, P., and Tversky, A. (1982). *Judgement Under Uncertainty: Heuristics and Biases.* New York: Cambridge University Press.

Kahneman, D., and Tversky, A. (1972). Subjective probability: A judgment of representativeness. *Cognitive Psychology,* 3: 430-454.

Kahneman, D., and Tversky, A. (1979). Prospect theory: An analysis of decision under risk. *Econometrica,* 47(2): 263-291.

Kalaska, J. F., Cohen, D. A. D., Prud'homme, M., and Hyde, M. L. (1990). Parietal area 5 neuronal activity encodes movement kinematics, not movement dynamics. *Experimental Brain Research,* 80(2): 351-364.

Kalaska, J. F., and Hyde, M. L. (1985). Area 4 and area 5: Differences between the load direction-dependent discharge variability of cells during active postural fixation. *Experimental Brain Research,* 59(1): 197-202.

Kamenica, E. (2008). Contextual inference in markets: on the informational content of product lines. *American Economic Review,* 98(5): 2127-2149.

Kelly, R. M., and Strick, P. L. (2003). Cerebellar loops with motor cortex and prefrontal cortex of a nonhuman primate. *Journal of Neuroscience,* 23(23): 8432-8444.

Kelly, R. M., and Strick, P. L. (2004). Macro-architecture of basal ganglia loops with the cerebral cortex: use of rabies virus to reveal multisynaptic circuits. *Progress in Brain Research*, 143: 449-459.

Kennerley, S. W., Dahmubed, A. F., Lara, A. H., and Wallis, J. D. (2009). Neurons in the frontal lobe encode the value of multiple decision variables. *Journal of Cognitive Neuroscience*, 21(6): 1162-1178.

Kennerley, S. W., and Wallis, J. D. (2009a). Evaluating choices by single neurons in the frontal lobe: outcome value encoded across multiple decision variables. *European Journal of Neuroscience*, 29: 2061-2073.

Kennerley, S. W., and Wallis, J. D. (2009b). Reward-dependent modulation of working memory in lateral prefrontal cortex. *Journal of Neuroscience*, 29(10): 3259-3270.

Kepecs, A., Uchida, N., Zariwala, H. A., and Mainen, Z. F. (2008). Neural correlates, computation and behavioural impact of decision confidence. *Nature*, 455: 227-231.

Killen, S. S., Brown, J. A., and Gamperl, A. K. (2007). The effect of prey density on foraging mode selection in juvenile lumpfish: balancing food intake with the metabolic cost of foraging. *Journal of Animal Ecology*, 76(4): 814-825.

Kim, J. N., and Shadlen, M. N. (1999). Neural correlates of a decision in the dorsolateral prefrontal cortex of the macaque. *Neuron*, 24: 415.

Kim, S., Hwang, J., and Lee, D. (2008). Prefrontal coding of temporally discounted values during intertemporal choice. *Neuron*, 59(3): 522.

Kitchener, R. F. (1986). *Piaget's Theory of Knowledge*. New Haven: Yale University Press.

Klein, J. T., Deaner, R. O., and Platt, M. L. (2008). Neural correlates of social target value in macaque parietal cortex. *Current Biology*, 18(6): 419-424.

Knutson, B., Adams, C. M., Fong, G. W., and Hommer, D. (2001a). Anticipation of increasing monetary reward selectively recruits nucleus accumbens. *Journal of Neuroscience*, 21(16): RC159.

Knutson, B., Fong, G. W., Adams, C. M., Varer, J. L., and Hommer, D. (2001b). Dissociation of reward anticipation and outcome with event-related fMRI. *Neuroreport*, 12(17): 3683-3687.

Knutson, B., Fong, G. W., Bennett, S. M., Adams, C. M., and Hommer, D. (2003). A region of mesial prefrontal cortex tracks monetarily rewarding outcomes: Characterization with rapid event-related fMRI. *Neuroimage*, 18(2): 263-72.

Knutson, B., Taylor, J., Kaufman, M., Peterson, R., and Glover, G. (2005). Distributed neural representation of expected value. *Journal of Neuroscience*, 25(19): 4806-4812.

Kobayashi, S., and Schultz, W. (2008). Influence of reward delays on responses of dopamine neurons. *Journal of Neuroscience*, 28(31): 7837-7846.

Komendatov, A. O., and Canavier, C. C. (2002). Electrical coupling between model midbrain dopamine neurons: Effects on firing pattern and synchrony. *Journal of Neurophysiology*, 87: 1526-1541.

Kőszegi, B., and Rabin, M. (2006). A model of reference-dependent preferences. *Quarterly Journal of Economics*, 121(4): 1133-1165.

Kőszegi, B., and Rabin, M. (2007). Reference-dependent risk attitudes. *American Economic Review*, 97(4): 1047-1073.

Kőszegi, B., and Rabin, M. (2009). Reference-dependent consumption plans. *American Economic Review*, 99(3): 909-936.

Krauzlis, R. J. (2005). The control of voluntary eye movements: new perspectives. *Neuroscientist*, 11: 124-137.

Krebs, J. R., and Davies, N. B. (1997). *Behavioral Ecology*, 4th edition. MA: Blackwell Science, Ltd.

Kreps, D. M. (1990). *A Course in Microeconomic Theory*, 1st ed. Princeton, NJ: Princeton University Press.

Kreps, D. M., and Porteus, E. L. (1978). Temporal resolution of uncertainty and dynamic choice theory. *Econometrica*, 46: 185-200.

Kreps, D. M., and Porteus, E. L. (1979). Dynamic choice theory and dynamic programming. *Econometrica*, 47: 91-100.

Kringelbach, M. L., and Berridge, K. C. (eds.). (2009). *Pleasures of the Brain*. New York: Oxford University Press.

Krug, K., Cumming, B. G., and Parker, A. J. (2004). Comparing perceptual signals of single V5/MT neurons in two binocular depth tasks. *Journal of Neurophysiology*, 92: 1586-1596.

Kuypers, H. G. J. M. (1960). Central cortical projections to motor and somatosensory cell groups. *Brain*, 83: 161-184.

Lakshminaryanan, V., Chen, M. K., and Santos, L. R. (2008). Endowment effect in capuchin monkeys. *Philosophical Transactions of the Royal Society: Biological Sciences*, 363(1511): 3837-3844.

Laibson, D. (1997). Golden eggs and hyperbolic discounting. *Quarterly Journal of Economics*, 62: 443-477.

Laplace, P. S. (1814; 1951). *Essai philosophique sur les probabilities* (Philosophical Essay on Probabilities), F. W. Truscott and F. L. Emory (trans.). New York: Dover.

Lau, B., and Glimcher, P. W. (2005). Dynamic response-by-response models of matching behavior in rhesus monkeys. *Journal of the Experimental Analysis of Behavior*, 84(3): 555-579.

Lau, B., and Glimcher, P. W. (2007). Action and outcome encoding in the primate caudate nucleus. *Journal of Neuroscience*, 27(52): 14502-14514.

Lau, B., and Glimcher, P. W. (2008). Value representations in the primate striatum during matching behavior. *Neuron*, 58: 451-463.

Lau, B., and Salzman, C. D. (2009). The rhythms of learning. *Nature Neuroscience*, 12(6): 675-676.

LeDoux, J. E. (2000). Emotion circuits in the brain. *Annual Review of Neuroscience*, 23: 155-184.

LeDoux, J. E. (2007). The amygdala. *Current Biology*, 17(20): R868-R874.

Lee, P., and Hal, W. C. (1995). Interlaminar connections of the superior colliculus in the tree shrew. II. Projections from the superficial gray to the optic layer. *Visual Neuroscience*, 12: 573-588.

Lee, C., Rohrer, W. H., and Sparks, D. L. (1988). Population coding of saccadic eye movements by neurons in the superior colliculus. *Nature*, 332: 357-360.

Leigh, R. J., and Zee, D. S. (2006). *The Neurology of Eye Movements*, 4th ed. New York: Oxford University Press.

Levy, I., Snell, J., Nelson, A. J., Rustichini, A., and Glimcher, P. W. (2010). The neural representation of subjective value under risk and ambiguity. *Journal of Neurophysiology*, 103(2): 1036-1047.

Liu, F., and Wang, X-J. (2008). A common cortical crcuit mechanism for perceptual categorical discrimination and veridical judgment. *PLoS Computational Biology*, 4(12): 1-14.

Lo, C. C., and Wang, X. J. (2006). Cortico-basal ganglia circuit mechanism for a decision threshold in reaction time tasks. *Nature Neuroscience*, 9(7): 956-963.

Loewenstein, G. (1987). Anticipation and the valuation of delayed consumption. *Economic Journal*, 97(387): 666-684.

Loewenstein, Y. (2008). Robustness of learning that is based on covariance-driven synaptic plasticity. *PLoS Computational Biology*, 4(3): e1000007.

Loewenstein, Y., Prelec, D., and Seung, H. S. (2009). Operant matching as a Nash equilibrium of an intertemporal game. *Neural Computation*, 21(10): 2755-2773.

Logothetis, N. K., and Wandell, B. A. (2004). Interpreting the BOLD signal. *Annual Review of Physiology*, 66: 735-769.

Loomes, G., and Sugden, R. (1982). Regret theory: An alternative theory of rational choice under uncertainty. *Economic Journal*, 92: 805-824.

Louie, K. L., and Glimcher, P. W. (2010). Separating value from choice: delay discounting activity in the lateral intraparietal area. *Journal of Neuroscience*, 30(26): 5498-5507.

Lucas, R. (2008). Discussion. In: A. Caplin and A. Schotter (eds.), *The Foundations of Positive and Normative Economics*. Conference at New York University's Center for Experimental Social Science, 25-26 April, New York.

Ma, W. J., Beck, J. M., Latham, P. E., and Pouget, A. (2006). Bayesian inference with probabilistic population codes. *Nature Neuroscience*, 9: 1432-1438.

Mach, E. (1897; 1984). *Beiträge zur Analyse der Empfindungen* (Contributions to the Analysis of the Sensations), C. M. Williams (trans.). LaSalle, IL: Open Court.

Mackel, R., Iriki, A., Jorum, E., and Asanuma, H. (1991). Neurons of the pretectal area convey spinal input to the motor thalamus of the cat. *Experimental Brain Research*, 84(1): 12-24.

Macmillan, N. A., and Creelman, C. D. (2005). *Detection Theory: A User's Guide*, 2nd ed. Mahwah, NJ: Lawrence Erlbaum Associates.

Mainen, Z. F., and Sejnowski, T. J. (1995). Reliability of spike timing in neocortical neurons. *Science*, 268(5216): 1503-1506.

Margolis, E. B., Lock, H., Hjelmstad, G. O., and Fields, H. L. (2006). The ventral tegmental area revisited: Is there an electrophysiological marker for dopaminergic neurons? *Journal of Physiology*, 577: 907-924.

Matell, M. S., Meck, W. H., and Nicolelis, M. A. L. (2003). Integration of behavior and timing: Anatomically separate systems or distributed processing? In: W. H. Meck (ed.), *Functional and Neural Mechanisms of Interval Timing*. Boca Raton, FL: CRC Press, pp. 371-391.

Matsumoto, M., and Hikosaka, O. (2007). Lateral habenula as a source of negative reward signals in dopamine neurons. *Nature*, 447: 1111-1115.

Matsumoto, M., and Hikosaka, O. (2009a). Two types of dopamine neuron distinctly convey positive and negative motivational signals. *Nature*, 459: 837-842.

Matsumoto, M., and Hikosaka, O. (2009b). Representation of negative motivational value in the primate lateral habenula. *Nature Neuroscience*, 12(1): 77-84.

McAdams, C. J., and Maunsell, J. H. (1999). Effects of attention on the reliability of individual neurons in monkey visual cortex. *Neuron*, 23: 765-773.

McClintock, B. (1950). The origin and behavior of mutable loci in maize. *Proceedings of the National Academy of Sciences USA*, 36(6): 344-355.

McClintock, B. (1983). *The Significance of Responses of the Genome to Challenge*. Nobel Prize Lecture presented at Carnegie Institution of Washington, Cold Spring Harbor Laboratory, Cold Spring Harbor, NY. Retrieved online October 10, 2009 from: http://nobelprize.org/nobel_prizes/medicine/laureates/1983/mcclintock-lecture.html.

McClure, S. M., Li, J., Tomlin, D., Cypert, K. S., Montague, L. M., and Montague, P. R. (2004). Neural correlates of behavioral preference for culturally familiar drinks. *Neuron*, 44: 379-387.

McCoy, A. N., and Platt, M. L. (2005). Expectations and outcomes: Decision making in the primate brain. *Journal of Comparative Physiology A: Neuroethology, Sensory, Neural and Behavioral Physiology*, 191(3): 201-211.

McCulloch, W. S., and Pitts, W. H. (1943). A logical calculus of the ideas immanent in nervous activity. *Bulletin of Mathematical Biophysics*, 5: 115-133.

McFadden, D. (1974). Conditional logit analysis of qualitative choice behavior. In: P. Zarembka (ed.), *Frontier in Econometrics*. New York: Academic Press, pp. 105-142.

McFadden, D. L. (2000). *Economic Choices*. Nobel Prize Lecture presented at Stockholm University, Stockholm, Sweden. Full text of speech retrieved October 24, 2008, from: http://nobelprize.org/nobel_prizes/economics/laureates/2000/mcfadden-lecture.html

McFadden, D. L. (2005). Revealed stochastic preference: a synthesis. *Economic Theory*, 26: 245-264.

Meier, J. D., Aflalo, T. N., Kastner, S., and Graziano, M. S. A. (2008). Complex organization of human primary motor cortex: A high-resolution fMRI study. *Journal of Neurophysiology*, 100: 1800-1812.

Mendel, J. G. (1866; 1901). *Versuche über Pflanzenhybriden Verhandlungen des naturforschenden Vereines in Brünn, Bd. IV für das Jahr, Abhandlungen*: 3-47. For the English translation, see: C. T. Druery and W. Bateson (1901). Experiments in plant hybridization. *Journal of the Royal Horticultural Society*, 26: 1-32.

Metcalfe, N. B., and Ure, S. E. (1995). Diurnal variation in flight performance and hence potential predation risk in small birds. *Proceedings of the Royal Society of London B* 261: 395-400.

Mirenowiez, J. and Schultz, W. (1994). Importance of unpredictability for reward responses in primate dopamine neurons. *Journal of Neurophysiology*, 72: 1024-1027.

Morrison, S. E., and Salzman, C. D. (2009). The convergence of information about rewarding and aversive stimuli in single neurons. *Journal of Neuroscience*, 29(37): 11471-11483.

Montague, P. R., Dayan, P., Person, C., and Sejnowski, T. J. (1995). Bee foraging in uncertain environments using predictive Hebbian learning. *Nature*, 377: 725-728.

Montague, P. R., Dayan, P., and Sejnowski, T. J. (1996). A framework for mesencephalic dopamine systems based on predictive Hebbian learning. *Journal of Neuroscience*, 16(5): 1936-1947.

Moore, G. P., Perkel, D. H., and Segundo, J. P. (1966). Statistical analysis and functional interpretation of neuronal spike data. *Annual Review of Physiology*, 28: 493-522.

Mountcastle, V. B. (1998). *Perceptual Neuroscience: The Cerebral Cortex*. Cambridge, MA: Harvard University Press.

Mountcastle, V. B. (2005). *The Sensory Hand: Neural Mechanisms of Somatic Sensation*. Cambridge, MA: Harvard University Press.

Movshon, J. A., and Newsome, W. T. (1992). Neural foundations of visual motion perception. *Current Directions in Psychological Science*, 1: 35-39.

Movshon, J. A., and Newsome, W. T. (1996). Visual response properties of striate cortical neurons projecting to area MT in macaque monkeys. *Journal of Neuroscience*, 16(23): 7733-7741.

Movshon, J. A., Thompson, I. D., and Tolhurst, D. J. (1978a). Spatial summation in the receptive fields of simple cells in the cat's striate cortex. *Journal of Physiology*, 283: 53-77.

Movshon, J. A., Thompson, I. D., and Tolhurst, D. J. (1978b). Receptive field organization of complex cells in the cat's striate cortex. *Journal of Physiology*, 283: 79-99.

Nagel, E. (1961). The *Structure of Science: Problems in the Logic of Scientific Explanation*. New York: Harcourt, Brace & World.

Nagel, T. (1998). Reductionism and antireductionism. In: G. R. Bock and J. A. Goode (eds.), *The Limits of Reductionism in Biology*. New York: Wiley.

Nakamura, K., Matsumoto, M., and Hikosaka, O. (2008). Reward-dependent modulation of neuronal activity in the primate dorsal raphe nucleus. *Journal of Neuroscience*, 28(20): 5331-5343.

Nash, J. F. (1950). Equilibrium points in n-person games. *Proceedings of the National Academy of Sciences USA*, 36: 48-49.

Nash, J. F. (1951). Non-cooperative games. *Annals of Mathematics*, 54: 286-295.

Neuringer, A. (2002). Operant variability: evidence, functions, theory. *Psychonomic Bulletin Review*, 9: 672-705.

Newsome, W. T., Britten, K. H., and Movshon, J. A. (1989). Neuronal correlates of a perceptual decision. *Nature*, 341(6237): 52-54.

Newsome, W. T., Britten, K. H., Salzman, C. D., and Movshon, J. A. (1990). Neuronal mechanisms of motion perception. *Cold Spring Harbor Symposia on Quantitative Biology*, Vol. LV: pp. 697-705.

Nickle, B., and Robinson, P. R. (2007). The opsins of the vertebrate retina: insights from structural, biochemical, and evolutionary studies. *Cellular and Molecular Life Sciences*, 64: 2917-2932.

Nieuwenheys, R. (1985). *Chemoarchitecture of the Brain*. New York: Springer.

Niv, Y., Daw, N. D., Joel, D., and Dayan, P. (2007). Tonic dopamine: Opportunity costs and the control of response vigor. *Psychopharmacology (Berlin)*, 191(3): 507-520.

Niv, Y., Dinstein, I., Malach, R., and Heeger, D. J. (2008). BOLD and spiking activity. *Nature Neuroscience*, 11: 523-524.

Niv, Y., Duff, M. O., and Dayan, P. (2005). Dopamine, uncertainty and TD learning. *Behavioral and Brain Functions*, 1: 6.

Ohki, K., Chung, S., Ch'ng, Y. H., Kara, P., and Reid, R. C. (2005). Functional imaging with cellular resolution reveals precise microarchitecture in visual cortex. *Nature*, 433: 597-603.

O'Doherty, J. P., Buchanan, T. W., Seymour, B., and Dolan, R. J. (2006). Predictive neural coding of reward preference involves dissociable responses in human ventral midbrain and ventral striatum. *Neuron*, 49(1): 157-166.

O'Doherty, J. P., Critchley, H. D., Deichmann, R., and Dolan, R. J. (2003). Dissociating valence of outcome from behavioral control in human orbital and ventral prefrontal cortices. *Journal of Neuroscience*, 23: 7931-7939.

O'Doherty, J. P., Deichmann, R., Critchley, H. D., and Dolan, R. J. (2002). Neural responses during anticipation of a primary taste reward. *Neuron*, 33(5): 815-826.

Ozen, G., Helms, M. C., and Hall, W. C. (2003). The intracollicular neuronal network. In: W. C. Hall and A. Moschovakis (eds.), *The Superior Colliculus: New Approaches for Studying Sensorimotor Integration*. Boca Raton, FL: CRC Press, pp. 147-158.

Padoa-Schioppa, C. (2009). Range-adapting representation of economic value in the orbitofrontal cortex. *Journal of Neuroscience*, 29: 14004-14014.

Padoa-Schioppa, C., and Assad, J. A. (2006). Neurons in the orbitofrontal cortex encode economic value. *Nature*, 441(7090): 223-226.

Padoa-Schioppa, C., and Assad, J. A. (2008). The representation of economic value in the orbitofrontal cortex is invariant for changes of menu. *Nature Neuroscience*, 11(1): 95-102.

Palmer, J., Huk, A. C. and Shadlen, M. N. (2005). The effect of stimulus strength on the speed and accuracy of a perceptual decision. *Journal of Vision*, 5 (5): 376-404.

Pareto, V. (1906; 1971). *Manuel d'économie politique* (Manual of Political Economy), A. S. Schwier (trans.). New York: Augustus M. Kelley.

Parker, A. J., and Newsome, W. T. (1998). Sense and the single neuron: Probing the physiology of perception. *Annual Review of Neuroscience*, 21: 227-277.

Pascal, B. (1623-1662; 1948). *Great Shorter Works of Pascal*, E. Cailliet and J. C. Blankenagel (trans.). Philadelphia: Westminster Press.

Pascal, B. (1670; 1966). *Pensées*, A. J. Kraisheime (trans.). New York: Penguin Books.

Pascual-Leone, A., Meyer, K., Treyer, V., and Fehr, E. (2006). Diminishing reciprocal fairness by disrupting the right prefrontal cortex. *Science*, 314(5800): 829-832.

Paulus, M. P., and Frank, L. R. (2003). Ventromedial prefrontal cortex activation is critical for preference judgements. *NeuroReport*, 14: 1311-1315.

Pavlov, I. P. (1927). *Conditioned Reflexes: An Investigation of the Physiological Activity of the Cerebral Cortex*. New York: Dover.

Payne, J. W., Bettman, J. R., and Johnson, E. J. (1992). Behavioral decision research: A constructive processing perspective. *Annual Reviews of Psychology*, 43: 87-131.

Payne, J. W., Bettman, J. R., and Johnson, E. J. (1993). *The Adaptive Decision Maker*. Massachusetts: Cambridge University Press.

Penfield, W., and Rasmussen, T. (1950). *The Cerebral Cortex of Man*. New York: Macmillan.

Penton-Voak, I. S., Perrett, D. I, Castles, D. I, Kobayashi, T., Burt, D. M., Murray, L. K., and Minamisawa, R. (1999). Menstrual cycle alters face preference. *Nature*, 399: 741-742.

Perrett, D. I., Lee, K. J., Penton-Voak, I. S., Rowland, D., Yoshikawa, S., Burt, D. M., Henzi, S. P., Castles, D. L., and Akamatsu, S. (1998). Effects of sexual dimorphism on facial attractiveness. *Nature*, 394: 884-887.

Phelps, E. A. (2002). The cognitive neuroscience of emotion. In: M. S. Gazzaniga, R. B. Ivry, and G. R. Mangun (eds.), *Cognitive Neuroscience: The Biology of Mind*, 2nd ed. New York: Norton, pp. 537-576.

Phelps, E. A. (2006). Emotion and cognition: Insights from studies of the human amygdala. *Annual Review of Psychology*, 24(57): 27-53.

Phelps, E. A. (2008). The study of emotion in neuroeconomics. In: P. W. Glimcher, C. F. Camerer, E. Fehr, and R. A. Poldrack (eds.), *Neuroeconomics: Decision Making and the Brain*. London: Academic Press, pp. 145-173.

Plassmann, H., O'Doherty, J., and Rangel, A. (2007). Orbitofrontal cortex encodes willingness to pay in everyday economic transactions. *Journal of Neuroscience,* 27(37): 9984-9988.

Platt, M. L., and Glimcher, P. W. (1998). Response fields of intraparietal neurons quantified with multiple saccadic targets. *Experimental Brain Research,* 121(1): 65-75.

Platt, M. L., and Glimcher, P. W. (1999). Neural correlates of decision variables in parietal cortex. *Nature,* 400: 233-238.

Platt, M. L., Lau, B., and Glimcher, P. W. (2004). Situating the superior colliculus within the gaze control network. In: W. C. Hall and A. Moschovakis (eds.), *The Superior Colliculus: New Approaches for Studying Sensorimotor Integration.* Boca Raton, FL: CRC Press.

Plott, C., and Zeiler, K. (2005). The willingness to pay/willingness to accept gap, the 'endowment effect,' subject misconceptions and experimental procedures for eliciting valuations. *American Economic Review,* 95(3): 530-545.

Plott, C., and Zeiler, K. (2007). Exchange asymmetries incorrectly interpreted as evidence of endowment effect theory and prospect theory. *American Economic Review,* 97(4): 1449-1466.

Popper, K. (1959). *The Logic of Scientific Discovery.* London: Hutchinson & Co. Reprinted London: Routledge, 2002.

Prelec, D. (1998). The probability weighting function. *Econometrica,* 66(3): 497-527.

Preuschoff, K., Bossaerts, P., and Quartz, S. R. (2006). Neural differentiation of expected reward and risk in human subcortical structures. *Neuron,* 51: 381-390.

Rangel, A. (2008). The computation and comparison of value in goal-directed choice. In: P. W. Glimcher, C. F. Camerer, E. Fehr, and R. A. Poldrack (eds.), *Neuroeconomics: Decision Making and the Brain.* London: Academic Press, pp. 145-173.

Ratcliff, R. (1978). A theory of memory retrieval. *Psychological Review,* 85: 59-108.

Ratcliff, R. (1980). A note on modeling accumulation of information when the rate of accumulation changes over time. *Journal of Mathematical Psychology,* 21: 178-184.

Redgrave, P., and Gurney, K. (2006). Opinion: The short-latency dopamine signal: A role in discovering actions? *Nature Reviews Neuroscience,* 7: 967-975.

Redgrave, P., Prescott, T. J., and Gurney, K. (1999). Is the short latency dopamine burst too short to signal reinforcement error? *Trends in Neurosciences,* 22: 146-151.

Rescorla, R. A., & Wagner, A. R. (1972). A theory of Pavlovian conditioning: Variations in the effectiveness of reinforcement and nonreinforcement. In: A. H. Black and W. F. Prokasy (eds.), *Classical Conditioning II: Current Research and Theory.* New York: Appleton Century Crofts, pp. 64-99.

Reynolds, J. H., and Heeger, D. J. (2009). The normalization model of attention. *Neuron*, 61: 168-185.

Reynolds, J. N., and Wickens, J. R. (2002). Dopamine-dependent plasticity of corticostriatal synapses. *Neural Networks*, 15: 507-521.

Richman, S. E., and Lovvorn, J. R. (2009). Predator size, prey size and threshold food densities of diving ducks: Does a common prey base support fewer large animals? *Journal of Animal Ecology*, 78(5): 1033-1042.

Robinson, B. L., and McAlpine, D. (2009). Gain control mechanisms in the auditory pathway. *Current Opinion in Neurobiology*, 19: 402-407.

Robinson, D. A. (1972). Eye movements evoked by collicular stimulation in the alert monkey. *Vision Research*, 12: 1795-1808.

Robinson, D. L., and Jarvis, C. D. (1974). Superior colliculus neurons studied during head and eye movements of the behaving monkey. *Journal of Neurophysiology*, 37: 533-540.

Rodieck, R. W., Kiang, N. Y. S, and Gerstein, G. L. (1962). Some quantitative methods for the study of spontaneous activity of single neurons. *Biophysics Journal*, 2: 351-368.

Roitman, J. D., and Shadlen, M. N. (2002). Response of neurons in the lateral intraparietal area during a combined visual discrimination reaction time task. *Nature Neuroscience*, 22(21): 9475-9489.

Rubinstein, A. (2008). Comments on neuroeconomics. In: A. Caplin and A. Schotter (eds.), *The Foundations of Positive and Normative Economics*. Conference at New York University's Center for Experimental Social Science, New York, 25-26 April.

Samejima, K., Ueda, Y., Doya, K., and Kimura, M. (2005). Representation of action-specific reward values in the striatum. *Science*, 310(5752): 1337-1340.

Samuelson, P. A. (1937). A note on measurement of utility. *Review of Economic Studies*, 4: 155-161.

Samuelson, P. A. (1938). A note on the pure theory of consumer's behaviour. *Economica*, 51(17): 61–71.

Santos, L. R., and Lakshminarayanan, V. (2008). Innate constraints on judgment and decision-making? Insights from children and non-human primates. In: P. Carruthers, S. Laurence, and S. Stich (eds.), *The Innate Mind: Foundations and the Future*. Oxford, UK: Oxford University Press, pp. 293-310.

Savage, L. J. (1954). *Foundations of Statistics*. New York: John Wiley & Sons, Inc.

Schall, J. D., Morel, A., King, D. J., and Bullier, J. (1995a). Topography of visual cortex connections with frontal eye field in macaque: convergence and segregation of processing streams. *Journal of Neuroscience*, 15: 4464-4487.

Schall, J. D., Hanes, D. P., Thompson, K. G., and King, D. J. (1995b). Saccade target selection in frontal eye field of macaque. I. Visual and premovement activation. *Journal of Neuroscience*, 15: 6905-6918.

Schall, J. D., and Thompson, K. G. (1999). Neural selection and control of visually guided eye movements. *Annual Review of Neuroscience*, 22: 241-259.

Schlick, M. (1918; 1985). *General Theory of Knowledge*. Illinois: Open Court.

Schiller, P. H., Sandell, J. H., and Maunsell, J. H. (1987). The effect of frontal eye field and superior colliculus lesions on saccadic latencies in the rhesus monkey. *Journal of Neurophysiology*, 57(4): 1033-1049.

Schönberg, T., Daw, N. D., Joel, D., and O'Doherty, J. P. (2007). Reinforcement learning signals in the humans distinguish learners from nonlearners during reward-based decision making. *Journal of Neuroscience*, 27(47): 12860-12867.

Schultz, W. (1986). Responses of midbrain dopamine neurons to behavioral trigger stimuli in the monkey. *Journal of Neurophysiology*, 56(5): 1439-1461.

Schultz, W. (2000). Multiple reward signals in the brain. *Nature Reviews Neuroscience*, 1: 199-207.

Schultz, W. (2006). Behavioral theories and the neurophysiology of reward. *Annual Review of Psychology*, 57: 87-115.

Schultz, W. (2007). Multiple dopamine functions at different time courses. *Annual Review Neuroscience*, 30: 259-288.

Schultz, W., Dayan, P., and Montague, P. R. (1997). A neural substrate of prediction and reward. *Science*, 275(5306): 1593-1599.

Schwartz, O., and Simoncelli, E. P. (2001). Natural signal statistics and sensory gain control. *Nature Neuroscience*, 4(8): 819-825.

Selten, R. (1965). *Spieltheoretische Behandlung eines Oligopolmodells mit Nachfragetragheit* (An oligopoly model with demand inertia). *Zeitschrift für die gesamte Staatswissenschaft*, 12: 301-324.

Selten, R. (1975). Reexamination of perfectness concept for equilibrium points in extensive games. *International Journal of Game Theory*, 4: 25-55.

Selten, R. (1994). Multistage game models and delay supergames. Nobel Prize Lecture presented at Rheinische Friedrich-Wilhelms-Universität, Bonn, Germany. Full text of speech retrieved December 2008 from: http://nobelprize.org/nobel_prizes/economics/laureates/1994/selten-lecture.html

Shadlen, M. N., and Newsome, W. T. (1996). Motion perception: Seeing and deciding. *Proceedings of the National Academy of Sciences USA*, 93: 628-633.

Shadlen, M. N., and Newsome, W. T. (1998). The variable discharge of cortical neurons: implications for connectivity, computation, and information coding. *Journal of Neuroscience*, 18: 3870-3896.

Sherrington, C. S. (1947). *The Integrative Action of the Nervous System*. New Haven: Yale University Press.

Simoncelli, E. P., and Heeger, D. J. (1998). A model of neuronal responses in visual area MT. *Vision Research*, 38: 743-761.

Singer, T. (2007). The neuronal basis of empathy and fairness. *Novartis Foundation Symposium*, 278: 20-30; discussion 30-40, 89-96, 216-211.

Singer, T., Critchley, H. D., and Preuschoff, K. (2009). A common role of insula in feelings, empathy and uncertainty. *Trends in Cognitive Science*, 13(8): 334-340.

Sparks, D. L. (1978). Functional properties of neurons in the monkey superior colliculus: Coupling of neuronal activity and saccade onset. *Brain Resolution*, 156: 1-16.

Smith, J. M. (1982). *Evolution and the Theory of Games*. Cambridge: Cambridge University Press.

Simon, H. A. (1955). A behavioral model of rational choice. *Quarterly Journal of Economics*, 69(1): 99-118.

Simon, H. A. (1957). *Models of Man: Social and Rational*. New York: Wiley.

Simon, H. A. (1978). *Rational Decision Making in Business*. Nobel Memorial Prize Lecture presented at Carnegie-Mellon University, Pittsburgh, Pennsylvania. Full text of speech retrieved December 22, 2008, from: http://nobelprize. org/nobel_prizes/economics/laureates/1978/simon-lecture.html

Softky, W. R., and Koch, C. (1993). The highly irregular firing of cortical cells is inconsistent with temporal integration of random EPSP's. *Journal of Neuroscience*, 13: 334-350.

Sokol-Hessner, P., Hsu, M., Curley, N. G., Delgado, M. R., Camerer, C. F., and Phelps, E. A. (2009). Thinking like a trader selectively reduces individuals' loss aversion. *Proceedings of the National Academy of Sciences USA*, 106(13): 5035-5040.

Squire, L. R., and Kandel, E. R. (2009). *Memory: From Mind to Molecules*, 2nd ed. New York: Scientific American Library.

Squire, Bloom, McConnell, Roberts, Spitzer, and Zigmond. (2003). *Fundamental Neuroscience*, 2nd ed. New York: Academic Press.

Stephens, D. W., and Krebs, J. R. (1986). *Foraging Theory*. Princeton, NJ: Princeton University Press.

Stevens, C. F. (2003). Neurotransmitter release at central synapses. *Neuron*, 40(2): 381-388.

Stevens, S. S. (1951). *Handbook of Experimental Psychology*, 1st ed. New York: John Wiley & Sons Inc.

Stevens, S. S. (1961). To honor Fechner and repeal his law. *Science*, 133: 80-86.

Stevens, S. S. (1970). Neural events and the psychophysical law. *Science*, 170: 1043-1050.

Stevens, S. S. (1975). *Psychophysics: Introduction to its Perceptual, Neural and Social Prospects*, G. Stevens (ed.). New York: Wiley.

Sugden, R. (1993). An axiomatic foundation for regret theory. *Journal of Economic Theory*, 60: 159-180.

Sugrue, L. P., Corrado, G. S., and Newsome, W. T. (2004). Matching behavior and the representation of value in the parietal cortex. *Science*, 304: 1782-1787.

Sutton, R. S., and Barto, A. G. (1998). *Reinforcement Learning: An Introduction*. Massachusetts: MIT Press.

Tanji, J., and Evarts, E.V. (1976). Anticipatory activity of motor cortex neurons in relation to direction of an intended movement. *Journal of Neurophysiology*, 39(5): 1062-1068.

Teich, M. C., and Turcott, R. G. (1988). Multinomial pulse-number distributions for neural spikes in primary auditory fibers: theory. *Biological Cybernetics*, 59(2): 91-102.

Teller, D. Y., and Pugh, E. N., Jr. (1983). Linking propositions in color vision. In: J. D. Mollon & T. Sharpe (eds.), *Colour Vision: Physiology and Psychophysics*. New York: Academic Press, pp. 11-21.

Tepper, J. M., Koós, T., and Wilson, C. J. (2004). GABAergic microcircuits in the neostriatum. *Trends in Neurosciences*, 27(11): 662-669.

Tobler, P. N., Fiorillo, C. D., and Schultz, W. (2005). Adaptive coding of reward value by dopamine neurons. *Science*, 307: 1642-1645.

Tolhurst, D. J., Movshon, J. A., and Dean, A. F. (1983). The statistical reliability of signals in single neurons in cat and monkey striate cortex. *Vision Research*, 23: 775-785.

Tolhurst, D. J., Movshon, J. A., and Thompson, I. D. (1981). The dependence of response amplitude and variance of cat visual cortical neurones on stimulus contrast. *Experimental Brain Research*, 41: 414-419.

Tom, S. M., Fox, C. R., Trepel, C., and Poldrack, R. A. (2007). The neural basis of loss aversion in decision making under risk. *Science*, 315(5811): 515-518.

Treisman, A. (1982). Perceptual grouping and attention in visual search for features and for objects. *Journal of Experimental Psychology: Human Perception and Performance*, 8: 194-214.

Tremblay, L., and Schultz, W. (1999). Relative reward preference in primate orbitofrontal cortex. *Nature*, 398: 704-708.

Tversky, A., and Kahneman, D. (1974). Judgment under uncertainty: Heuristics and biases. *Science*, 185: 1124-1131.

Tversky, A., and Kahneman, D. (1981). The framing of decisions and the psychology of choice. *Science*, 211(4481): 453-458.

Tversky, A., and Kahneman, D. (1982). Judgments of and by representativeness. In: D. Kahneman, P. Slovic, and A. Tversky (eds.), *Judgment Under Uncertainty: Heuristics and Biases*. Cambridge, MA: Cambridge University Press, pp. 84-98.

Tversky, A., and Kahneman, D. (1983). Extensional vs. intuitive reasoning: The conjunction fallacy in probability judgment. *Psychological Review*, 90: 293-315.

Tversky, A., and Kahneman, D. (1986). Rational choice and the framing of decisions. *Journal of Business*, 59: 251-278.

Tversky, A., and Kahneman D. (1992). Advances in prospect theory: cumulative representation of uncertainty. *Journal of Risk and Uncertainty*, 5(4): 297-323.

Ungerleider, L. G., and Mishkin, M. (1982). Two cortical visual systems. In: D. J. Ingle, M. A. Goodale, and R. J. W. Mansfield (eds.), *Analysis of Visual Behavior*. Cambridge, MA: MIT Press, pp. 549-586.

Vandecasteele, M., Glowinski, J., and Venance, L. (2005). Electrical synapses between dopaminergic neurons of the substantia nigra pars compacta. *Journal of Neuroscience*, 25(2): 291-298.

Walker, A. E. (1940). A cytoarchitectural study of the prefrontal area of the macaque monkey. *Journal of Comparative Neurology*, 73: 59-86.

Wald, G., and Brown, P. K. (1956). Synthesis and bleaching of rhodopsin. *Nature*, 177(4500): 174-176.

Wald, G., and Brown, P. K. (1958). Human rhodopsin. *Science*, 127: 222-226.

Wald, G., and Brown, P. K. (1965). Human color vision and color blindness. *Cold Spring Harbor Symposium on Quantitative Biology*, 30: 345-361.

Wandell, B. A. (1995). *Foundations of Vision*. Sunderland, MA: Sinauer Associates.

Wang, X. J. (2002). Probabilistic decision making by slow reverberation in cortical circuits. *Neuron*, 36: 955-968.

Watson, J., and Crick, F. (1953). A structure of deoxyribonucleic acid. *Nature*, 171: 737-738.

Weber, E. H. (1834; 1996). *E. H. Weber: On the Tactile Senses* (with translation of *De Tactu*), H. E. Ross and D. J. Murray (trans. and eds.). New York: Experimental Psychology Society.

Webster, M. A., and De Valois, R. L. (1985). Relationship between spatial-frequency and orientation tuning of striate-cortex cells. *Journal of the Optical Society of America A*, 2(7): 1124-1132.

Werner, G., and Mountcastle, V. B. (1963). The variability of central neural activity in a sensory system, and its implications for the central reflection of sensory events. *Journal of Neurophysiology*, 26: 958-977.

Wickens, J. R. (1993). *A Theory of the Striatum*, 1st ed. Leeds: Pergamon Press.

Wickens, J. R., Begg, A. J., and Arbuthnott, G. W. (1996). Dopamine reverses the depression of rat cortico-striatal synapses which normally follows high frequency stimulation of cortex in vitro. *Neuroscience*, 70: 1-5.

Wickens, J. R., and Kotter, R. (1995). Cellular models of reinforcement. In J. C. Houk, J. L. Davis, and D. G. Beiser (eds.), *Models of Information Processing in Basal Ganglia*. Cambridge, MA: MIT Press, pp. 187-214.

Williams, S. M., and Goldman-Rakic, P. S. (1998). Widespread origin of the primate mesofrontal dopamine system. *Cerebral Cortex*, 8: 321-345.

Wilson, E. O. (1998). *Consilience: The Unity of Knowledge*. New York: Alfred A. Knopf, Inc.

Winston, J. S., O'Doherty, J., Kilner, J. M., Perrett, D. I., and Dolan, R. J. (2007). Brain systems for assessing facial attractiveness. *Neuropsychologia*, 45(1): 195-206.

Wise, R. A. (2008). Dopamine and reward: the anhedonia hypothesis 30 years on. *Neurotoxicity Research*, 14(2,3): 169-183.

Wise, R. A., and Rompre, P. P. (1989). Brain, dopamine and reward. Annual Review of Psychology, 40: 191-225.

Wolfe, J. (1998). Visual search. In: Pashler, H., ed. *Attention*. London: University College London Press.

Woolsey, C. N. (1952). Patterns of localization in sensory and motor areas of the cerebral cortex. In: *The Biology of Mental Health and Disease*. New York: Hoeber, pp. 192-206.

Wu, G., and Gonzalez, R. (1998). Common consequence effects in decision making under risk. *Journal of Risk and Uncertainty*, 16: 115-139.

Wunderlich, K., Rangel, A., and O'Doherty, J. P. (2009). Neural computations underlying action-based decision making in the human brain. *Proceedings of the National Academy of Sciences USA*, 106(40): 17199-17204.

van Beuzekom, D., and van Gisbergen, J. A. M. (2002). Interaction between visual and vestibular signals for the control of rapid eye movements. *Journal of Neurophysiology*, 88: 306-322.

van Gisbergen, J. A. M., van Opstal, A. J., and Tax, A. A. M. (1987). Collicular ensemble coding of saccades based on vector summation. *Neuroscience*, 21: 541.

von Bonin, G., and Bailey, P. (1947). *The Neocortex of Macaca mulatta*. Urbana, IL: University of Illinois Press.

von Economo, C. (1929). *Die Cytoarchitectonik der Hirnrinde des erwachsenen Menschen* (The cytoarchitectonics of the human cerebral cortex), S. Parker (trans.). New York: Oxford University Press.

von Neumann, J. V., and Morgenstern, O. (1944). *Theory of Games and Economic Behavior*. Princeton, NJ: Princeton University Press.

Yeung, N., Botvinick, M. M., and Cohen, J. D. (2004). The neural basis of error detection: Conflict monitoring and the error-related negativity. *Psychology Review*, 111(4): 931-959.

Zeki, S. M. (1974). Functional organization of a visual area in the posterior bank of the superior temporal sulcus of the rhesus monkey. *Journal of Physiology*, 236(3): 549-573.

Zhang, L., Doyon, W. M., Clark, J. J., Phillips, P. E., and Dani, J. A. (2009). Controls of tonic and phasic dopamine transmission in the dorsal and ventral striatum. *Molecular Pharmacology*, 76(2): 396-404.

Zigmond, M. J., Bloom, F. E., Landis, S. C., and Squire, L. R. (1999). *Fundamental Neuroscience*. San Diego: Academic Press.

Zoccolan, D., Cox, D. D., and DiCarlo, J. J. (2005). Multiple object response normalization in monkey inferotemporal cortex. *Journal of Neuroscience*, 25(36): 8150-8164.

Zohary, E., Shadlen, M. N., and Newsome, W. T. (1994). Correlated neuronal discharge rate and its implications for psychophysical performance. *Nature*, 370: 140-143.

Author Index

Subject Index

Printed in the USA/Agawam, MA
October 27, 2015

625399.035